AF571922

Psychoanalysis, Psychotherapy, and the New England Medical Scene, 1894–1944

Psychoanalysis, Psychotherapy and the New England Medical Scene, 1894-1944

GEORGE E. GIFFORD, JR.
EDITOR

Science History Publications/USA
New York 1978

Science History Publications/USA
a division of
Neale Watson Academic Publications, Inc.
156 Fifth Avenue, New York, New York 10010

Library of Congress Cataloging in Publication Data
Main entry under title:

Psychoanalysis, psychotherapy, and the New England medical scene, 1894–1944.

Includes bibliographies and index.
1. Psychiatry—United States—New England—History.
2. Psychoanalysis—United States—New England—History.
3. Psychotherapy—United States—New England—History.
I. Gifford, George Edmund. [DNLM: 1. Psychiatry—History—New England. 2. History of Medicine, 20th century—New England. WM11 AN25 P9]
RC443.P78 616.8′9′00974 77-22378
ISBN 0-88202-169-9

Designed and manufactured in the U.S.A.

THIS BOOK

IS DEDICATED

TO

JOHN Z. BOWERS

WHO

MADE IT POSSIBLE

"The truth is that medicine, professedly founded on observation, is as sensitive to outside influence, political, religious, philosophical, imaginative, as is the barometer to the changes of atmospheric density. Theoretically it ought to go on its own straightforward inductive path, without regard to changes of government or to fluctuations of public opinion. But . . . actually there is a closer relation between the medical sciences and the conditions of society and the general thought of the time, than would at first be suspected."

Oliver Wendell Holmes, *Medical Essays 1842–1882*
(Boston: Houghton Mifflin, 1891), p. 177.

"Forsan et haec olim meminisse iuvabit."
(It will perhaps be pleasant one day to look back on these events.)

Virgil, *The Aeneid.*

Contents

Beginnings at the Turn of the Century

Popular Psychotherapy Movements

"The Age of Putnam"

The 1920s and 1930s

Early Psychoanalysis in Boston

Preface

In 1958 when I came to the Peter Bent Brigham Hospital, Boston, Massachusetts, to do my residency in psychiatry, the third volume of Ernest Jones's *The Life and Work of Sigmund Freud*, had appeared. I read with particular interest the passages relating to Freud's visit to Clark University in 1909 and the "Boston School" of psychotherapy at the turn of the century. One of the people mentioned by Jones was George Arthur Waterman, M.D. This made a particular impression on me because I was seeing a patient who frequently talked about his psychotherapy sessions, as an adolescent, with Dr. Waterman—and what a magnetic person he had been. I began to collect material about Dr. Waterman; the little bits and pieces formed the biographical sketch of him that is now a paper in this symposium. It seemed to me that the lives of lesser known figures in psychiatry might more accurately reveal the manner in which the new psychodynamic ideas were accepted or rejected, integrated and assimilated into the medical mosaic of the time.

On April 25–26, 1967, I attended the conference on the history of psychiatry at Yale, which had been planned by George Mora and Jeanne Brand.[1] The symposium was actually a series of lectures on the methodology and problems of the history of psychiatry, and had limited participant interaction. With my paper on Waterman still in mind, I thought how productive it could have been for me to ask questions and hear those distinguished historians discuss the "Boston School," the interactions between its various members, and the social and intellectual focus which influenced early American psychiatry. It was then that I thought about a symposium to which both historians and those who participated in the events themselves would come together to discuss the "Boston School" from the turn of the century up to the general acceptance of psychodynamic theories in the United States. By juxtaposing young historians with special sensitivity to the social and intellectual forces, and those who could speak with knowledge from their own personal accounts, in the oral history tradition, it would be enriching for both parties.

It was at this time that a new group of young historians was making itself known and respected; they brought a new rigor and enthusiasm to both the history of psychology and psychiatry by applying the tools and insights of the social and intellectual historian to a specific area of interest. The scholarship evident in the section on the history of the behavioral sciences of the Cornell University Medical College (Payne Whitney Clinic) under the direction of Eric T. Carlson, M.D., was most impressive. With guidance from this center, Ph.D. candidates at Columbia University produced major works such as Norman Dain's *Concepts of Insanity in the United States, 1789–1865* (1964), Gerald C. Grob's *The State and the Mentally Ill, A History of the Worcester State Hospital in Massachusetts, 1830–1920* (1966), Barbara Sicherman's unpublished doctoral thesis, "A Quest for Mental Health in America, 1880–1917" (1967), and Dorothy Ross's *G. Stanley Hall, the Psychologist as Prophet* (1972).

Other young historians also made equally distinguished contributions. John C. Burnham's thesis at Stanford, "Psychoanalysis in American Civilization before 1918" (1958), grew into *Psychoanalysis and American Medicine, 1894–1918 Medicine, Science and Culture* (1967). Nathan G. Hale, Jr., who received his Ph.D. from the University of California at Berkeley, produced major works in 1971: *James Jackson Putnam and Psychoanalysis, Letters between Putnam and Sigmund Freud, Ernest Jones, William James, Sandor Ferenczi, and Morton Prince, 1877–1917* and *Freud and the Americans: the Beginnings of Psychoanalysis in the United States, 1876–1917*. In 1975 appeared *Morton Prince, Psychotherapy and Multiple Personality: Selected Essays*. At Harvard, Ruth B. Kaplan published *Psychiatry and Community in Nineteenth Century America* (1969).

The history of psychology also had a flowering at the University of New Hampshire under Robert I. Watson.[2,3] In 1968, under the cochairmanship of Watson and Joseph Brožek of Lehigh University, a group sponsored by the National Science Foundation met at the University of New Hampshire and established The International Society for the History of Behavioral and Social Sciences—Cheiron. As early as 1965, Watson and Dr. Eric T. Carlson of Cornell Medical College had founded the *Journal of the History of the Behavioral Sciences*, edited originally by Watson and now by his former Ph.D. student Barbara Ross. This journal has been most effective in stimulating and publishing the material on the history of psychology. Not only were young historians writing on the history of psychology and psychiatry, psychologists and psychiatrists, too, continued to make major contributions to the history of their professions. The psychologists David Rapaport and David Shakow wrote *Freud's Influence in American Psychology* (1968), and the psychiatrist Henri F. Ellenberger wrote his monumental work, *The Discovery of the Unconscious, the History of the Evolution of Dynamic Psychiatry* (1970).

As these areas of interest in the history of psychology and psychiatry were developing around the country, so were they also at Harvard. In 1964 Richard J. Wolfe came to the Francis A. Countway Library as curator of rare books. After the Harvard Medical Library and the Boston Medical Library pooled resources to become the Countway, Richard Wolfe defined his job so that he played a vital part in a history of medicine program, not merely as the keeper of old books. His creative enthusiasm was infectious. The Countway had inherited from the Boston Medical Library one of the first collections in phrenology as well as the papers of Drs. Morton Prince and Isador Coriat. In 1965 the late Dr. Marian C. Putnam had donated the papers and letters of her father, James Jackson Putnam, to the Countway; these were then edited for publication by Nathan G. Hale, Jr. In 1971 I myself was appointed consultant to the historical collections at the Francis A. Countway Library of Medicine, and it has been a happy chore to help build the history of psychiatry archives.[4]

At the Yale symposium I shared my thoughts about a symposium on the "Boston School" with Richard Wolfe. We talked about it from time to time, and after the publication of Hale's *James Jackson Putnam and Psychoanalysis*, we began to plan in earnest. At this time, Dr. Otto Marx, who was visiting professor of the history of medicine at Harvard and teaching a course on the history of psychiatry, joined us in our talks. At the same time, Dr. Sanford Gifford, librarian of the Boston Psychoanalytic Society and Institute, became interested in the Emmanuel Movement from some scrapbooks, collected by Coriat from 1898 to 1943, bequeathed to the Boston Psychoanalytic Society and Institute, and deposited in the Countway, and he, too, became a member of our informal committee. Starting in 1970, we all worked to plan the program, which would include both the professional historians and those who had "lived" the history. At one point we had the advice of David Musto of Yale in our planning sessions.

We decided that the symposium would be entitled, "Psychoanalysis, Psychotherapy and the New England Medical Scene, 1894–1944" and would bring together a group of eminent medical, social, and intellectual historians, historically oriented psychiatrists and psychologists, and related specialists who would review and discuss the developments of psychotherapy in the New England region from 1894, when William James noticed Freud's early work on hysteria, through the intervening events of the next fifty years.[5] The symposium would encompass the late 1890s, when William James, Boris Sidis, Morton Prince, G. Stanley Hall, and Adolf Meyer, assimilating their exposure to German clinical psychology and French clinical neurology and psychiatry, would establish a pattern of close ties between the university and the state hospital, such as that between Clark University and the Worcester State Hospital. It would consider the New England medical scene with its strong local tradition of medical psychotherapy; the social and cultural trends in an "age of reform" with the religious and political movements and the social and intellectual background of New England; and the critical decade and a half before the First World War when the psychotherapy movements coincided with the development of several medical psychotherapeutic schools. Finally it would deal with the founding of the Boston Psychoanalytic Society in 1928, its reorganization in 1933, the arrival of European analysts—part of the great intellectual migration before World War II[6]—and their influence on the local psychoanalytic scene. A concluding panel discussion, "Early Psychoanalysis in Boston," brought rich recollections from the psychoanalysts themselves.

The symposium was held April 12–14, 1973, at the Jimmy Fund Auditorium, 35 Binney Street, Boston. It was supported by two grants, one from the Francis G. Wickes Foundation, Inc., to the Francis A. Countway Library of Medicine and one from the Ella Lyman Cabot Trust to the Boston Psychoanalytic Society and Institute, Inc. Other funds were contributed by Mr. William King of Lincoln, Massachusetts, Mrs. Morton Peabody Prince of Boston, Massachusetts, Mrs. Merrill Moore of Squantum, Massachusetts, and the late John A.P. Millet of New York, New York. Videotapes of the symposium were made and copies have been deposited in the Countway Library and the Boston Psychoanalytic Society.

A group of distinguished invited participants gave depth to the discussions: John A. Abbott, M.D., S. Spafford Ackerly, M.D., J. Sanbourne Bockoven, M.D., G. Colket Caner, M.D., Jean A. Curran, M.D., Henry M. Fox, M.D., Bardwell H. Flower, M.D., Frank Fremont-Smith, M.D., Mrs. Francis C. Hall (Mrs. Stanley A. Cobb), Leston L. Havens, M.D., Edna Heidbreder, Ph.D., William Malamud, Sr., M.D., John A.P. Millet, M.D., Miss Lillian Saltman, and Robert I. Watson, Ph.D. Otto Marx, M.D., Jeanne Brand, Ph.D., Sanford Gifford, M.D., William Malamud, Jr., M.D., and George E. Gardner, M.D. presided at the sessions.

The editing of the symposium was facilitated by two grants to George E. Gifford, Jr., one from the William F. Milton Fund, Harvard Medical School (1974) and another from the Josiah Macy Jr. Foundation (1976). These funds were used to collect illustrations for this book and to employ two editors who helped prepare the manuscripts for publication: Joseph D. Elder and Deborah W. Miller.

The original program of the symposium has been altered for this book; two papers were invited additions: Benjamin C. Riggs's paper on his father, "Austen Fox Riggs: Pioneer in the Psychotherapy of the Neuroses" and Milton Greenblatt's "Fifty Years of Research Contributions at the Massachusetts Mental Health Center" (Boston Psychopathic Hospital), which had been presented at the semicentenary celebration of that hospital in 1962. The paper by Professor Kenneth S. Lynn of Johns Hopkins was deleted since it was of a general background nature and not specifically related to the topic of this book. Most appropriately, Sanford Gifford added an introduction to the panel discussion, "Psychoanalysis in Boston: Innocence and Experience" (which he also organized). He also edited the panel discussion and did biographical sketches of the early psychoanalysts. Rose Jacobowitz, executive editor of Neale Watson Academic Publications, Inc., with her quick mind and sharp eye, prepared the manuscript for publication.

A good symposium should be greater than the sum of its parts in illuminating the theme of the program, to warrant publication.[7] We feel that this collection meets that criterion.

George E. Gifford, Jr., M.D.
Cambridge, Massachusetts

References

1 George Mora and Jeanne L. Brand, *Psychiatry and its History, Methodological Problems in Research* (Springfield, Mass.: Charles C. Thomas, 1970).

2 Robert I. Watson, Sr., "The History of Psychology as a Specialty: A Personal View of its First 15 Years," *Journal of the History of Behavioral Science, 11* (1975), 5–14.

3 Eric T. Carlson and Robert I. Watson, "Editorial, the Birthday of a Journal," *Journal of the History of the Behavioral Sciences, 1* (1965), 3.

4 George E. Gifford, Jr., "Why Putnam Now?" *Harvard Medical Alumni Bulletin*, vol. 46, no. 4, March/April 1972, pp. 32–33.

5 William James, Abstract of Freud, *Psychological Review, 1* (1894), 199. See John C. Burnham, *Psychoanalysis and American Medicine, 1894–1918: Medicine, Science, and Culture*, Psychological Issues, Monograph 20 (New York: International Universities Press, 1967), p. 5.

6 Donald Fleming and Bernard Bailyn, *The Intellectual Migration* (Cambridge, Mass.: Harvard University Press, 1969).

7 Cyril E. Blake and Carol Orr, "E plurubus unum, symposia and publishers," *Scholarly Publishing*, University of Toronto Press, vol. 5, no. 2, January 1974, pp. 145–152.

Introduction

In the last several years some American psychiatrists have been taking stock of their theoretical commitments and their historical roots.[1] E. Fuller Torrey, in *Death of Psychiatry*, contends that the medical model for psychiatry is dying and must soon give way to a "neo-educational" model in which psychiatrists function not as physicians, but as "tutors, educators, counselors."[2] Others see just the opposite. Hagop Akiskal and William T. McKinney, Jr., in an article in *Archives of General Psychiatry*, report that the "psychodynamic" model which has traditionally dominated North American psychiatric thought is readily losing ground to the medical model.[3] Psychiatrists trained before 1970 continue to view emotional and behavioral problems as ramifications of familial or social conflicts; those trained after 1970 tend to ascribe these problems to chemical or hereditary factors. Most recently, Miriam Siegler and Humphrey Osmond, in *Models of Madness, Models of Medicine*, have divided the present psychiatric approaches into eight models: medical, moral, impaired, psychoanalytic, social, psychedelic, conspiratorial, family interaction.[4] Clearly, psychiatrists of all persuasions can agree with Peter Amacher, Freud's biographer, who wrote of psychoanalysis after World War II:

> Psychoanalysis was no longer equated with Freud's thought, but his influence remained. The libidinous inflow of excitation was no longer taken as the sole motive power for the symptoms of mental illness but was one among several drives given equal theoretical status. Yet much of Freud's description of infantile psychosexual development as the primary determinant of adult psychology was incorporated into more complex theories. Above all, his general view of the unconscious remained influential. Most psychoanalytic theories included the unconscious as the sum of processes that, while not observable consciously, determine conscious thought and are organized so as to satisfy needs, although the needs are not necessarily consciously recognized. While the psychoanalytic hegemony over American psychiatry and the medical hegemony over psychotherapy began to break up in the 1960's, there was, by 1970, no clear indication of how this would affect the influence of Freud's thought.[5]

As Amacher indicates, the psychoanalytic paradigm is waning in influence, psychiatry having been subjected to more compelling theories in the last decade or so. To the historian, the process is inevitable: medicine is a constantly evolving or regressing system that mirrors all the social forces of its time and place. As we are now witnessing the rise of new psychiatric paradigms and the demise of others, perhaps it is historically important to return to the turn of the century and review the social and intellectual forces then—when the organic model was yielding to the psychodynamic and psychoanalytic models. In New England, the years 1894–1944 rather precisely encompass the shifting viewpoints within American psychiatry.

Why were these years chosen as the inclusive dates of this symposium? Dates in the history of ideas tend to be arbitrary and simplistic; however, 1894 was undeniably a hallmark in the history of American psychiatry. It was on May 16, 1894, that S. Weir Mitchell addressed the American Medico-Psychological Association denouncing the psychiatrists of that time:

> Once we spoke of asylums with respect; it is not so now. We, neurologists, think you have fallen behind us, and this opinion is gaining ground outside of our own ranks, and is in part at least, your own fault....Where [are] your careful scientific reports?...You live alone uncriticized, unquestioned out of the healthy conflicts and honest rivalries which keep us [neurologists] up to the mark of the fullest competence.[6]

Severe criticism of the old asylum system of American psychiatry came in the same year that Freud's ideas were first noted in an American journal; William James noticed Freud's early work on hysteria in *Psychological Review*.[7] In the following half-century, S. Weir Mitchell's admonitions were heeded and psychodynamic theories rose to the zenith of their influence.

Why should the shift be seen most clearly in New England? Many of the historical and social factors peculiar to New England affected the changing nature of psychiatry. Its religious and philosophical antecedents,[4] emphasis on social reform,[6] and the rise of scientific psychology as an academic discipline[2] all provided fertile soil for less than orthodox expressions. Within the medical community, interaction with European psychiatry,[3] a tradition of medical psychotherapy,[5] a history of medical eclecticism, which engendered respect for differing medical viewpoints,[7] and serious interest in neurology, which showed increasing fascination with "problems of the mind,"[2] made New England a suitable medium for the germination of new ideas and approaches.

Boris Sidis, Morton Prince, and J.J. Putnam were part of that pioneer generation of New England physicians who established neurology on a firm professional footing in the United States. At a time when medicine considered insanity a disease of the brain, neurologists boldly claimed competence in the field of mental as well as neurological disorders. They worked in private offices or in hospitals, rather than in the insane asylums run by hospital superintendents, who frequently adhered rigidly to the concept of brain pathology. The patients in the asylums were, for the most part, psychotic, whereas patients seen by the neurologists in their offices were more often neurotic. Many of the symptoms were diagnosed as "neurasthenia," a term popularized by George M. Beard,[8] but which earlier had been described by E.H. van Deusen in his patients at Boston City and Massachusetts General hospitals.[9]

Scientific psychology as an academic discipline with a concomitant interest in clinical problems was established early in New England. It was G. Stanley Hall, the academic psychologist and president of Clark University, who was instrumental in bringing Adolf Meyer to Worcester State Hospital in 1895.[10] Graduate students in psychology were instructed there and Meyer was also appointed docent in psychiatry at Clark, establishing mutual ties between the theoretical and practical spheres. At Harvard, psychologists William James and Hugo Munsterberg were part of the "Boston Group," whose leader was J.J. Putnam and whose other members were: Josiah Royce, George A. Waterman, Boris Sidis, Morton Prince, and Edward Cowles.[11] Later they were joined by Adolf Meyer. They met regularly to discuss patients and assess ideas stemming from the European literature, including those of Charcot, Janet, Bergson, and Freud. Again psychologists and psychiatrists reinforced one another.

European psychiatry took hold readily in New England—the most famous example being the visit of Sigmund Freud, Carl Jung, and Sandor Ferenczi in 1909. A decade earlier, however, G. Stanley Hall had asked Auguste Forel, Adolf Meyer's old teacher in Zurich, to attend the Clark Decennial celebration in 1899. Forel's paper, "Hypnotism and Cerebral Activity,"[12] alluded to the work of Breuer and Freud, relating the partial successes of therapies using hypnosis, while describing his own attempts at suggestion therapy. Pierre Janet arrived in the United States to lecture on psychopathology in 1904 at the International Congress during the Great Universal Exposition at St. Louis, Missouri, under the chairmanship of Edward Cowles of McLean Hospital. (Adolf Meyer was secretary of the section.[13]) His itinerary included a visit to Boston, and in 1906 Harvard University invited him to give a series of fifteen lectures on hysteria. Not until the late 1930s was there another influx of European psychiatrists—many of them German-Jewish intellectuals, such as the Deutsches and the Bibrings, who fled their homeland and settled in Boston.

New England boasted a strong tradition of academic psychology that influenced psychotherapy, as well as academic philosophers who significantly influenced these early leaders by advocating a pragmatic behavioral approach.[14] J.J. Putnam was influenced by both Josiah Royce and a New England background steeped in transcendentalism. Adolf Meyer was influenced by John Dewey, George H. Meade, Charles Horton Cooley, Charles S. Peirce, and William James. To continue the chain further, Peirce was also a mentor for William James, G. Stanley Hall, and E.E. Southard.[15]

As early as 1853, Pliny Earle was appointed professor of psychological medicine at the Berkshire Medical Institution in Pittsfield, Massachusetts—probably the first time in the United States that a chair of this kind had been established, thereby recognizing the study of mental disorders as an appropriate part of medical education.[16] Indeed, in New England the Industrial Revolution had actually produced the first significant patient population.[17] An indication of concerted interest in psychological aspects of medicine was the Shattuck Lecture of 1895, read before the Massachusetts Medical Society on June 11, by Robert T. Edes, professor of medicine at Harvard. Titled "The New England Invalid," it contained this statement:

> It is held by Breuer and Freud that the essential part of the action of mental and moral shock in the production of hysteria lies in the absence of the appropriate motor reaction, as, for instance, when a lower official received from his superior an insult which he could not resent. The correctness of this view seemed to be demonstrated by the result that when the history of the affair was completely elaborated by hypnotism and fully talked over, the hysterical symptoms disappeared.[18]

This whole tradition of medical psychotherapy set the stage for the integration of the psychoanalytic tradition into the medical institutional structure. Psychoanalytic leaders became a part of the academic medical community, a harbinger of psychiatry's future status. The new interest in psychotherapeutics extended to the social reform movements, such as the social work movement, the organized religion of the Emmanuel Movement, and the developing field of child psychiatry and juvenile delinquency.

Fortunately, strong medical eclecticism decreased polarization between the physiological and psychological schools, and instead encouraged cooperative study. The pioneer research of Walter Bradford Cannon on the physiological correlates of emotion brought together the psychological and organic approaches. The investigations of Otto Folin, John C. Whitehorn, and William G. Lennox developed more completely such symbiotic viewpoints and, most important, diverse approaches were tolerantly supported by hospital administrators.

For example, E.E. Southard, a neuropathologist, encouraged the work of staff members with different inclinations, both somatic and psychotherapeutic. This tradition at the Boston Psychopathic continued under Macfie Campbell and Harry Solomon. Strong psychiatry departments were promoted in general hospitals in Boston, such as the department formed by Stanley Cobb at the Massachusetts General Hospital, and those at the Peter Bent Brigham and Boston City hospitals. In 1939, at the Peter Bent Brigham, John Romano pioneered the teaching of psychiatric residents in a purely medical setting. Analysts themselves were interested in the psychiatric aspects of medical problems—Felix Deutsch became involved in psychosomatic medicine as did Henry Fox, John Nemiah, and Erich Lindemann.

There have been a few general histories or surveys of American psychiatry,[19] but this symposium is unique in that it is the only time in which social and intellectual historians and historians of psychology and psychiatry, along with some of the participants in the history making, came together to analyze the underpinnings and the development of American psychiatry in a specific locality within a specific era. This symposium is meant to be a provocative rather than a definitive history of the period 1894 to 1944, yet its focus is distinctly on psychoanalysis and psychotherapy as it was in New England.

Included are different types of historical styles: the intellectual and social historians Daniel Aaron, Dorothy Ross, Norman Dain, Nathan Hale, Jr.; the historians of psychology and psychiatry—John C. Burnham, Barbara Ross, David Shakow, Barbara Sicherman; and the historically oriented psychiatrists, psychologists, and social workers—Julius Silberger, Jr., Sanford Gifford, Eunice Allan, Otto Marx, Henri Ellenberger, and George E. Gifford, Jr. Finally, there is a group of immediate disciples and children: Fox on Meyer, Myerson on Myerson, Gardner on Healy, Riggs on Riggs, Millet on Riggs, Sharpley on Fuller, McHoward on Austin Riggs. Ostensibly to some historical purists this violates the canons of the trade, and subjects the contributors to being labeled "sentimental," "uncritical," "anecdotal," and "filiopietistic"—but can any historian claim "uncritical perspective" and be "truly evaluative"?

We realize that there are gaps within this presentation; there is little material on significant figures, such as Hugo Munsterberg, Boris Sidis, Adolf Meyer, Stanley Cobb, Vernon L. Briggs. At present these individuals have not received their proper historical notice.

The purpose of this symposium was to examine the forces that affected the acceptance, rejection, and final assimilation of the psychodynamic paradigm into the New England medical scene. As Oliver Wendell Holmes said:

> The truth is that medicine, professedly founded on observation, is as sensitive to outside influence, political, religious, philosophical, imaginative, as is the barometer to the changes of atmospheric density. Theoretically it ought to go on its own straightforward inductive path, without regard to changes of government or to fluctuations of public opinion. But...actually there is a closer relation between the medical sciences and the condition of society and the general thought of the time, than would at first be suspected.[20]

References

[1] David F. Musto, "History and Psychiatry's Present State of Transition," *Archives of General Psychiatry, 23:11* (1970), 385–392.

[2] E. Fuller Torrey, *Death of Psychiatry* (Radnor, Pennsylvania: Chilton, 1974).

[3] Hagop S. Akiskal and William T. McKinney, Jr., "Overview of Recent Research in Depression," *Archives of General Psychiatry, 32:3* (1975), 285–305.

[4] Miriam Siegler and Humphrey Osmond, *Models of Madness, Models of Medicine* (New York: Macmillan, 1974).

[5] Peter Amacher, "Sigmund Freud" in *Dictionary of Scientific Biography*, vol. V, pp. 180–181 (New York: Charles Scribner, 1972).

[6] S. Weir Mitchell, Address before the American Medico-Psychological Association, May 16, 1894.

[7] William James, *Psychological Review, 1* (1894), 199. See John C. Burnham, *Psychoanalysis and American Medicine 1894–1918: Medicine, Science, and Culture.* Psychological Issues, monograph 20, vol. V, no. 4, p. 5.

[8] George M. Beard, "Neurasthenia or Nervous Exhaustion," *Boston Medical and Surgical Journal, 3* (1869), 217.

[9] E.H. van Deusen, "Observations on a Form of Nervous Prostration (neurasthesias) Culminating in Insanity," *American Journal of Insanity, 25* (1869), 445–461. See Barbara Sicherman, "The Uses of a Diagnosis: Doctors, Patients, and Neurasthenia," *Journal of*

the History of Medicine and Allied Sciences, 32:1 (1977), 33–54.

10 Dorothy Ross, *G. Stanley Hall: The Psychologist as Prophet* (Chicago: University of Chicago Press, 1972), p. 381.

11 Fred A. Mettler, "Presidents in the First Fifty Years," *Centennial Anniversary Volume of the American Neurological Association*, edited by Derek Denny-Brown (New York: Springer, 1975), p. 89.

12 Ross, *Ibid.*, p. 382.

13 Henri F. Ellenberger, *The Discovery of the Unconscious* (New York: Basic Books, 1970), p. 344.

14 Bruce Kuklick, *The Rise of American Philosophy, Cambridge, Massachusetts: 1860–1930* (New Haven: Yale University Press, 1977).

15 Thomas C. Cadwallader, "Peirce as an Experimental Psychologist," *Transactions of the Charles S. Peirce Society*, Summer 1975, vol. XI, no. 3, pp. 167–186.

16 James Boardley and McGehee Harvey, "Psychiatry," *Two Centuries of American Medicine 1776–1976* (Philadelphia: W.B. Saunders, 1976), p. 732.

17 John S. Haller and Robin S. Haller, "The Nervous Century," *The Physician and Sexuality in Victorian America* (Urbana: University of Illinois Press, 1974), pp. 3–43.

18 Robert T. Edes, *The New England Invalid* (Boston: Clapp, 1895), p. 16.

19 Jerome M. Schneck, "United States of America," *World History of Psychiatry*, edited by John G. Howells (New York: Brunner-Mazel, 1975), pp. 432–475. James Boardley and McGehee Harvey, *Ibid.*, pp. 727–749. J.K. Hall, G.K. Zilborg, and H.A. Bunker, *One Hundred Years of American Psychiatry* (New York: Columbia University Press, 1944). Jerome M. Schneck, *A History of Psychiatry* (Springfield: Charles C. Thomas, 1960). Nolen D.C. Lewis, "American Psychiatry from its Beginnings to World War II," *American Handbook of Psychiatry*, vol. II, edited by Silvano Arieti (New York: Basic Books, 1959). John A.P. Millet, "Psychoanalysis in the United States," *Psychoanalytic Pioneers*, edited by Franz Alexander, Samuel Eisenstein, and Martin Grotjahn (New York: Basic Books, 1966), pp. 546–596. Clarence Obendorf, *A History of Psychoanalysis in America* (New York: Grune & Stratton, 1953).

20 Oliver Wendell Holmes, *Medical Essays 1842–1882* (Boston: Houghton Mifflin, 1891), p. 177.

Beginnings at the Turn of the Century

Boston at the Turn of the Century

DANIEL AARON

Cultural historians surveying the city of Boston at the end of the nineteenth century have tended to picture it as a decorous but devitalized community living off its financial and intellectual principal. This view is simplistic and partial, for Boston (like most major American cities between 1880 and 1900) was neither dull nor tepid; Boston exhibited its own forms of energy. But there is enough truth in the indictment to make it stick.

First, a few statistics and reminders. In 1900 the city numbered about a half-million inhabitants, almost two-thirds of them of recent foreign stock. Citizens of Irish descent predominated, but some 30,000 Jews (the latest influx from Russia and Austria-Hungary) flavored the melting pot. In all, twenty-five nationalities were represented in the North End.[1]

The denizens who swarmed in the Boston ghetto—particularly the recent arrivals from Southern and Eastern Europe—did not strike many old-stock Americans as suitable material for "amalgamation." When Frederick Jackson Turner accidentally wandered into Salem Street one day in 1887, the young visitor was more revolted than fascinated by "the swarthy sons and daughters of Israel" and elbowed his way out of "this mess of oriental noise and squalor" to the comforting haven of Old North Church.[2] Four years after Turner's misadventure in that ghetto, a group of Proper Bostonians ("wearied," in the words of Barbara Solomon, "of the burdens of humanitarianism") organized the Immigration Restriction League "to save the nation from foreign infiltration."[3] With the frontier virtually closed, as Turner himself announced in 1893, it was clear to the leaders of the league that Boston, along with other cities on the Eastern seaboard, faced a grave problem: the accumulation of "the objectionable races" in urban pockets. By this time the local gentry had already pretty well lost what tenuous connection they once might have had with immigrant Boston by enclosing themselves within the precincts of Beacon Hill and the Back Bay.[4]

A small number of liberal reformers, almost all of them born outside the Hub, did concern themselves with the plight of the slum dwellers and invidiously contrasted the well-being of the inhabitants of Commonwealth Avenue with the miseries of the tenement people in the North and South Ends. The majority of the old families, however, did not share the social attitudes of the new philanthropists any more than they did the moral and civic concerns of the antebellum reformers. Between 1882 and 1894, the last of these Boston worthies—Emerson, James Freeman Clarke, Bronson Alcott, Lowell, Whittier, Dr. Holmes, and Elizabeth Peabody—passed from the scene. Julia Ward Howe, Thomas Wentworth Higginson, and Edward Everett Hale lingered on for a decade or more, but in 1900 they were anachronisms who despised the ideals and manners of the reigning Boston society. Mrs. Howe referred slightingly to "society men" who mistook "the aristocracy of position for the aristocracy of character." Hale contrasted Boston's leaders of the 1840s—men who had "discovered the Columbia River or traded for fur with the Indians, or split off an iceberg in Labrador and sent it to Havana or Calcutta"[5] with latter-day Bostonians whose adventures were confined to unlocking boxes in safety-deposit vaults and clipping coupons. He might have added that they had cut themselves off from Boston's foreign constituency, which was to dominate city politics by 1900 (Boston elected its first Irish mayor in 1884), and played second fiddle to aggressive capitalists in less tradition-bound centers of the country.[6]

When and why did the fatal change occur? Most historians agree that the decline set in gradually and see the shift from self-assurance to "complacency and fulfillment" as coming after the Civil War. For a brief period the war held out a hope that men of Henry Adams's generation and class would assume the political leadership once enjoyed by their forebears before President Jackson's rise to power. Politicians more adroit than they in the art of machine politics and more at ease with the immigrant masses ended that possibility.[7] After New York decisively blocked Boston's bid for financial and industrial hegemony, the Brahmin class turned from business enterprise to civic custodial functions. They disparaged commerce, excluded parvenus, and disdained the aspirations of materialistic democracy. In the words of Frederic Jaher, the "established class . . . feared to confront new wealth, new relationships and innovations in technological techniques or social structure." Unsuccessful in the competition with bolder entrepreneurs from other regions and of humbler origins, the Boston patriciate fell back on social and cultural preoccupations. They became, in effect, the custodians of culture as well as of money.[8]

Boston's economic demotion did not cancel out its significance as a commercial or financial center. All the same, the city advanced less spectacularly than its rivals during the last decades of the century. Scions of the enterprising men who built factories and who financed and constructed western railroads no longer took chances. As business ability ceased to be a requisite for social recognition, it became harder for aspiring newcomers to penetrate the barricades erected by the old families. To quote Jaher again: "Class values rationalized class failures in commerce and Brahmin defeats strengthened resistance to the demands of competitive commercial life. As a result, many potential magnates practiced their entrepreneurial skills in other fields."[8] Nationally known Bostonians in the late nineteenth century were not commonly the sons of rich businessmen who had retreated from the competitive struggle. They were more likely to be activists like Oliver Wendell Holmes, Jr., or Charles Eliot, or Henry Cabot Lodge—Bostonians who were readier than most of the other menfolk in their clan to accommodate themselves to the values and assumptions of the industrial age.[9]

In the fine arts and the life of the mind, *fin de siècle* Boston (despite the vigor and genius of a handful of intellectuals) no longer deserved its title of America's Athens. Although H.G. Wells discovered nothing base or cruel or stupid in the Boston mentality of 1906, he pronounced it ineffectual and backward-looking, correct and imitative. He saw in it, he said, a "terrifying unanimity of aesthetic discrimination." In place of outstanding figures, it offered "a chorus of indistinguishable culture."[10] Another and more recent commentator from England makes the same point in a different way. According to Martin Green, the clubby and nerveless inheritors of New England's modest flowering reduced literature to its "social functions" and lied to themselves and the world. A few "aesthetes"—Henry Adams, Bay Lodge (the Senator's son), Trumbull Stickney—saved themselves by exile but gained their freedom at the price of vitality. The failure of the literary community could be traced in their lives, in their excessive dependence upon traditional culture, and in their inability to immerse themselves in the contemporary.[11]

William Dean Howells, that cool outsider charmed and flattered by old Boston yet never relinquishing his resentment against its snobberies, moved to New York City in 1889, an act signifying his recognition of New York's preeminence as a literary center. Howells noted "critical, fastidious" Boston's distaste for vulgarity in literature and architecture (he shared some of that feeling himself), but he was drawn to the robust culture of vulgar cities like New York.[12] Henry James winced at vulgarity even more perceptibly than his friend Howells, but he also felt the chill of Boston for all its serenity and decency. The Back Bay in particular evoked a quality of vacancy he never sensed in the Boston he had briefly but intensively known in the early sixties. Old Boston might have lacked "the parks and palaces and institutions" taken for granted by the new, but James missed the "uplifting *idea*," the "aptitude for the finer curiosity." Recollections of Wendell Phillips's antislavery eloquence, of Emerson lecturing in some "primitive" lecture hall, conveyed to him "more of the consciousness of literature and of history than all the promiscuous bustle of the Florentine palace by Copley Square."[13]

To James and other critics, Boston may have seemed a relic—a community sustained only by its past—but to less exacting observers, the city was far from dead. No other American city equaled the quality and number of its educational facilities, its public and private libraries, its impressive museums. If New York superseded it as a publishing center, Boston publishing more than merely survived. The *Atlantic* underwent a face lifting between 1898 and 1900 thanks to its new editor, Walter Hines Page. Houghton Mifflin and Little, Brown branched out and supplemented their standard lists of "household favorites" with best-selling historical novels and romances.[14]

Visitors to Boston were impressed by the variety of its cultural life, the high place Bostonians still accorded to "high thinking," their devotion to music and the fine arts, their tolerance for a genteel heterodoxy—even a mild bohemianism—if it did not clash with any public truths. To be sure, Boston was stronger in orchestras than in composers, in museums than in artists, in libraries than in distinguished writers, but in 1900 it exercised a strong if not dominant influence on American cultural life.

We are likely to forget this as we read the sardonic or despairing comments of Boston's detractors in the closing years of the century or the books and essays memorializing the city's past glories. It is easy to overlook the attraction Boston continued to have for passionate pilgrims from all over the United States. Howard Mumford Jones in *The Age of Energy* quotes a passage from a novel published in 1901. It records a young Southern woman's first impressions of Boston:

> Scanning the faces of pedestrians on the Boylston Street Mall, the little bride remarked, with some relief, that they did not look altogether inhuman. But the shop-fronts, with their enormous plate-glass windows, mosaiced [*sic*] in gorgeous costumes, deep-toned Oriental rugs, or glittering Japanese screens, seemed visions of impossible splendor. The squareness of the streets, the absence of trees, the vista of colossal stone palaces along Arlington, the carved animals over the windows of the Natural History Build-

ing, the terraced steps of the Institute, the air-hung pyramids of Trinity's towers, and, more than all, the stupendous white fortress of the Public Library dominating Copley Square, oppressed her with a sense of magnificence, of civilization, of the power of the North, of the presence of man, which belied every generalization of her rustic, untutored youth. It was her first revelation of a real city.[15]

This was one outsider's view. Another was Santayana's. His Boston/Cambridge (as he wrote to William James in 1900) was marked by "an unintelligent sanctimonious and often disingenuous Protestantism which is thoroughly alien and repulsive to me."[16] But the Protestant legacy (an amalgam of Puritanism, Unitarianism, and transcendentalism) that was so sterile to Santayana may have some bearing on the themes to be touched on in this symposium.

Ten years after Santayana complained to William James, Sigmund Freud observed in a letter to James Jackson Putnam: "I understand that all important intellectual movements have originated in Boston."[17] We can imagine how Santayana would have responded to this remark, but Freud's dubious generalization at least suggests an interesting question.

Is there any discernible connection between Boston's cultural condition in the late nineties and the founding of the Boston Psychoanalytic Society? I have been talking about a city that had lost its former dynamism, whose potency (to paraphrase what Santayana said of his Last Puritan) had petered out; a city where culture had become imitative, bland, introspective—where museums and collectors abounded but where there was little visual art. This is the city, Van Wyck Brooks observed, that had ceased to attract outsiders and had even repelled its own gifted children. This is the same Boston once renowned for its cranks and faddists of all persuasions. And this is the Boston whose most famous authors—in their own special sense—were psychologists. (The French critic Regis Michaud called Hawthorne the Conan Doyle of the conscience.)

Keep in mind, too, that the descendants of antebellum Boston leaders were not the comparatively integrated persons their fathers were, that they apparently felt qualms about their ineffectuality and constantly drew invidious contrasts between Boston's idyllic childhood and its jejune maturity. Is it entirely fortuitous, then, that a proper Bostonian like Dr. James Jackson Putnam should find in the doctrines of Sigmund Freud support for his theory (I quote Professor Nathan G. Hale, Jr.) "of internal conflict and alienation as major factors in nervous disorder?"[18]

According to Professor Hale, Putnam—like many other physicians of New England—encountered "the morbidly sensitive conscience that drove patients to pathological self-reproach." (Santayana's phrase for this state of mind was "the agonized conscience.") And as we read Putnam's analyses of children who tried but failed to conform to the expectations of others, who were unsuccessful competitors in games or business, who were unsustained by strong personal directives or by religious faith, and who adopted attitudes "of secrecy, shame, hostility or superiority" toward their critics or admirers,[19] are we not having spelled out for us what Henry Adams called in a letter to Henry James the "Type-Bourgeois-bostonien?" Was there any group in any American city at this time for whom the symbol of the Super Ego—the Puritan Paterfamilias, the monitory Ancestor—had such a compelling and enduring presence?

It need only be said in conclusion that if Henry Adams was describing himself and his spiritual kinsmen, he did not subsume all of Boston in that definition. There were others like William James and Putnam who retained something of the courage and independence and confidence of the older Boston. Like their friends or patients, they also felt anxiety—even at times despair—and could not be accused as their master, Emerson, was with disposing too easily of the problem of evil. But like him they were not slaves to memory or prisoners of the past. Both science and religion confirmed their confidence in the possibilities of spiritual freedom.

References

1 Arthur Mann, *Yankee Reformers in the Urban Age* (Cambridge, Mass., 1954), pp. 1–5.

2 Quoted in D. Aaron, "Communism and the Jewish Writer," in *The Ghetto Beyond*, ed. P.I. Rose (New York, 1969), p. 268. From a letter by F.J. Turner to Ellen Turner, June 30, 1887, in the Turner Papers, the Huntington Library.

3 Barbara M. Solomon, *Ancestors and Immigrants* (Cambridge, Mass., 1956), p. 104.

4 Mann, *Yankee Reformers*, p. 5.

5 *Ibid.*, pp. 11–23.

6 F.C. Jaher, "Boston Brahmins in the Age of Industrial Capitalism," in *The Age of Industrialism in America* (New York, 1968), p. 197.

7 G.M. Fredrickson, *The Inner Civil War* (New York, 1965).

8 F.C. Jaher, "Boston Brahmins," pp. 202, 215, and *passim*. See also Bainbridge Bunting, *Houses of Boston's Back Bay* (Cambridge, Mass., 1967), pp. 15–17.

9 Jaher, "Boston Brahmins," pp. 243, 214–215.

10 Quoted in Bunting, *Houses of Boston's Back Bay*, p. 17–18.

[11] Martin Green, *The Problem of Boston* (London, 1966), pp. 142–163.

[12] Van Wyck Brooks, *New England: Indian Summer, 1865–1915* (New York, 1940), p. 379.

[13] Henry James, *The American Scene* (New York and London, 1907), pp. 239–240. The "Florentine palace" is the Boston Public Library.

[14] Henry May, *The End of American Innocence* (New York, 1959), pp. 54–55.

[15] H.M. Jones, *The Age of Energy. Varieties of American Experience, 1865–1915* (New York, 1970), p. 194.

[16] Quoted in Brooks, *New England*, p. 441.

[17] Quoted in Nathan G. Hale, Jr., ed., *James Jackson Putnam and Psychoanalysis* (Cambridge, Mass., 1971), p. 101.

[18] *Ibid.*, p. 51.

[19] *Ibid.*, pp. 51–52.

William James: A Prime Mover of the Psychoanalytic Movement in America

BARBARA ROSS

William James has frequently been cited as a moralist, philosopher, essayist, man of letters, physiologist, and psychologist; seldom, however, is he included among the psychoanalytic pioneers. Nevertheless, James was one of the powerful individual personalities who contributed to the development of psychoanalysis and psychotherapy in its early days, at a time when few were willing to do so.

Revolutionary intellectual forces were at work in the late nineteenth century as a number of perspectives converged. One movement was dedicated to restoring a type of economic individualism and political democracy as well as a kind of morality and civic purity that was widely believed to have existed earlier in America and to have been destroyed by the great corporations and the corrupt political machine.[1]

William James was a proponent of rugged individualism and recognized the important role of the energies of men in their struggle for survival. He epitomized the practical pioneer spirit, the sense of personal responsibility, and a profound distaste for American institutions. He did not respect civilization with its "herding and branding, licensing and degree-giving, authorizing and appointing, and in general regulating and administering by system the lives of human beings."[2] He did not like political questions being focused for him; the same was true of philosophical issues.[3] James's constant wish was that all ideas, including his own, be viewed as only approaches to the truth, and that all possibilities be heard.[4]

The prevailing views in science in the latter half of the nineteenth century were positivistic and materialistic; the intellectual populace prided itself on its love of "Science and Facts." Although James respected the careful procedures of empirical science, he was not in accord with its contempt for all metaphysics. He was vehemently against *authoritarian* science, which, he believed, forced reduction of the world to isolated and particular phenomena that had no ulterior connections. "Love is dead," he wrote, "or at any rate seems weak and shallow wherever science has taken possession."[5] Dickinson S. Miller said of James: "His attitude was incomparably superior to that of naturalistic philosophers who continue to play their favorite chess-game of theory without even considering what provision is to be made for the religious nature and needs of mankind, what reconstruction is possible in the devastated region."[6]

Naturalism was in need of an airing, in James's opinion. The major faults that he found with scientists were their overwhelming need for order and their tendency to perceive the world selectively. He criticized them for invoking the authority of science when dealing with ultimate problems.[7] He preferred instead to search for relations among the chaos that did not attract the typical scientist's attention.[8] His mind was always sympathetic, as he saw men and women trying to stifle faiths natural and joyful to them at the dictates of the scientific code.[9]

At the same time, psychologists, self-conscious about the status of their discipline and wanting to emulate the natural sciences, turned to laboratory psychology in the tradition of German experimentalism. They sought exactness and measurement, applied physical and mathematical laws to psychic facts, and emphasized the external conditions of psychic life. James could not be bound by these criteria. His interest went further than that of most of psychology's adherents; it proceeded to the regions of men's aspirations, and their sense of support for these aspirations.[10]

A chief part of James's function, it appears, was to protest in psychology, as in his life, against artificial analyses, the excesses and mechanical crudities of the analytical spirit (for example, associationism), and to make others feel the uniqueness, the individuality of psychic facts.[11] He disputed the subject matter, aims, and methods of psychology with Ladd, Cattell, and other leading figures in American psychology.

James was called an "impressionist" in psychology by G. Stanley Hall, his former student. In a review of the monumental work, *The Principles of Psychology*,[12] Hall criticized James's mixture of science and metaphysics and his lack of the experimental spirit. However, Hall described the book as "altogether stimulating and suggestive, and showing great industry and versatility...Its very inconsistencies and incoherences not only reflect but greatly magnify all the unrest, distraction, and conflicts of the present hour." Hall referred to James as "a veritable storm-bird, fascinated by problems most impossible of solution, and surest where specialists and experts in his own field are most in doubt."[13]

Early in 1890, James wrote to Sully, an English friend: "It seems to me that psychology is like physics before Galileo's time, not a single *ele-*

mentary law yet caught a glimpse of. A great chance for some future psychologue to make a greater name than Newton's."[14] James did not have the temperament of the true laboratory man.[15] He advised Howison[16] in 1891 to "...give up the notion of having a laboratory of *original research.* My private impression," he wrote, "is that that business is being overstocked in America, and that the results are not proportionate to the money expended. I refer especially to 'exact' work like that of Wundt's laboratory."[17] Several years later James saw no improvement: "The results that come from all this laboratory work seem to me to grow more and more disappointing and trivial."[18] James felt that there was little point in such preoccupation with measurement without the development of imaginative assumptions or interesting hypotheses.

The provisional and hypothetical nature of the foundations of scientific psychology were obvious to James, and it led him to disavow any finality of psychology as a natural science,[19] and he pleaded with his colleagues to do the same. Realizing that he was living in a time of transition and confusion in the discipline, he was attuned to any and all information that might contribute to clarifying some of the issues. Most frequently, he promoted ideas and movements that were unpopular among the scientific community—hypnosis, psychical research,[20] and the study of abnormal psychology in general. James hoped that studies of abnormal phenomena might throw light on the central constitution and deeper causes of human nature.[21]

James was inspired by the writings of the Scottish School and the German Idealist movement, which in the latter part of the nineteenth century had lost ground to the positivist, naturalist, and materialist philosophies.[22] French and English psychology, which was not in such sharp opposition to the old metaphysical conceptions, appealed to James; those who followed in that tradition never ceased to employ self-observation, and were interested in investigation of higher psychic functions rather than in theories of sensation and psychometry.

James's metaphysics was pluralistic; he dealt with a multitude of mental states, stressed the dynamic in the interpretation of mental life, and emphasized the pathology of the mind.[23] He referred to his psychology as "functional," by which he meant that the clinical conceptions, "though they may be vaguer than the analytic ones (associationist), are certainly more adequate, give the concreter picture of the way the whole mind works, and are of far more urgent practical importance."[24] Functional or clinical psychology as pursued by Janet and others was assuredly most worthy of study, James argued. That approach, which emphasized apparently "mystical" phenomena and the subconscious, was the unpopular one held by only a minority of American academic psychologists.

In his presidential address before the American Psychological Association in 1894, James repeated his earlier condemnations of laboratory psychology, and discussed the phenomenon of dissociation of consciousness, which, he said, "surely throws more new light on human nature than the work of all the psychophysical laboratories put together."[25] He disputed the associationist position, denounced "soul-doctrines" such as Ladd's, suggested that transcendental philosophers dabble some in psychology, and finally, "to make the unlucky presidential hour more gossipy," announced that he was giving up the position taken in the *Principles* regarding consciousness. He said, "I see...better now than then that my proposal to designate mental states merely by their cognitive functions leads to a somewhat strained way of talking of some emotional states. I am willing, consequently, henceforward, that mental contents should be called complex, just as their objects are, and this even in psychology." He advised his colleagues that not till they had "laid bare more of the nature of that altogether unique kind of complexity in unity which mental states involve; not till then, I say, will psychology reach any real benefit from the conciliatory spirit of which I have done what I can to set an example."[26]

James was trying to persuade his fellow psychologists to change their ways; he felt they would profit by attending to the work coming out of other areas, particularly the studies of extramarginal or subliminal consciousness. His comments were not confined to psychologists, however. He attacked medical men, neurologists, physiologists, or any who were predisposed to champion natural science, a mechanistic explanation, or an oversimplified approach to mental disorders. He tried to direct them into a broader conception of the study of human nature than those held by the individual factions. This broader conception should include a consideration of the studies of phenomena such as hypnosis, hallucinations, trancelike states, demoniacal possession, psychical research, and automatic writing. He wrote that he wanted to get the medical profession out of "its conceited ignorance of such matters which everywhere and at all times played a vital part in human history."[27] "No part of the unclassed residuum," he said, "has usually been treated with a more contemptuous scientific disregard than the mass of phenomena generally called *mystical*. Physiology will have nothing to do with them. Orthodox psychology turns its back upon them. Medicine sweeps them out."[28]

As in so many realms, James held left-wing beliefs even within the party of the supernaturalists. He preferred to include the supernatural in the same realm of fact with the natural. He proposed a pluralistic mysticism and an experimental supernaturalism.[29]

Despite the negative scientific and medical attitude toward "mystical" phenomena, James read the available works and published extensive accounts. He was an avid reader in several languages. In 1868 he wrote a lengthy review of Liébault's *Du Sommeil et des États analogues, considérés surtout au point de vue de l'action du Moral sur le Physique*.[30] Essentially, Liébault proposed that artificial or "magnetic" sleep be enlisted in the service of therapeutics used by physicians. Although James was concerned that Liébault was led to "some curious theories," he recommended the book, because he believed that many observations promised to be of scientific importance, and that practitioners would find in it "a great many sagacious practical hints."

In the same year, when discussing Claude Bernard's report of the state of general physiology in France,[31] James focused on the difficulties of the medical student, who, he suggested, was called upon to master a considerable amount of science of which the applications were not developed.

In his 1869 review of *Planchette: or the Despair of Science*,[32] James showed interest in applying scientific method to abnormal psychology, and urged vigorous study of a few test cases of alleged spiritistic phenomena.

James demonstrated both his objectivity and promotion of interest in all kinds of evidence and ideas, however unpopular, by his willingness to gather information in America for the Census of Hallucinations, an idea of Edmund Guerney's. James wrote letters to the editors of the *American Journal of Psychology* and *The Open Court* asking their cooperation in soliciting canvassers.[33] He expected that the census would help to settle the issues regarding the truth of such phenomena. When the report was completed, James asked that science give a fair hearing to the results. He hoped the readers would appreciate the candor of the committee, and see how earnestly they sought to eliminate all that might add specious color, as distinguished from real weight, to their side.[34]

A "notable" book on the subject of hallucinations was Parrish's *Ueber die Trugwahrnehmung*. About it James wrote: "One may find reference to everything, important and unimportant, that in recent years has been written on hallucinations from either the medical or the psychological point of view." According to James, Parrish's theory of the hallucinatory process, that it is always an incident of "dissociated" conditions of consciousness, was "most important."[35]

Little escaped James's attention, including the work of several Frenchmen on déjà vu, which, according to Lalande, was too widespread to be pathological. He proposed a theory based on subliminal or "unconscious" telepathic perception, and suggested that the key to paramnesia must be sought in the existence of a double perception, unconscious at first and then conscious.[36]

Janet's work on hysteria, in the tradition of Charcot, drew the most admiration from James. In "The Hidden Self" James noted Janet's and Binet's studies on hypnotism, hysteria, and multiple personality, and predicted that the reports would provoke controversy and stimulate observation.[37] In a lengthy article several years later, James reviewed Janet's position and said that every psychologist should be acquainted with the material.[38] Of Janet's monograph, *Histoire d'une Idée Fixe*, he said: "The article is full of acute psychology...and is of course most instructive practically."[39]

James's interest in hysteria and related subjects was high in the nineties, yet he did not appear terribly impressed with Breuer's and Freud's initial work. He wrote that F.W.H. Myers, a British researcher in psychical phenomena, had stated many years before that hysteria was a disease of the hypnotic stratum, and that the article, which James *did* say was "important," was "a comment on Myers's dictum" and "an independent corroboration of Janet's views." Breuer and Freud, James concluded, "make then (apparently) a new connection with the principal consciousness...and the sufferer gets well. Janet's Marcella...would be a case in point."[40] At the time of Freud's visit to Clark University, when most American psychiatrists and psychologists were still not receptive to dynamic considerations, James wrote to Flournoy, after having talked with Freud at Clark, that he hoped Freud and his pupils would push their ideas to their utmost limits.[41] Hale submits that James was perhaps the first American to notice the work of Breuer and Freud.[42]

James was aware of the work being done in abnormal psychology in many countries, and saw relationships among the so-called "mystical" phenomena not so clearly seen by others. He commented on Bernheim's work, which contended that "all hysteric anaesthesias were mental and the resultant of 'auto-suggestion' analogous in all points to the systematized anaesthesias which suggestion produced in hypnotic subjects." James ended his article with the comment: "One is reminded of Mr. Myers's phrase that hysteria is a 'disease of the hypnotic stratum.' "[43]

Myers's discovery of an extramarginal or subliminal consciousness was seen by James as the most important step forward in psychology. Classical psychology, he believed, was only an extract of something infinitely more complex than was previously suspected.[44]

James's ability to synthesize various information about mystical phenomena is also seen in his article on Wernicke's studies of disordered mental functions. "In many respects there are analogies between patients with delusions and cases of hysteria such as those that Janet, Breuer and Freud have explored," he wrote, "and this would suggest that it might be well to search for parasitic systems of subconscious ideas as a possible source of some of the trouble in the former cases. In one way ('disintegration of personality') Wernicke's 'sejunction' formula coincides with Janet's, yet Wernicke ignores altogether the notion of subconscious ideas; and indeed it is evident that if they exist we need quite new methods of finding them out." Wernicke's hypothesis of sejunction opened "a new era of interpretation in mental psychology," which was a "great service." James expressed the hope that the book would be translated "without loss of time."[45]

James continued to promote Janet's and similar viewpoints. He replied to Peirce's, Von Schrenk's, and Landmann's writings in which Guerney, Janet, Binet, and others were criticized. Peirce's essays "brought out no new facts, and their alternative hypotheses," it seemed to James, carried matters "backwards rather than forwards."[46] And of Morselli's book on an experimental examination of consciousness James wrote, "We get almost the whole of Wundt's physiological psychology...It is only one more instance to add to the number which prove affinity between the Italian and German turn of mind...An Englishman or Frenchman would have lightened the burden by throwing out much of the only hypothetically practical matter."[47] He was convinced the French were doing the best work,[48] and their studies on subliminal phenomena took on great significance in his own theorizing.

James's attention was not confined to work being done in foreign countries. American psychiatrists and others were taken to task for holding too narrow a perspective in their consideration of abnormal states. Dr. Isaac Ray was criticized for being concerned with sending patients to asylums and for attending to legal issues "rather than making fresh discoveries."[49] Maudsley, who suggested that the insane were not flexible enough to be held responsible for their acts, was another with whom James took issue. The matter, he argued, was one of public policy, and Hammond's pamphlet on the subject published a year before reflected a "truer, if less merciful view."[50]

Asylums in America were described by James as inflicted with "bad and sodden routine with resigned officials and an ignorant public." When Clifford Beers requested James's opinion as to the advisability and feasibility of a national society for the improvement of conditions among the insane, James responded: "Such an improvement is one of the most crying needs of civilization...As mediator between officials, patients, and the public conscience, a society such as you sketch is absolutely required, and the sooner it gets under way the better."[51] James gave time and counsel to further the organization of the Mental Hygiene Committee; he even departed from his fixed policy at this late time in his life "of keeping out of Committees and Societies,"[52] and became one of the twelve charter members. Furthermore, at one point the continuance of the society was made possible only by a timely $1,000 loan from James to Beers.[53]

James held views on many subjects and presented them with force and vigor. He wanted to see psychologists and psychiatrists deal with the facts of personal functioning. He recognized the poorer chance for definiteness and measurability with this emphasis, but was more interested in gains in the possiblity of treatment. He believed that the value of psychological knowledge rested in the power of applying general principles to real life situations.

The "thought healing," "moral treatment," or "mental therapeutics" movements of the latter part of the nineteenth century captured James's attention. Such developments were not taken seriously by American academic or scientific psychologists, nor by most neurologists and medical men. Even though the movements incurred the "enmity of the trades union wing" of the medical profession,[54] James not only was seriously interested, but also became a strong supporter. Such movements were "important, interesting, and had both a speculative and practical side."[55] He realized that there were inherent failures and deceptions; the fact remained, however, that the spread of these ideas was due to "practical fruits." Although the treatment of neuroses and everyday emotional problems developed as somewhat independent movements, he saw relationships among them and these other seemingly peripheral movements.

James noted that the findings of the studies on subliminal and other abnormal matters reflected attempts to apply the use of spiritual participation for psychotherapeutic purposes. The Emmanuel Movement was one example of "moral" treatment. Proponents employed faith and suggestion and the strengthening of the will, and recognized hypnosis, suggestion, and persuasion as legitimate methods of psychotherapy. The aim of the Emmanuel Movement was to inculcate suggestions from the scriptures in accordance with the principle that a temporary dissociation of the personality allowed ready acceptance of faith-laden ideas by the subconscious. In this manner, the universality of suggestion as a mechanism operating through the subconscious was stressed.[56]

The real problems of reconciling religion and psychiatry in their common therapeutic goals drew attention from exponents in both fields. "Both disciplines taught methods for attaining serenity and peace of mind; both charged themselves with the task of resolving basic concepts of psychotherapy with correlative ones from the Christian doctrine of redemption and Judaic concepts of the 'revelation of God's working in history.' From a theological point of view the possibility arose that 'inner conflict' could be incorporated in the doctrine of sin, and healing (trust and acceptance) in the doctrine of grace."[57] James held the conviction that most metaphysical healing seemed to involve something like the telepathic action of one subliminal self upon another.[58] In *The Varieties of Religious Experience* James wrote that "the subconscious may be the mediating link between the human and the divine." He also noted that the subconscious, however designated, was one of the fundamental verities of the mental healers. When he reviewed Whipple's *Philosophy of Mental Healing* he said: "It is but just to our American mind-curers of the various sects to say that for years past the notion that all sorts of morbid symptoms may spring from subconscious fixed ideas, such as old fears, griefs, and remorses, has been the basis of their treatment."[59]

Once again, promulgating a nonpopular point of view, James made a speech in 1898 to oppose a bill regarding licensing of medical practitioners. The bill attempted to abolish the faith curers by requiring them to become Doctors of Medicine. James's speech, given at the State House, was published in the *Banner of Light*.[60] He referred to the incident in a letter to Putnam: "If you think I *enjoy* that sort of thing you are mistaken. I never did anything that required as much moral effort in my life."[61] But moral effort expended by James seemed always to be replenished.

Although James's influence on the development of psychotherapy and psychiatry is not always directly discernible,[62] through the power of his personality and writing he was chiefly responsible in his time for advancing European ideas in psychology and related areas. He has often been praised for his early attention to the contributions that nineteenth century medicine made to psychological knowledge; his sympathetic references to the French neurologists, to Guerney's and Myers' work in England, and to similar viewpoints aroused much interest in America. After many years of struggling with such phenomena as the "mystical," he did his utmost to make the doctrine of the subconscious respectable.

It appears that James's ideas made an impression and were realized by some of his students and colleagues. Among the former were G. Stanley Hall, Morton Prince, and Boris Sidis. W.A. White, who was a student of Sidis's, attributed an especially important role to Hall, James, and Sidis in influencing psychiatric thinking in this country.[63] Otto Marx wrote that James's and Janet's orientation might have been at least partially responsible for drawing Prince toward academic psychology, and that it might have been due to James's influence that Prince retained a nondoctrinaire approach. As was true of James, Prince focused on exceptional psychological phenomena, recognized that "cures" could be effected by any mode of therapy, psychoanalysis included, and helped to make psychotherapeutic efforts more generally acceptable.[64] He was noted among the "greats" by James in *The Varieties of Religious Experience*: "The wonderful explorations by Binet, Janet, Breuer, Freud, Mason, Prince, and others, of the subliminal consciousness of patients with hysteria . . . have revealed to us whole systems of underground life."[65]

James's importance in the professional development of William Healy, who founded the Juvenile Psychopathic Institute in Chicago, is recognized by George Gardner in another paper in this collection and, as Hale has suggested, it is possible that James Jackson Putnam would not have taken up psychoanalysis without the influence of William James.[66]

About a year and a half before his death, James was referred to as "a philosopher-psychologist, temperamentally interested in mysticism, professionally engaged in philosophy, and temporarily assuming the role of a psychologist...the spoiled child of American psychology, exempt from all serious criticism, and the beau ideal of a large and cultured circle . . . [who] since the publication of his *Principles of Psychology*, has apparently relaxed the intellectual inhibition which every man should exert over his desires . . . "[67] James was hardly exempt from criticism; his preference for the unusual and his tendency toward nonconformity evoked sharp criticism from many directions. He had a strong intellectual conscience, however, which did not allow him to acquiesce for the sake of being agreeable. To exert inhibitions over his beliefs would have been uncharacteristic. A friend wrote to him in 1902, "Your glorious freedom from any inhibitory impulse seems admirably illustrative of what...God had in mind when he started to make man in his image and hadn't made a botch of it."[68]

James must certainly be considered among those powerful individuals in New England who contributed to the development of psychotherapy. His good fortune of having had liberal and well-to-do parents allowed him to have a liberal education, exposure to many of the outstanding intellectuals in diverse areas, and the opportunity to travel extensively. His ability to read and speak several languages was, no doubt, an important factor in his role as harbinger of foreign ideas to Americans. He read, studied, assimilated, and passed on to psychologists, psychiatrists, others in the medical field, and the public at large all the information on the subject of the abnormal that he believed to be important, whether he was in complete accord with it or not. And, as has been demonstrated, he supported controversial and nonpopular issues at a time when few were willing to do so.

James laid much of the groundwork that compelled psychologists and others to initiate research into dynamic processes and mental disorders and that led to an interest in psychoanalytic thought in particular and to psychotherapy in general.

References

1 Richard Hofstadter, *The Age of Reform* (New York: Random House, 1955).

2 Ralph B. Perry, ed., *The Thought and Character of William James* (2 vols.; Boston: Little, Brown, 1935), II, 267. James wrote an article entitled "The Ph.D. Octopus," in the *Harvard Monthly, 36* (1903), 1–9, in which he he expressed concern with the growing emphasis on the doctor's degree as un-American.

3 *Ibid.*, I, 624.

4 D.S. Miller, *Journal of Philosophy, 24* (1924), 204.

5 Henry James, ed., *Letters of William James* (2 vols.; Boston: Atlantic Monthly Press; London: Longmans, Green, 1920), I, 337ff.

6 Miller, *Journal of Philosophy, 24* (1924), 205. Miller was a personal and close friend of James who nevertheless was the leader of the opposition to James's emphasis on the primacy of the will.

7 James, note (unsigned) on the *Revue Philosophique, Nation, 22* (March 2, 1876), 147.

8 William James, *The Varieties of Religious Experience: A Study in Human Nature* (New York and London: Longmans, Green, 1902), p. 438.

9 Miller, *Journal of Philosophy, 24* (1924), 206.

10 *Ibid.*, p. 204.

11 *Ibid.*, p. 206.

12 William James, *The Principles of Psychology* (New York: Holt, 1890).

[13] G.S. Hall, *American Journal of Psychology, 3* (1891), 585–591.

[14] Perry, *Thought and Character of William James*, II, 113.

[15] Despite his later aversion to laboratory psychology, James wrote: "I, myself, 'founded' the instruction in experimental psychology at Harvard in 1874–5, or 1876...For a long series of years the laboratory was in two rooms of the Scientific School building, which at last became choked with apparatus, so that a change was necessary. I then, in 1890, resolved on an altogether new departure, raised several thousand dollars, fitted up Dana Hall, and introduced laboratory exercises as a regular part of the undergraduate psychology-course." *Ibid.*, II, 13ff. Original published in *Science*, N.S., II (1895), 626.

[16] G.H. Howison was a friend and a member of the Boston Philosophical Club to which James also belonged in Boston.

[17] Perry, *Thought and Character of William James*, II, 116.

[18] *Letters of William James*, II, 54.

[19] O. Kraushaar, "Lotze's Influence on the Psychology of William James," *Psychological Review, 43* (1936), 235–257.

[20] In James's view, critics of psychical research such as G. Stanley Hall "were obeying the dictates of a theoretic creed." William James, *American Journal of Psychology, 1* (1887), p. 128ff.

[21] Perry, *Thought and Character of William James*, II, 157.

[22] *Ibid.*, I, 464.

[23] *Ibid.*, II, 156.

[24] *Ibid.*, II, 51.

[25] James, "The Knowing of Things Together," *Psychological Review, 2* (1895), 114.

[26] *Ibid.*, p. 124.

[27] *Letters of William James*, II, 57.

[28] James, "The Hidden Self," *Scribner's Magazine, 7* (1890), 361–373.

[29] *Thought and Character of William James*, II, 332ff.

[30] James, review (unsigned) on Moral Medication, *Nation, 7* (July 16, 1868), 50–52.

[31] James, review (unsigned) of Claude Bernard's *Rapport sur le Progrès et la Marche de la Physiologie générale en France, North American Review, 107* (1868), 322–328.

[32] James, *Boston Daily Advertiser*, March 10, 1869.

[33] James, letter to the editor, *American Journal of Psychology, 3* (1890), 292; letter to the editor, *Open Court, 4* (May 22, 1890), 2437–2440.

[34] James, review of (H. Sidgwick, A. Johnson, et al.) "Report on the Census of Hallucinations," *Psychological Review, 2* (1895), 69–75.

[35] James, *Psychological Review, 2* (1895), 65–67. James added a footnote (p. 65): "Herr P. expressly bases his theory on that of the hallucinatory process given in *Principles of Psychology*, II, ii.ff."

36 James, notice of A. Lalande, *Des Paramnésies, Psychological Review, 1* (1894), 94–95; notice of B. Bourdon, *La Reconnaissance des Phenomènes Nouveaux, ibid.*, 317; notice of J. Le Lorrain, *A Propos de la Paramnésie, ibid.*

37 James, "The Hidden Self," *Scribner's Magazine, 7* (1890), 361–373.

38 James, notice of P. Janet, *État Mental des Hysteriques and L'Amnésie Continue, Psychological Review, 1* (1894), 195–199.

39 James, notice of P. Janet, *Histoire d'une Idée Fixe, Psychological Review, 1* (1894), 315–316.

40 James, notice of J. Breuer and S. Freud, *Ueber den Psychischen Mechanismus Hysterischer Phänomene, Psychological Review, 1* (1894), 199.

41 Henry James, *Letters of William James*, II, 327.

42 Nathan G. Hale, Jr., *James Jackson Putnam and Psychoanalysis* (Cambridge, Mass.: Harvard University Press, 1971) p. 67.

43 James, notice of H. Bernheim, *Psychical Nature of Hysterical Unilateral Amblyopia, etc., Psychological Review, 1* (1894), 93–94.

44 Perry, *Thought and Character of William James*, II, 168, and James, *Varieties of Religious Experience*, p. 120.

45 James, notice of C. Wernicke, *Grundriss der Psychiatrie, Psychological Review, 4* (1897), 225–227.

46 James, notice of A.H. Peirce, *Subliminal Self*, F. Podmore, *Reply*, F. Von Schrenk-Notzing, *Ueber Spaltung der Persönlichkeit*, and S. Landmann, *Die Mehrheit geistiger Persönlichkeiten, Psychological Review, 3* (1896), 682–684.

47 James, notice of E. Morselli, *Manuale della Semejotica della Malattie Mentali, Psychological Review, 3* (1896), 679–681.

48 Perry, *Thought and Character of William James*, II, 121.

49 James, review (unsigned) of I. Ray, *Contributions to Mental Pathology, Atlantic Monthly, 31* (1873), 748–750.

50 James, review (unsigned) of H. Maudsley, *Responsibility in Mental Disease, Atlantic Monthly, 34* (1874), 364–365.

51 *Letters of William James*, II, 274.

52 *Ibid.*, 273.

53 J.K. Hall, ed., *One Hundred Years of American Psychiatry* (New York: Columbia University Press, 1944), p. 359.

54 Walter Bromberg, *Man Above Humanity* (Philadelphia: Lippincott, 1954), p. 141.

55 James, notice of L.E. Whipple, *Philosophy of Mental Healing, Psychological Review, 1* (1894), 199–200. Also, Hale, *James Jackson Putnam and Psychoanalysis*, p. 67.

56 Bromberg, *Man Above Humanity*, pp. 140–141.

57 *Ibid.*, p. 142.

58 Both James and Janet struggled with the reconciliation of scientific and religious sentiment, and both were intrigued with "occult" matters of "mystical" phenomena.

59 James, review of Leander E. Whipple, *The Philosophy of Mental Healing: A Practical Exposition of Natural Restorative Power* (New York: Metaphysical Publishing Co., 1893), *Psychological Review, 1* (1894), 199–200.

60 *Banner of Light*, March 12, 1898.

61 Nathan G. Hale, Jr., *James Jackson Putnam and Psychoanalysis* (Cambridge, Mass.: Harvard University Press, 1971), p. 71.

62 See Otto M. Marx, "American Psychiatry Without William James," *Bulletin of the History of Medicine, 42* (1968), No. 1.

63 Hall, *One Hundred Years of American Psychiatry*, p. 297.

64 Otto M. Marx, "Morton Prince and the Dissociation of a Personality," *Journal of the History of the Behavioral Sciences, 6* (1970), 129, 128.

65 James, *Varieties of Religious Experience*, p. 235.

66 Hale, *James Jackson Putnam and Psychoanalysis*, p. 67.

67 L. Witmer, *Psychological Clinic, 2* (1909), 289–299. See also *The Thought and Character of William James*, II, 153.

68 B. Wendell, in *Thought and Character of William James*, II, 341.

G. Stanley Hall

DOROTHY ROSS

In his own lifetime, Stanley Hall was never at the center of intellectual or cultural affairs in Boston, and he was always keenly aware of that fact.[1] He was born in 1844 in a small village in northwestern Massachusetts, of nine generations of modest Congregational ancestors. His father was a farmer, and, as often happened with young men on the farms who had to work off time before they were free to leave, Stanley was almost twenty when he enrolled in nearby Williams College. Though he went on to Union Theological Seminary in New York, and then spent a year in Germany, he still felt somewhat the provincial when he arrived in Boston in 1876 to study psychology with William James. He never managed to assume easy relations with James, James's impressive father and the intellectual milieu in Cambridge, a group closely knit by ties of family and acquaintance, for he was already the kind of person who felt constantly threatened, martyred, and abused. Consequently, most of the young Cambridge men never got closer than to regard him, as Henry P. Bowditch remarked, as a kind of "queer genius."

His relations with William James, the teacher to whom he owned so much, grew particularly tortuous as their individual careers developed. In 1878, after taking a Ph.D. degree with James in psychology, the first such degree awarded in this country, Hall returned to Berlin and Leipzig for two more years of study, making himself one of the most widely, if not deeply, schooled Americans in the new field of physiological psychology. But when he came back again to America, now with a wife expecting their first child, he could barely support himself with academic odds and ends. In only a few more years the reform of American colleges and universities would create a burgeoning market for new Ph.D.'s with some scientific expertise, but Hall was still some years ahead of his time. Finally in 1884, at the age of forty, he was appointed professor of psychology and pedagogy at Johns Hopkins University, then the apex of America's educational system.

But Hall's new eminence did not quiet his anxieties. He began to champion what he called a "strictly scientific" psychology, as opposed to the kind of armchair psychology practiced by James and the older philosophically oriented theorists. Although he himself had severe doubts about an empirical psychology limited only to the narrow range of laboratory experimentation that was then available—indeed precisely because he did distrust such a narrow framework—he attacked James and the philosophical psychologists, cleverly and mercilessly. He was determined to make psychology a rigorous science and to capture the leadership of the new profession from that height.

When, in 1887, Hall left Hopkins to become the founding president of Clark University in Worcester, Massachusetts, he had still another and nearer base from which to challenge James. Hall hoped to make Clark University into a solely graduate institution, dedicated to advanced scientific research. For its first few years of operation, from 1889 to 1892, he came very close to fulfilling his ideal, with an exceptionally talented group of young scientists, including Albert A. Michelson in physics, H.H. Donaldson in physiology, Franklin P. Mall in neuroanatomy, and Franz Boas in anthropology. Hall was unable to keep this band together, however, and, as seemed often to be the case with him, the circumstances under which he lost his brilliant faculty led to personal recriminations and quarrels that seriously damaged his reputation in the academic world. Before and after this turning point at Clark in 1892, Hall continued to quarrel publicly with James, and now with Harvard too, about issues of rivalry between their institutions. Hall let it be known that he considered Clark a far more "advanced" institution than Harvard, a contention that James was hardly ready to admit. Things came to such an impasse that Robert M. Yerkes, the animal psychologist, recalled that when he was at Harvard around the turn of the century, he was "given to understand that it was either indiscreet or bad form for a Harvard psychologist to try to cultivate friendly professional relations with G. Stanley Hall and his Clark associates."

During the late 1890s and the first two decades of the twentieth century, Hall largely withdrew from psychological combat into the tiny institution at Clark, which he had managed to salvage, and which he ran during all those years on an annual budget of $28,000 (except for separate library funds). Beleaguered, the victim of the hostilities from his colleagues that he himself had set off, Hall also gave up the attempt to formulate a strictly scientific psychology. He turned his interest to subjects his psychological colleagues considered marginal and heretical, but which he felt to be of genuine moment in the lives of people—sexuality, psychopathology, the study of child development, and adolescence. The man who brought Freud to America in 1909 was decidedly a maverick, whose actions were always suspect to his professional peers, and whose cherished institution clung precariously to existence.

Yet Stanley Hall also managed to preserve in himself and in Clark University genuine intellectual values, and the high quality of some of the work done there was appreciated elsewhere. One of the impressive intellectual events sponsored by Hall was the conference he arranged at Clark in 1899 to celebrate the tenth anniversary of the founding of the university. He brought five distinguished foreign scientists to Clark: Santiago Ramón y Cajal, of the University of Madrid, whose work in histology was one of the principal sources of the neurone theory; Antonio Mosso of the University of Milan, pioneer student of physiology and development; August Forel, professor of psychiatry at Basel and director of the Bürgholzli Asylum; Emile Picard, professor of mathematics at the University of Paris; and Ludwig Boltzmann, professor of theoretical physics at the University of Vienna. Clearly, Hall had a talent for recognizing intellectual quality. When the twentieth anniversary of Clark drew near, in 1909, he wanted to arrange a conference of equal distinction.

Hall recognized the rising interest in the subject of psychotherapy in Boston and Cambridge, and although he was still largely cut off from Boston psychological and medical circles, he followed with interest the new literature on psychotherapy. Since he read widely in German, he was aware of Freud's work with Breuer on hysteria as early as 1899, and there are references to Freud's work in his books and lectures in the years following. With typical aplomb, Hall apparently sensed that this was the right moment to upstage Boston and to make a major intellectual coup, both for himself and for Freud. This is undoubtedly part of what Freud sensed when he remarked later that "there was a touch of the 'King-maker' about [Hall]." Hall brought to Clark for the 1909 conference other distinguished European and American scholars, and spoke of Freud as representing "the psychology of the future." The conference proved to be a turning point not only in Freud's life, but in the receptiveness of America to psychoanalysis.

But this is only one part of the story of Hall's relationship to Freud and to the development of psychoanalysis and psychotherapy in America. Another part concerns his interest in sexuality. As Nathan Hale has shown us so brilliantly in his book, *Freud and the Americans*,[2] many of those who early appreciated the power of Freud's ideas were peculiarly sensitive to the ways in which American morality had inhibited sexuality and thereby crippled personality. Hall, too, was a victim of what Hale has termed "civilized morality." He initially believed that Freud's understanding of the importance of sexuality in psychic life was one of his principal accomplishments, but came later to retreat somewhat, and to criticize what he regarded as Freud's undue emphasis on sexuality. I might add that at some point during this shifting attachment to Freud, Hall underwent a partial psychoanalysis, though his analyst remains anonymous.[3]

But perhaps the most important factor in Hall's sympathetic attitude toward psychoanalysis was his devotion to genetic psychology. When, in the middle 1890s, he gave up the attempt to follow a rigorously scientific psychology, he began to work out his own version of a genetic psychology. He had always been attracted to evolutionary ideas, and had become impressed with the developmental approach through his studies of historical religious criticism, and of Hegel, Comte, and Herbert Spencer —that is, through the many sources of historical and evolutionary consciousness in the nineteenth century prior to Darwin. His serious studies of Darwin and biology only confirmed an outlook which he had long been forming.

Darwin enabled Hall to formulate a psychology based on the central role of instincts, or, as Hall called them, "feeling-instincts." These feeling-instincts, he believed, were native to the individual, but were acquired through experience in the long history of the race. As each individual develops, these instincts appear in sequence. Ontogeny recapitulates phylogeny. Hall studied this process in the context of individual development and thus came to concepts *somewhat* similar to Freud's; he talked, for example, about repression, reversion, and sublimation, which he called irradiation. The result of these processes, he believed, was a psyche that "seems built layer upon layer of partly isolated yet strangely interacting strata," a psyche in which much of the dynamic structure is unconscious and ill coordinated, yet acts powerfully on behavior. These unconscious layers, Hall said, revealed themselves in "the many-voiced comments, the sense of assent and dissent, pleasure and pain, the elation of strength or the esthetic responses, the play of intuitions, the impulses to do or not to do, automatic tensions or contractions" that run along beneath the conscious stream of images; and, he added, the "mild or incipient insanities which anyone that is honest and has true self-knowledge will...confess to recognizing in his own soul . . . " Hall obviously was sensitive to the troubled workings of his own mind. Evolutionary and biological conceptions allowed him to see these many, strangely interacting layers as deposits from past developmental stages. Unlike Freud, however, Hall traced these stages to the distant racial past and not to the dynamics of the living individual. He concluded that what was needed to understand the psyche was, quite literally, an "archeology of mind."

Hall was thus in a position to recognize the power of Freud's genetic theory, to appreciate the clarity it brought to processes he had only vaguely sensed, but also to distort it by assimilating it into his own phylogentically oriented geneticism. His own theory allows us to recognize the importance of biological evolutionary ideas, as forming a cultural matrix from which Freud himself drew and which also prepared the way for the acceptance of psychoanalysis.

Hall provides us, then, with a fascinating mixture of blindness and perspicuity, of overreaching ambition and stoic failure, of debilitating personal problems and skewed perspectives all turned into genuine insight and intellectual courage. It is really quite fitting that such a man should have brought Freud to America.

References

1 The reader is referred to Dorothy Ross, *G. Stanley Hall: The Psychologist as Prophet* (Chicago: University of Chicago Press, 1972) for a more extended account of this subject and for references to the sources on which this essay is based. Hall's own account of his life is given in his *Life and Confessions of a Psychologist* (New York: D. Appleton, 1923). Hall's major work is a kind of compendium of his many interests and ideas: *Adolescence*, 2 vols. (New York: D. Appleton, 1904).

2 Nathan G. Hale, Jr., *Freud and the Americans: The Beginnings of Psychoanalysis in the United States, 1876–1917* (London: Oxford University Press, 1971).

3 Dr. Robert H. Sharpley reported to the conference that he was told by the son of Dr. Solomon Fuller that Dr. Fuller, the black neurologist, treated Hall for many years. Dr. Greta Bibring reported that Dr. Isador Coriat had told her that Hall's analysis had been conducted by someone who was not a real psychoanalyst.

The Contributions of the Worcester State Hospital and Post-Hall Clark University to Psychoanalysis

DAVID SHAKOW

My presentation will deal briefly with the Worcester State Hospital and Clark University in the period before I had personal experience with these institutions, and then return for a much fuller discussion of them in my own days. I shall also consider certain related aspects of the Boston scene with which I have been personally acquainted, but which appear to me to have been overlooked. Such an approach seems unavoidable if I am to consider some not unimportant features of psychoanalytic developments, both in the natural geographic hinterland of Boston, and in the artificial hinterland of neglect produced by the selective practices of historians.

We must keep in mind that this "back country" is the third city in New England and the second in Massachusetts. It had its own important institutions, institutions that played at least some role in the development of psychoanalysis, and that reached even beyond New England. In my time there (the twenties through the forties) it used to be said that Worcester had only three significant institutions: the Worcester Art Museum (particularly in the Taylor period), the Worcester Polytechnic Institute, and the Worcester State Hospital (particularly under William A. Bryan as superintendent). Their respective boards of trustees consisted mainly of interlocking directorates from among the first families of Worcester. Although Clark University had similar persons on its board, they did not appear so deeply committed to Clark—the poor man's college which their sons did not attend. (Of course, few of their sons attended Polytech, but that presumably stemmed from the fact that it provided training only for engineers.) This may have been true mainly because the university was so strongly identified with Jonas Clark, an outsider from Hubbardston. However, only the hospital and Clark are relevant and I shall briefly discuss the hospital in the Meyer period (1895–1902) and Clark in the Hall period (1888–1920). I shall devote most of my time to the hospital in the Bryan period (1921–1946), examine Clark in the Willoughby period (1926–1936), comment on the Boston Psychopathic Hospital in the Wells period (1922–1938), and close with an attempt to evaluate some of the factors I believe to have been neglected in the consideration of the history of psychoanalysis and its influence.

My initial involvement with psychoanalysis started around the age of fifteen—this was before our country had entered World War I—when I was a member of a nature-study-hiking-discussion group at a settlement house on the Lower East Side of New York. The "club" was a favorite of the head worker, Howard Bradstreet, a scion of that very early Massachusetts Puritan family which included Simon and Anne. At one of our meetings he told us about a revolution in ways of thinking about man which had resulted from the work of "Yungenfroid." His remarks intrigued me, so after the meeting I headed straight for the Seward Park Public Library—that incalculably important wellspring of intellectual development in our neighborhood—to get hold of some books by this author. But a search in the card catalogue under *Y* yielded nothing. At some cost to my self-esteem, I was finally reduced to inquiring of the librarian at the desk whether they had any books by Yungenfroid. Fortunately for me, she was—to use the old-fashioned but peculiarly appropriate term from introspective psychology—analytic rather than synthetic in type. This enabled her to disengage the "Freud" and "Jung" from the gestalt and refer me to the proper shelves. (I have distinguished company in this type of telescoped misunderstanding. Faulkner apparently did not disentangle the constituent parts of "damyankee" until he was a grown man!) In some way Jung got lost in the shuffle, which is perhaps not surprising since *Dreams*, *Psychopathology*, and *Wit* were enough to keep any youngster my age occupied!

From this early period, even though James, through Dewey, soon entered my life and became my permanent hero, I have maintained a deep and abiding interest in Freudian theory. The Jamesian influence led me to Harvard, where I obtained all my collegiate and postcollegiate education.

Despite the fact that there were no formal courses in Freud or personality while I was an undergraduate at Harvard (1921–1924), Freud was much in the air. I seem to remember mention of Freud in Floyd Allport's course in social psychology, which used as one of its texts a book of Hunter's containing a brief section on Freud. But mostly during my earlier undergraduate years it was William McDougall who gave Freud prominence. In two of the several courses I had with him, he read to us (in dull fashion, I might add; it always seemed to me that McDougall was much more comfortable in his teaching when he had a manuscript before him for support) from the manuscripts of two of his yet unpublished books: *Outline of Psychology* McDougall (1923) and *Outline of Abnormal Psychology* McDougall (1926). In both, despite the ambivalence with which he was presented, Freud played a most important role, for he was the constant foil against whom McDougall developed his own theories, particularly those on instinct. Indeed, it was McDougall who held, in the preface to his *Outline of Abnormal Psychology* (p. viii), that "Freud has done more for the advancement of psychology than any student since Aristotle." (This is in part corroborated by the eighteen lines given to Freud in the index to this volume as compared with those for the runners-up: ten for Jung, seven for Prince, and six for Janet.) I might point out that this judgment was expressed about a quarter century before that of Boring (1950:743), who, besides considering Freud one of the four "greats" of psychology's history—along with Darwin, Helmholtz, and James—characterized him as the "greatest originator of all."

In my later college years, 1923 and 1924, I was strongly influenced by my experiences at the Boston Psychopathic Hospital. These included Macfie Campbell's college seminar on "Psychology of Belief," which was heavily psychoanalytic in flavor, and the courses and opportunities for personal contact with one of the less appreciated early American influences in the spread of Freudian thinking—Fred Wells.

Such were some of the early psychoanalytic influences on a Harvard psychology student, especially on one interested in psychopathology, during the early 1920s.

The essential implications of my presentation will become evident as I go along. My major point will be to raise a question about the tendency of some psychoanalytic historians, particularly those medically oriented, to limit themselves altogether too much to obvious, direct lines of descent represented in more or less official persons and theories, particularly medical ones, and not to recognize sufficiently the lesser but gradual channeling effect of the nonmedical and related, if indirectly involved, persons and theories. I have in mind such interrelated factors as the role of conceptions rather than rigorous concepts in the spread of psychoanalysis, the role of the generally dynamic, the role of teachers and researchers, and the influence of certain minor aspects of the *Zeitgeist*.

Worcester State Hospital: the Meyer Period (1895–1902)

In 1895, Adolf Meyer (1866–1950), then at Kankakee, Illinois, accepted the invitation of Superintendent Quinby to come to Worcester, nominally as pathologist, but mainly as "guide, philosopher, and friend" (Meyer 1951:58) to the staff to supervise their work and, in an atmosphere of freedom, to develop research, therapy, and training there. This appointment laid the ground for one of the truly important developments in psychiatry and psychopathology of this century.

I suppose that the Meyer period at the Worcester State Hospital, the second of the three golden ages of the hospital, is in the present context important mainly for the excellent psychiatric training Meyer provided. It was probably the broadest and most complete in the United States at that time, and it helped to develop many future leaders in psychiatry. Among these was a young junior physician who was to become an outstanding psychoanalyst, particularly significant in Boston, Isador Coriat. Coriat spent five years at Worcester (1900–1905), only the first of two of which were under Meyer. The other persons important nationally to psychoanalytic and dynamic psychiatry were George H. Kirby, A.M. Barrett, and George M. Kline.

Meyer (1951:80) indicated that he considered his Worcester period "one of the soundest and in a way the most solidly useful phase" of his work, one in which he "collected the most lastingly valuable and most substantial material." In the context of our present topic, however, Meyer's most direct influence in relation to psychoanalysis came later, during his New York and Baltimore periods.

Clark University: the Hall Period (1888–1920)

Clark under Hall (1844–1924) has naturally received considerable attention in the historical literature on psychoanalysis, particularly in Dorothy Ross's (1972) outstanding biography. I merely wish to add a few comments about three aspects of Hall's influence as it touches upon psychoanalysis: his influence on some of his students, his contribution through the Clark twentieth anniversary meeting, and the impact made by the journals he founded and administered. Of his many distinguished doctoral students, I wish particularly to mention two, Lewis Terman and Phyllis Blanchard.

Terman, whose opinions about Freud over a span of approximately fifty years are available to us, wrote in a personal communication to David Rapaport (February 24, 1956, quoted in Shakow and Rapaport 1964:70–71):

> My first interest in Freud was aroused by some lectures given by Stanley Hall at Clark University in 1904–05. However, the first reading I did on psychoanalysis was when the lectures were published that were given at Clark University in 1909 by Freud and others...I read and reread them. From that time until perhaps 1935 or so, I read a good many books on psychoanalysis, at least one magazine, and comments and articles by psychologists who ranged from favorable to most unfavorable in their attitude toward Freudianism.

In his autobiography, written in 1930, Terman (1932:330) said:

> The Freudian concepts, even when their validity has been discounted about 90 percent, nevertheless constitute one of the two most important contributions to modern psychology, mental tests being the other.

Neale Miller (personal communication, January 1956) reports that while he was at Stanford in 1931–32 Terman made him aware of the importance of Freud's theory. Terman himself, in the letter already referred to, indicates that he subsequently took an even stronger position. He discovered evidence for, and a method of corroborating, Freudian observation and theories:

> My estimate now would be that Freudian psychology does not have to be discounted to the extent of 90 percent. In fact I think that Freud and other analysts, however much they may have differed on specific points, have left a terrific imprint upon modern psychology. What seemed 50 years ago so speculative regarding the part played by the subconscious has now become generally accepted and commonplace—the concepts of repression, the Oedipus complex in the broad sense of that term, overcompensation, and the subconscious factors in human motivation. The hundreds of projective techniques that have been devised, or at least many of them, are based on concepts that Freud and his associates developed 50 or more years ago. I may add that I have been much interested in biographies which draw upon psychoanalytic concepts. Such biographers have probably gone too far in applying psychoanalytic concepts, but in my opinion the lives of many great men cannot be understood without some knowledge of the Freudian School. There are a good many persons in my large group of gifted subjects whose lives I have followed from childhood who could serve as good examples of early subconscious influences.

It is difficult to overestimate the impact that a teacher of Terman's standing had in disseminating Freudian views during his long teaching life.

Phyllis Blanchard (1895–) is perhaps the one Clark student of Hall's who subsequently identified herself most clearly with psychoanalysis. During her long years at the Philadelphia Child Guidance Clinic under Fred Allen, she held the Freudian fort in that strongly Rankian clinic. She was a charter member of the Philadelphia Association for Psychoanalysis, and has published much on problems of child and adolescent guidance, reading disabilities, and personality, generally from a psychoanalytic point of view.

The place of teachers of psychology—which most of the Clark students became—in the spread of Freudian notions is most important.

But perhaps Hall's single most significant contribution was his organization of the conference celebrating the twentieth anniversary of Clark's founding. The meetings centered on psychology, in which Freud and his colleagues played a central role. The conference was important for psychoanalysis and for its spread in the United States. Fred Wells, who attended, made some astute observations that come from a typescript copy he sent me of the talk "Psychoclinical Recollections," that he gave a short time before his death, at the meetings of the New England Psychological Association, November 9–10, 1962. "To memory, it was the next morning while walking behind Freud to the lecture hall, when I overheard a remark that Freud and Jung 'hadn't completed their psychoanalyses of each other yet.' " If Wells's hints about what he overheard and Billinsky's (1969) account of his conversation with Jung are to be taken at all seriously, perhaps Freud deserves as much credit for dealing with his own more chronic psychological problems (Eissler, 1971: 245–247) as he gave James for handling his acute angina attack.

The last area of Hall's influence relates to the journals he founded and administered. These were receptive to psychoanalytic, psychoanalytically oriented, and generally psychodynamic material, and played a considerable role particularly in keeping psychologists aware of psychoanalysis.

Worcester State Hospital: the Bryan Period (1921–1946)

During three periods the Worcester State Hospital programs were so notable that they deserve to be characterized as "golden ages." The first was under Samuel B. Woodward, who was superintendent from 1833 to 1846 and the second was under Adolf Meyer, who served as director of clinics and pathologist from 1896 to 1902. In 1921 the hospital entered its third period when William A. Bryan (1883–1944) became superintendent. (Although he departed for the Norwich, Connecticut State Hospital in 1940, his influence continued to be felt at least through 1946 when I left, so I am considering that whole quarter-century as the Bryan era.)

Bryan was probably one of the greatest state hospital superintendents in American history; this is reflected only in part by his *Administrative Psychiatry (1936)*, the first volume ever written on psychiatric administration. Most of the credit for the rise of Worcester's prestige during Bryan's incumbency is rightly his. Despite some weaknesses, he had the strengths of the "big idea" man, the ability to formulate and carry out new ideas and to deal with the broad general aspects of problems related to institutions. What made him so superb a leader and his regime so notable was in large part his readiness to experiment and his awareness that detail was not his forte. He appointed able persons to head the various departments and, with rare exceptions, had the sense to leave them alone.

Education was a central part of the Worcester enterprise, permeating all aspects of its activity. The members of the staff considered the institution to be a small-scale graduate school (Shakow 1972). The students, who were regarded as an extension of the staff, came from different sections of the country and from a great variety of fields and educational institutions. At Worcester they had close contact with students and staff not only in their own professional areas but in others as well. During the year, and especially in the summer, the hospital was host to students of nursing, medicine, social work, psychiatry, psychology, occupational therapy, theology, biochemistry, and statistics, with an occasional sociology or anthropology student thrown in for good measure. The constant professional interactions among them constituted an enormous educational force.

I will first consider the intramural aspects of our program that involved psychoanalysis, and then go on to deal with some of the extramural influences. Among the intramural factors, I shall examine the part played by the analysts on our staff, the dynamic-analytically oriented staff members, the preanalytic staff members and students, and even the antianalytic staff members. For the extramural factors, I shall attempt to appraise those psychoanalytic influences from the outside, whether continuing, periodic, or only occasional.

Intramural Psychoanalytic Influences

In a period when psychoanalysis was burgeoning and was probably the only theoretically consistent underpinning for psychiatric practice, it is not surprising that many persons influenced by this point of view became, in one way or another, a part of the Worcester scene. But in order for these influences to flourish, receptive soil was necessary. This was liberally provided by the openness of the setting created by Bryan, and by the impact of various individuals who gravitated to and helped mold the Worcester environment. There were senior persons who at the time either were well-qualified analysts, or were acquiring the necessary training and experience to become so. There were, as well, several members of groups who had been subjected to vigorous analytic and dynamic thinking, individuals who had had a history of personal analysis in the past, a psychological group that used investigative techniques based on dynamic principles such as the Rorschach and the TAT, and many others who had in numerous ways been touched by psychoanalytic thought. And there were also, of course, the junior physicians and the psychiatric trainees, many of whom were going into Boston for personal analysis, and the social work students, mainly from Smith College, whose academic training was so fundamentally psychoanalytic. The library, which had a good representation of psychoanalytic monographs and journals, made its contribution, too. The very opposition of the few antianalytic staff members only served to point up the importance of psychoanalysis.

Analysts

Lewis B. Hill (1894–1958). To begin with, there were the analysts at Worcester. The first of these I shall consider is Lewis Hill, though during his period at Worcester he was actually in a preanalytic stage. Hill came to Worcester from the Foxboro, Massachusetts State Hospital in late 1924 to serve as assistant superintendent under Bryan. This promotion was one of the series of steps routinely made by the Department of Mental Diseases for the eventual appointment of promising candidates to the superintendency of a state mental institution in the Commonwealth. Hill had taken his medical degree at the University of Virginia and his residency at Highland Hospital in Asheville, North Carolina, and had had a postgraduate period at the Boston Psychopathic Hospital before joining the staff at Foxboro. I was already at Worcester, between undergraduate and graduate study, when he arrived. We became quite friendly because of a common enthusiasm for tennis and a sharing of similar intellectual interests in an environment that had not as yet developed the richness that was later to characterize it.

One of the topics we discussed endlessly was psychoanalysis: Hill's position was generally antagonistic; mine generally favorable. As part of his responsibilities as assistant superintendent (Worcester at that time did not have a clinical director) and as a natural outgrowth of his remarkable teaching ability, he did much of the clinical teaching at the hospital for several groups of students—psychiatric, social work, theological, and psychological—as well as older and younger staff members. In this role he was most effective and a particularly great favorite with the students.

Upon my return to graduate work the following fall, I continued to spend occasional weekends with the Hills. During one of these visits Hill somewhat shamefacedly admitted to me that he had undertaken an analysis with Ray Willoughby. Willoughby, then at Clark, was the only analytically experienced person in Worcester at this time. This was the beginning of Hill's actual involvement with psychoanalysis. From this first experience, he went on to analyses with Clara Thompson and subsequently, in Budapest, with Ferenczi. His major psychoanalytic period was spent in the Baltimore-Washington area; as clinical director at the Sheppard and Enoch Pratt Hospital, and as a major teacher, analyst, training analyst, and president of the Washington-Baltimore group. He also served as president of the American Psychoanalytic Association in 1940.

But more directly relevant to our present purposes is Hill's most valuable contribution, his profound influence on the Worcester atmosphere, particularly his dynamic teaching of the staff, the theological students at the hospital, and the social work group from Smith. Anton Boisen, for instance, leaped at the opportunity offered by Hill's openness and sympathy for the theological trainees, and took advantage of his pedagogical skill to recruit him as the major teacher for his group. The authorities at Smith also recognized early what a pearl they had in Hill as a teacher and took full advantage of his extraordinary talent.

Earl Zinn (1889–1964). Zinn came to Worcester through John Dollard in the fall of 1933. When Dollard, who had previously spent two summers at the hospital, approached Bryan about the possibility of Zinn's joining the staff, Bryan, with his characteristic receptivity to new approaches, welcomed him and provided the facilities he needed. From 1922 to 1929 Zinn had been executive secretary of the Committee for Research on Sex Problems of the Division of Medical Sciences, National Research Council (Zinn 1924), and then, until 1931, director of a foundation-supported "Committee for the Study of Personality." Sometime during this period he apparently was analyzed by L. Pierce Clark. In 1931 and 1932 both he and Dollard had gone to Berlin, where they were analyzed by Hanns Sachs. Subsequently, on the basis of his combined interest in psychoanalysis and previous graduate work in psychology both at Clark University and with Watson at Johns Hopkins, he decided to undertake an objective study of psychoanalysis. In order to achieve this goal, Zinn recorded a psychoanalysis verbatim. This was, I believe, the first attempt to use such a detailed approach to the study of the course of a psychoanalysis. In those early days the best technical equipment he could develop was to join up two dictaphones, which recorded alternately. In the adjoining room, where these machines were located, his secretary replaced the completed cylinders when necessary during the analytic hour. The communicating microphone was hidden in the head of the couch used by the patient and transmitted what both the patient and the analyst said. The research patient was an obsessive-compulsive person who lived in the city of Worcester and who was willing to participate in the project, knowing that he was being recorded, because he was able to obtain his analysis without cost.

In addition, Zinn analyzed Hugh Carmichael and me. (I might say that I had over 450 hours of analysis with him from November 1933 to December 1935 at $1.50 an hour. Thus, you can see that the advantages and convenience of a "house analyst" are in many ways *calculable*, as well as *incalculable*!)

Zinn attended many of our staff conferences, and provided an analytic viewpoint to the discussions. Much more important, however, he conducted a staff seminar on the recorded case of one of our schizophrenic patients whom he was also analyzing. When Zinn left in December 1935, arrangements were made to transfer this patient to the Yale Clinic so that Zinn could continue his therapeutic-recording work with him. The recorded case is now in the files of Yale University.

Zinn further enriched our program by his memorandum about the possible contribution of psychoanalysis to our extensive schizophrenia research program (Shakow 1972). The memorandum was part of the very substantial report by the Committee on Coordination set up by the directors in 1934 (Shakow 1972:86–87) to take stock of the past, present, and future of this program. In his statement Zinn took exception to Freud's rather negative therapeutic attitude toward psychoanalysis with psychotics, but built upon Freud's theoretical contributions. On the basis of his own analysis of the schizophrenic patient, he believed there was much to justify psychoanalysis with schizophrenics and urged the appointment of a full-time analyst to the research staff. He emphasized that the appointment of someone merely verbally acquainted with psychoanalysis would be neither sufficient nor effective.

Géza Róheim (1891–1953). Some three years after Zinn left Worcester, we acquired our second "house analyst," the gifted anthropologist-analyst, Géza Róheim. Róheim was a childhood friend of Morton Jellinek, our biometrician, and it was through him that he came to Worcester during the Hitler hegira. Róheim and Melanie Klein apparently were analyzed by Ferenczi during the same period (*ca.* 1915–16), and I surmise that Jellinek was also analyzed by Ferenczi at about that time. The maneuvers we had to go through in those Hitlerite days to make it possible for Róheim to come to us were most complicated. As was the case with several others of our staff whom we recruited directly from Europe, it was necessary, in order to get around immigration restrictions, to appoint him to a "professorship" at the hospital.

Again, Bryan was receptive and supported what we asked of him. Róheim was provided with office space for his analytic work and writing, and an apartment for his wife and himself. But what was probably even more important to him was the space set aside in the basement directly beneath the hospital library for the scholarly books he had brought with him. Though most substantial in number, they were undoubtedly only part of the "magnificent" library Balint (1954) mentions in his obituary.

Róheim came to the hospital in 1938 and left in 1940 to settle in New York, where he lived, taught, and practiced until his death in 1953.

Having been analyzed by both Zinn and Róheim, I am able to compare their styles: Zinn was gentle, tentative, hypothesis-proposing; Róheim, quite the opposite. Perhaps it was Róheim's far more extensive psychoanalytic experience that led to his firm self-assuredness. He was markedly gruff, candid, and outspoken in his opinions and interpretations. Although I was presumably carrying on a "control analysis" with him, he would persist in disregarding what I had to say about my patient. Rather, he analyzed what associations *I* had to the material the patient provided.

In his personal life, he took advantage of being close to Lake Quinsigamond, the original course for the Harvard-Yale boat races, to maintain his expertness as a sculler. He was also an accomplished swordsman, though I do not remember any special opportunities to use this skill at Worcester!

The sketch of Róheim by LaBarre (1966:272–281) in *Psychoanalytic Pioneers* gives some notion of the man, based as it is largely on the obituaries by Balint (1954) and by Spitz (1953). However, it neglects entirely his Worcester period, as does the sketch by Münsterberger and Domhoff (1968).

Róheim made many contributions to our research, in part by making himself available to staff members for discussions rather than in more formal ways. Perhaps his greatest contribution was in analyzing several members of the staff, among others Saul Rosenzweig, Benjamin Simon, and myself. Aside from this, he gave occasional lectures to the staff and served as the role model of the devoted scholar who provided a new slant on psychoanalysis.

Analytically Oriented (Dynamic) Personnel

A most important aspect of the psychoanalytic influence at Worcester was represented in the contributions of a variety of groups and persons. These provided much of the ongoing psychoanalytic climate that characterized the hospital in the period during which I was associated with it.

The Schilder Group. There were, to start with, what might be called the Schilderians—persons who had studied with Schilder in Vienna for varying lengths of time.

The earliest of these at Worcester was S. Spafford Ackerly, who, after serving first as assistant physician at the hospital in 1926–27, left to spend the following year in Vienna with Schilder. He then returned to Worcester to head the Child Guidance Clinic and serve as the hospital's clinical director from 1928 to 1930. In 1930 he left to join Healy in carrying out a study of delinquency centered at the Yale Institute of Human Relations. Ackerly was a member of the Boston Psychoanalytical Society in the early days, 1930–1932, but when the society set up standards to conform with those of the constitution of the "American" for a constituent society, Ackerly, with his characteristic gentlemanliness and grace, led most of the ten older members who had not sought further training and were not qualified according to the new standards to resign "in order that the Boston Society might meet the new standards of the American" (Hendrick 1961:38). After his return from Vienna, Ackerly, in his quiet way, helped to influence the direction of interest toward psychoanalysis in the early days of the period we are considering.

William Malamud, who obtained his experience with Schilder during his two years abroad in 1924–1926, had also attended meetings of the Boston Psychoanalytical Society, while he was at Foxboro, in the same period as Ackerly, before the society became a constituent society (Hendrik 1961:10). He did not become associated with the Worcester State Hospital until almost a decade after Ackerly left. In 1939, he left the assistant directorship of the Iowa Psychopathic Hospital to become clinical director at Worcester, where he stayed until 1946. Again, though not officially an analyst, he represented an analytic-dynamic point of view, as is reflected in his *Outlines of General Psychopathology* (Malamud 1935). As clinical director, Malamud presided not only at the staff conferences of the hospital's general services, but also those of the Schizophrenia Research Service. At these, in his characteristic dynamic style, he defended a dynamic point of view in the interpretation of cases.

David Rothschild was another of this group who, while abroad in 1925–1927, had had some training with Schilder. He joined the Worcester staff as clinical director in 1946 when Malamud left, and held that post for ten years. However, he was in and out at Worcester unofficially, particularly during Malamud's time, and was active in the Massachusetts Society for Psychiatric Research. In such contacts he exercised a lesser influence on the Worcester scene.

The Sapir Group. Another group which in several ways exercised influence on the development of a dynamic climate at the hospital was composed of the persons associated with Edward Sapir (1885–1939) during his Yale period (1931–1939).

Early in this period (1932–33) Sapir conducted an international seminar on "The Impact of Culture on Personality," supported by the Rockefeller Foundation. John Dollard served as assistant to Sapir in the program. The tenor of the seminar was psychodynamic and in part psychoanalytic. The members of the seminar were recruited from countries in various parts of the world, particularly from Europe and Asia, with only one member to a country, I believe. Some remained in the United States; others returned to their native countries. From the Sapir group we obtained one of our most valuable staff members, that eminent psychiatrist Andras Angyal, who had represented Hungary. Several members of the seminar group paid occasional visits to Worcester: Bingham Dai, the Chinese representative, who from 1934 on was a professor on the faculty of Duke University; Beck, the German representative, who returned to Germany and was killed in the holocaust; the Japanese representative (whose name I do not remember), who went back to Japan. (Others who did not get to Worcester from this unusual group were Robert E. Marjolin, the distinguished member of the European Economic Community and professor at the Sorbonne, and Max Weinreich of Yivo fame, from Vilna, who represented Russia.)

But from this group it was Dollard, who spent relatively extended periods with us, whose impact on our staff was the greatest psychoanalytically. The actual periods that Dollard and his first wife, Victorine, spent at Worcester were the summers of 1931 and 1932. At the hospital the Dollards were on their own, free to immerse themselves in patient material as they wished. They carried out numerous case studies, and to some extent participated in staff conferences. If I remember correctly, they studied one case intensively, which they made part of the hospital record. They had many informal contacts with members of the staff, who considered them as representatives of the psychoanalytic point of view. One product of Dollard's Worcester experience is to be found in a paper he wrote for the *American Journal of Sociology* (1934).

The Boisen Group. Another group that considerably influenced the Worcester scene in the dynamic direction was that headed by Anton Boisen (1876–1965). Boisen had been brought to the hospital by Bryan in the spring of 1924 to serve as Protestant chaplain, but his main interest was in personality work with patients. Earlier he had suffered a schizophrenic breakdown, which led to his coming to the Boston area to study psychology and social work, mostly at Harvard. (We took two courses together at Harvard, both at the Boston Psychopathic Hospital. One was under Wells on the Stanford-Binet, in which Boisen and I practiced this intelligence scale on each other; the second was the seminar under Campbell on the "Psychology of Belief.")

The appointment of Boisen was another instance of Bryan's liberal approach. Some of the psychiatrists on the staff manifested considerable opposition, mostly evidenced in subtle forms of lack of cooperation. This presumably stemmed from their resistance to a clergyman, especially one who had had a psychosis, working with patients.

It was at Worcester that Boisen initiated the pastoral-training program which has spread worldwide. During the first year of his appointment, 1924–25, he worked toward laying the groundwork for the program. Training actually began in the summer of 1925, when his two major students were Philip Guiles and Flanders Dunbar. For most of that year I was at Worcester between undergraduate and graduate study, and my room was next to Boisen's office off Appleton 4 Ward. This permitted considerable mutual contact for many discussions of his program. He had an excellent psychological library, much of it analytic. I remember particularly Kempf's *Psychopathology*, which the hospital library did not own. This volume was particularly intriguing to me, for a variety of reasons!

A good deal of Boisen's time during the first year was spent in intensive interviewing of patients and the writing up of their case histories in great detail. He bound these individually and later used them most effectively with his students. If I were to attempt to characterize Boisen's general approach, I would say that psychologically it had a Sullivanian cast with a heavy admixture of strict nineteenth century moralism and early twentieth century theological liberalism. (I am indebted to Saward Hiltner for this apt characterization.) He had a truly committed sense of mission. When Hill came to Worcester some half year after Boisen did, he was quite sympathetic and most helpful to him.

After that first summer of 1925, the pastoral training program grew quite rapidly in the succeeding summers—the periods during which the theologs came from their seminaries. Later on, I believe, some were employed throughout the year.

For our present purposes, the important contribution of this group was the dynamic influences that characterized Boisen's own approach and those of his assistants and students. After the first few years of the program, his formal teaching schedule with the theologs, which had been constantly growing, involved persons like Hill, Healy, Harry Stack Sullivan, and Dunbar—who by this time had gone on to take her medical and psychiatric work—as well as many other distinguished persons in related fields.

It should be recognized that Boisen's dynamic-psychoanalytic approach (in a religious context, of course) and his insistence on practical work with patients in mental institutions, rather than in prisons or general hospitals, were in part responsible for the break with Richard Cabot, one of the original mainstays of the program. This resulted in the formation of the two separate pastoral counseling groups.

E. Morton Jellinek (1890–1963). Jellinek was at Worcester as chief of biometrics for the Schizophrenia Research Service from 1931 to 1939. During this period he had immeasurable impact on the Research Service, but he also contributed significantly to the rest of the hospital. Jellinek was probably the most gifted person associated with the hospital during its third golden age.

Early in 1931 Roy G. Hoskins, the director of research, had met Jellinek in Boston, where he had recently returned from Honduras to report to Zemurray, the head of the United Fruit Company. Hoskins was much impressed not only with Jellinek's obvious statistical expertise, but also with his psychological sophistication and interest in schizophrenia. He appeared an ideal person to recruit for the developing schizophrenia research program.

Jellinek's background had indeed been broad. He had spent the immediately preceding years in agricultural field work in Africa with Elder and Dempster (1920–1925), and in Honduras working for the United Fruit Company as assistant director of research (1926–1930). In these positions he had been using Fisherian and similar small-sample statistical techniques to lay out experimental plantations for the study of a variety of plant growth factors. He introduced these statistical techniques to our research, which, I believe, made us the earliest group to use small-sample techniques in the human field, at least in relation to psychopathology.

But it was his experiences prior to those I have mentioned that are most pertinent in the present context. Jellinek, a native of Budapest, seems to have been interested in anthropology and psychoanalysis quite early. He was analyzed by Ferenczi either before the first World War began or, as I have suggested earlier, around 1916, when Ferenczi returned from the war and analyzed Róheim and Melanie Klein. His deepest involvement in psychoanalysis apparently extended for approximately the decade from 1909 to 1920, when he left Hungary. I assume this from the psychoanalytic journals he had subscribed to and which he presented to me while we were together at Worcester. (These consisted of issues of *Imago* from 1912 to 1920, the full file of six volumes of the *Jahrbücher* (1909–1914), and numerous volumes by Freud and other early psychoanalysts issued by Franz Deuticke in the years between 1911 and 1917.) An obituary (Bacon 1963) indicates that he had presented a paper at the Second International Psycho-Analytical Congress, held in Nuremberg in 1910, "immediately preceding Sigmund Freud on the platform." This paper may have been the one "On the Origin of Footwear" (1917).

Jellinek had taken an M.Ed. degree at Leipzig in 1914, and from 1915 to 1920 had been biometrician at the Government School in Budapest. With the takeover of the Hungarian government by Bela Kun, he had gone first to Africa, from there to Central America, and then to Worcester.

Jellinek made his influence felt in relation to psychoanalysis because of his obvious knowledge of the field, the respect in which he was universally held as a competent biometrician, his broad culture, and his rare sense and intelligence. If "Bunky," as he was without exception called, felt positive toward psychoanalysis, then presumably psychoanalysis was indeed important and worth paying attention to. His high opinion of psychoanalysis is reflected in what he wrote about psychoanalysis in his capacity as chairman, in the Report of the Committee on Coordination of Research (November 1934), from which I have already paraphrased Zinn's memorandum:

> Discussion of the psychoanalytic approach to schizophrenia problems requires a small book in itself. We are not undertaking to condense it into a few pages; indeed, we shall not touch on the subject at all. It is in our case really not necessary because there is hardly a man on this research who would take exception to its inclusion into our activities.
>
> We wish to say that we urgently recommend hiring a competent psychoanalyst. We are not favorable to psychoanalysis by "educated readers." This standpoint is clearly expressed by Mr. Zinn, whose memorandum we are attaching.
>
> The reason that we gave these few words a separate chapter heading and have not included them into the chapter on psychiatry, is symbolical. We do not wish to regard psychoanalysis as a psychatric technique but as a distinct science of mental disorders. It is probably the only science in this field which is properly rounded out and conceptualized. It definitely forms a *Weltanschauung*, a thing that cannot be said of any other psychiatry. [p. 66]

The Psychology Group. Another important psychoanalytic influence came from the fairly substantial psychology group at the hospital, particularly as represented by Saul Rosenzweig and myself.

Rosenzweig was at the hospital from 1934 to 1943, and during the latter part of this period (1938–1943) was an affiliate professor at Clark. I believe he was the first from the hospital since the time of Adolf Meyer and Samuel Orton to hold such an appointment. He came to the hospital Psychology Department directly from that oasis of personality and psychoanalytic research, Henry A. Murray's Psychological Clinic, where he had been one of its outstanding members. While at Harvard he had taken his three degrees with great distinction, and had served at the Psychological Clinic as research assistant from 1929 to 1934.

He was deeply interested in personality theory and psychoanalysis, on which he had published a number of papers. While at Worcester he continued his publishing and also lectured widely, especially on frustration theory and repression (Rosenzweig 1943*a*, 1944). He viewed psychoanalysis as an important school of psychology and was a strong advocate of making psychoanalysis experimental. (See his correspondence with Freud in 1934 and further comments in Shakow and Rapaport 1964:129–131).

Rosenzweig continued his psychoanalytic research while at Worcester, tying it into the ongoing research on schizophrenia. He was among the most productive members of the research team, and collaborated not only with the other psychologists but also with the endocrinologists on the staff. On the one hand, he continued some of his research on repression and frustration, and wrote on theoretical problems in psychoanalysis. On the other, he participated in studies of the effects of sex hormones (Rosenzweig and Freeman 1942), new projective devices (1942), and the role of sibling death in schizophrenia (1943*b*).

During this period he was analyzed by Róheim, taught dynamic psychology and supervised several students in this area at Clark, and made substantial plans for the establishment of a periodical on experimental psychopathology, which was to have a strong psychoanalytic flavor. Although the plans for the journal were close to fruition, the contemporary development of another publication (ultimately, *Psychosomatic Medicine*), jointly sponsored by the National Research Council and the Macy Foundation, which provided the financial support, made its abandonment justifiable. Despite the enormous amount of work Rosenzweig had put into the project, he graciously made this decision.

As for myself, I have already indicated my early involvement in psychoanalysis. Aside from my associations with Hill, Zinn, and Róheim, which I have mentioned, I continued my interest in psychoanalysis in directing the research and clinical work of the Department of Psychology, in my own researches, and in my activities on the Councils of the Research Service and of the hospital as a whole. My research included such studies as the objective investigation of hypnotically induced complexes (Huston, Shakow, and Erickson 1934), studies in mirror behavior (Rosenzweig and Shakow 1937*a*), auditory apperception (Shakow and Rosenzweig 1940; Shakow, Rosenzweig, and Hollander 1966), and play technique (Rosenzweig and Shakow 1937*b*), as well as involvement in a number of studies dealing with projective techniques. I also prepared one of the papers for Allport's symposium on analyzed psychologists (1940). During my last period at Worcester, I spent several years "analyzing" a schizophrenic young man, at times with, and at times without, concurrent physiological studies.

The Psychology Department as a whole contained other members who had had contact with psychoanalysis, whether through personal analysis or through some degree of training. But in their work, perhaps most of the members of the department—staff and students alike, because of the techniques they used, many of a projective nature—were in constant contact with psychoanalysis. The psychodynamic point of view generally predominated, though several other theoretical views were represented—Lewinian, gestalt, behavioristic, and functional.

Other Senior Staff. A further influence toward the psychoanalytic direction at Worcester stemmed from a number of members of the senior staff who had not been trained in psychoanalysis at the time they were at the hospital, yet who did think dynamically. Subsequently they received such training. I have already discussed the earliest of these, Hill. But there were also three other such staff members: Hugh Carmichael, Minna Emch, and Ben Simon.

Carmichael served as psychiatrist on the Research Service from 1931 to 1934. From 1936 to 1940 he obtained his psychoanalytic training at the Psychoanalytic Institute of Chicago and subsequently became one of the prominent analysts in that area, serving as president of the Chicago Psychoanalytic Society from 1952 to 1954.

Emch was at Worcester on the House Service from 1932 to 1935, and after her return to Chicago took her training at the Psychoanalytic Institute of Chicago from 1937 to 1941. She also became one of Chicago's prominent psychoanalysts. She had special affinities with the Blitzten group.

Simon was at Worcester for a longer period, between 1934 and 1941, serving successively in posts from assistant physician through head of one of the House Services. From 1950 to 1954 he had his psychoanalytic training at the Boston Psychoanalytic Institute.

A most important member of the staff, whom I have already mentioned in association with the Sapir seminar, belongs to this group of senior staff. This was Andras Angyal, who played so significant a role in our schizophrenia research from 1933 to 1945. He came to us as a research fellow, then became a research psychiatrist, and finally served for a number of years as our resident director of research until he left in 1945. Although not an analyst, this outstanding proponent of holistic psychology (Angyal 1941, 1965) developed a system whose dynamics might very well be viewed as having parallels with analytic theory.

There were also a variety of other influences, less prominent, but equally dynamic. One of these was Samuel Hartwell, that premier director of the Worcester Child Guidance Clinic. He served in this capacity from 1929 to 1935, before going on to head the University of Buffalo Medical School psychiatry program. After engaging in rural general practice in Iowa for many years, he was led by the nature of the personality problems he was constantly facing to arrange to study child guidance with Healy at the Judge Baker Clinic. Against the context of his broad eclectic background, he carried on the work of the Worcester Clinic brilliantly in his own dynamic manner based on a philosophy not incompatible with psychoanalysis.

And there were also peripheral persons like Heinrich Bosshard, a Swiss, at the time a professor of German at Clark, who served as part-time librarian. He was an Adlerian, having been analyzed abroad by Sief. In the considerable time he spent at the hospital he helped to make us acquainted with Adlerian views.

Junior Staff and Students. We now come to a vital group—the junior staff and students. These persons are important because in an organization with high standards of selection and performance they play such an obvious role in establishing and maintaining a live and innovative atmosphere. Such was the situation at Worcester. This younger group was made up of able persons, many of whom later contributed much to psychiatry and psychoanalysis.

The more peculiarly psychoanalytic atmosphere came mostly from those psychiatric trainees who were simultaneously in personal analysis. A constant topic of conversation occupying the senior staff at the time related to when in professional training a personal analysis might best be introduced. More particularly, the question centered on whether it was or was not desirable to permit psychiatric residents to receive their personal analyses during their residency, because we had had bad experiences in some instances. The question was, of course, never answered satisfactorily, since individual differences were so great. Some residents were undoubtedly so seriously disturbed by analysis that they became quite ineffective in their relations with patients and in maintaining responsibility to them and personal discipline. Others became more effective generally, despite occasional lapses. And some did not seem to be affected at all. The solution we arrived at, as I remember, was to require a resident (or even a junior staff member) to apply for permission to undertake such treatment. The purported (and, to some extent, realistic) reason for such permission was that analysis involved considerable time off, or at least much rearrangement of schedules. Personal analyses could be obtained only in Boston, and the round trip of forty-odd miles, together with the analytic hour, took at least three hours. At the rate of three to five times a week, a considerable portion of the work week was consumed. (This was true even if some of the time was made up.) While it held for good weather, during the long Massachusetts winters the problem became even more acute and more serious; it could often mean half a day or longer out for one analytic hour.

If it is true that cost and suffering contribute to the effectiveness of psychoanalytic therapy, then I think our Worcester residents must have been well analyzed indeed. From my own safe and easy haven of analysis by "house analysts," I was especially sympathetic. Particularly during the icy and blustery days of winter with the only fair roads of the time (especially before Henry Ford had the turnpike improved in the region of the Wayside Inn), I would often imagine a resident on his eerie trip to his analyst, battling the elements, befogged and astray on the turnpike, crying out plaintively like Amy Lowell's Peter Rugg: "Boston—Boston—Will *no* one show me the way to Boston?"

Social Work Students. And then there were the social work students from Smith, who, after a summer at school, spent the rest of the year with us and again returned to school for a second summer to complete their training. The training at Smith was strongly analytic, which was, of course, reflected in their contacts with their supervisors and in their handling of cases. They, too, helped to add to the psychoanalytic flavor of the institution.

The students we later had from other schools of social work (Simmons and Boston University), who came in part time over the full year, were not quite as analytic as those from Smith, but they played a somewhat similar, if more attenuated, role.

Antianalytic Staff. Not to be dismissed is the influence of those who represented antipsychoanalytic views. These persons provided a foil against which to pose and to emphasize psychoanalysis. In particular, I can think of two psychiatrists who expressed such antagonism: Milton Harrington and Ewen Cameron.

Harrington, who was at Worcester during 1931–32, was strongly behavioristic and McDougallian (at the same time!) in his approach, and outspokenly antipsychoanalytic. Several of his publications attest to this (Harrington 1915, 1934).

Cameron, who was at Worcester from 1936 through 1938, was not so vehemently expressive in his antagonism to psychoanalysis. Mainly he appeared to consider psychoanalysis personally—how it might affect him. He was a terrific worker, starting early in the morning and working late into the evening. He believed that for himself analysis would result in the loss of this urge to work, and he was taking no chances!

Finally, there were numerous behavior supports for psychoanalysis in the environment; one instance of this was the library with its general journals and monographs in the various fields of mental health, which had much psychoanalytic material, but particularly its extensive holdings of psychoanalytic journals and monograph volumes dealing with psychoanalytic subjects.

Extramural Psychoanalytic Influences

As I indicated earlier, apart from the major factors that internally influenced the Worcester group analytically, many stemmed from outside the institution. Some of these were continuing ones, while others were merely occasional. However, they all served to contribute something to the general complex of influences.

One considerable source of continuing influence came from the visits paid by certain persons with an interest in psychoanalysis. Raymond Willoughby, about whom I shall have something more to say shortly, was one of these. During the time Willoughby was at Clark, from 1926 to 1936, but particularly during the years after I came to Worcester in 1928, there was much visiting, correspondence, and interchange of students between Clark and Worcester. Much of this interchange centered on psychoanalysis in one way or another—the several steps necessary to set up and standardize the Emotional Maturity Questionnaire, the abstracting of psychoanalytic and other articles for *Psychological Abstracts*, attendance at some of Willoughby's seminars on psychoanalysis, or the employment of Willoughby-associated Clark students as attendants. All the occasions are too numerous to mention.

Another influence of the same kind was that of Fred Wells, about whom I shall also say more shortly. The close rapport established between Wells and myself while I interned at the Boston Psychopathic Hospital continued throughout my period at Worcester. But particularly I wish to mention a course on Mental Adjustments that Wells came out from Boston to give us. It consisted of some eight to ten two-hour evening sessions discussing dynamic psychology and mental mechanisms, but built almost entirely around projected cartoons coming from the *New Yorker* and other humor magazines!

And then there were the meetings we attended in Boston, of the psychiatric associations—the Boston Society of Psychiatry and Neurology, the New England Society of Psychiatry, and occasionally those of the national societies. I remember in particular one meeting in the early thirties which several of us from Worcester attended because the speaker was Franz Alexander and his topic schizophrenia. He held forth at the Boston Society of Psychiatry and Neurology. I believe it was the meeting held in February 1931, with Abraham Myerson in the chair. My outstanding memory (in fact, practically the only one that has remained with me vividly) is the furor caused by Myerson's pronouncement during the discussion period about the need for cleaning out the Augean stables of psychiatry—unmistakably referring to psychoanalysis! I have not been able to locate a report containing such content. According to the abstract, which appears in the *Journal of Nervous and Mental Disease* for the February date—the only one reported at which Alexander spoke—the topic was the problem of therapy in schizophrenia as seen from a psychoanalytic standpoint. If this indeed was the meeting, then Tracy Putnam (1931), its reporter, must have had Bowdler as amanuensis when he wrote the abstract for the *Journal of Nervous and Mental Disease*, for I can find nothing of "stables" in the account! But at least my report suggests something of the heat that the topic of psychoanalysis engendered in those days.

Clark University: the Willoughby Period (1926–1936)

In the earlier decades of this century, psychoanalysis played a role at Clark during two periods. I have already considered one briefly, that of Hall (1888–1920). The second period, understandably much less well known, was during the decade 1926–1936. At that time, in the context of a strongly behavioristic atmosphere dominated by Walter Hunter, chairman of the Psychology Department, Raymond Willoughby in his quiet way brought to it, and to some extent to the university as a whole, a psychoanalytic flavor.

During the twenties and thirties there was, in contrast to the much larger group who were negative, a small group of psychologists in America who could on the whole be regarded as favorable to psychoanalysis. Among these were Raymond Willoughby, Phyllis Blanchard, Percival Symonds, Gardner Murphy, Harry Murray, J.F. Brown, Else Frenkel-Brunswik, and several others. From this group I shall deal only with Willoughby; only he and Murray meet our geographic criteria.

Although Willoughby died at forty-eight, he managed during his brief life to make a substantial contribution through amalgamating his own brand of psychoanalysis with academic psychology. Willoughby was one of the finest characters it has been my privilege to know. He had a remarkable inquiring mind, which was combined with genuine concern for people and the deepest social consciousness. His breadth of interests was amazing: anything human, whether an individual or a group, anything natural, from astronomy to zoology, fascinated him and led him to its study. Intellectual possessions, yes; material possessions, no. He was constantly divesting himself of any accumulated "things." Unfortunately for his family, this included money as well.

Willoughby was at Clark University from 1926 to 1936, and at Brown University from 1936 to 1940. These major periods of professional activity provided him with a number of different channels through which to make his influence felt. He was at first assistant editor and then associate editor of the newly established *Psychological Abstracts*, the only journal during this period that was being distributed as part of their dues to all members of the American Psychological Association. It eventually became the most important behavioral sciences abstract journal in the world. It was officially under the editorship of Walter Hunter, but Willoughby was the sole professional person devoting full time to it. In this capacity he had an unusual opportunity to make a broad range of psychological material available to psychologists. Because of his interest in psychoanalysis, stemming in part from his association with Terman at Stanford and his *Genetic Studies of Genius*, as well as the psychoanalysis he had undergone during his graduate years at Stanford with Moxon, he devoted substantial space to psychoanalytic authors and writings. His unusually broad view of psychology (which included the genetic, statistical, psychoanalytic, and personality fields) made him aware of the relative neglect of psychoanalysis by psychologists and the importance of clinical as well as experimental data. From the very first volume, Willoughby was mainly responsible for the growth of the *Abstracts* and for the high standards it achieved. During his tenure the number of annual abstracts increased from over 2,700 in Volume 1 to almost 7,000 in Volume 12. His avid lexicographic and conceptual interests led him to establish a cross-referenced index that is a model of its kind and has been most useful to several generations of psychologists. In this enterprise, psychoanalysis fared well indeed.

Related to his work on *Psychological Abstracts* is the yeoman job he did as a collaborator on Warren's *Dictionary of Psychology*, where he had much to do with providing the many psychoanalytic terms included.

Although he was not actually on the faculty of Clark University, where *Psychological Abstracts* was being edited during the first of his two academic periods, Willoughby carried on extensive informal teaching there. He held seminars for faculty and graduate students on psychoanalysis, giving it something of an original interpretation, frequently experimental in flavor. In addition, as the only psychoanalyst in Worcester at the time, he engaged in a heavy program of psychoanalytically oriented psychotherapy with students and with other Worcester residents. Through these contacts he greatly influenced a number of psychologists, many of whom subsequently held important university teaching positions. These included such persons as Robert Leeper, Mason Crook, J. McV. Hunt, and Clarence Graham. And, as Don Marquis has somewhere pointed out, one of the greatest opportunities afforded psychoanalysis for the spread of its ideas lies in university courses—both undergraduate and graduate—for psychologists. Further, as I have already noted, Willoughby made a considerable contribution by serving as Lewis Hill's original analyst.

His own publications along psychoanalytic lines fall into four categories. He wrote a few short papers on dreams (Willoughby 1929, 1933*b*), and an extensive paper which made a substantial psychodynamic contribution, "Magic and Cognate Phenomena" (Willoughby 1935). His work on the Emotional Maturity Scale (Willoughby 1932) combined his interests in psychometrics and personality. Because of its strong psychoanalytic orientation, in both conception and development, it was certainly the most sophisticated instrument of its kind at the time it was issued—and has probably remained so to this day. In addition, he wrote on psychoanalysis proper. An early report on the work he did between 1928 and 1930 (Willoughby 1931) describes an experiment with brief psychoanalysis in which he discusses and evaluates results of sixteen cases. This anticipation of the work of Alexander and French (1946) reflects Willoughby's characteristic inquiring and unorthodox attitude and his need to experiment with new approaches. He contributed another paper, this one dealing directly with psychoanalysis (Willoughby 1940), to "Psychoanalysis as Seen by Analyzed Psychologists," the symposium that Gordon Allport solicited and published in the *Journal of Abnormal Psychology* in the early forties.

Outstanding were Willoughby's reviews of books on psychoanalysis, in which he showed considerable objectivity and keen critical prowess. I cannot forbear quoting what he wrote in a review (Willoughby 1933*a*) of Melanie Klein's (1932) *Psycho-analysis of Children*. In it he refers to Jastrow's paper, "The House that Freud Built": "The recent animadversions of Jastrow [suggest that he] has not troubled to inform himself regarding the subject matter of his discourse, though he has displayed his characteristic acumen in discussing what he inferred from other discussions to be this matter." (See Hull on Jastrow in Shakow and Rapaport 1964:92). He concludes the review:

> The growing point of civilization is in the social sciences; the growing point of the social sciences is in psychology; and the growing point of psychology is in child analysis. This is the most important book ever written about child analysis, because it has been written by the most capable technician now alive. But it is too logically naïve, condensed, and even confused to be a wholly trustworthy guide. Another half century, perhaps.

If we are to judge by James Anthony's exciting (and excited) review of Frances Tustin's "Autism and Childhood Psychosis" in a recent issue of *Psychotherapy and Social Science Review*, perhaps we are slowly approaching this half-century goal.

Willoughby is perhaps outstanding because his influence, though effected largely through informal channels, helped substantially to keep psychoanalysis before students of psychology.

Boston Psychopathic Hospital (1922–1938)

I believe I was the first *resident* intern in psychology with Fred Wells at the Boston Psychopathic and my prejudices may be somewhat different from those of contemporary psychiatric contributors. I had two sets of experiences at the "Psycho:" one as a nonresident while an undergraduate at Harvard, which I have already mentioned; the other as resident intern in 1925–26, when I was receiving maintenance for half-time work while I carried on my first year of graduate work in psychology at Harvard.

Among the psychiatric residents who were there while I was resident were Geoffrey Biddle (with whom I shared a room), Ives Hendrick, and Edwin Gildea. There was much psychoanalytic talk in that ground-floor wing at the time. The staff during this period included Campbell, Bowman, and Wells. Jascha Kasanin was, I believe, a young instructor in psychiatry; at least this was where I first became acquainted with him. But it is mainly about Wells that I wish to make some comments. I believe his contribution to psychoanalysis has never received the recognition it deserves.

Frederick Lyman Wells (1884–1964), familiarly known as "Freddy," is, in the context of the point of view I have maintained, a much underestimated, unappreciated contributor to the psychoanalytic scene. At the time of his death in 1964 he was the last person alive of those in the famous photograph of most of the prominent attendants at the 1909 meeting at Clark University. (He was twenty-five at the time; Jung, the penultimate decedent, had died in 1961.) Wells was much concerned with dynamic psychology, going beyond the Freudian particularly into the anthropological. It seems that his extreme nonpartisanship, his general erudition (he was also an accomplished philologist), and his wide ranging interest in nature and in folkways would not let him remain within ordinary bounds. He nevertheless gave considerable space to Freudian topics in his books, and helped to spread Freudian influence by his independent articles on psychoanalytic themes. His reviews in the *Psychological Bulletin*, beginning in 1912 (a task taken over from Adolf Meyer and August Hoch), were among the main sources through which psychologists (and many psychiatrists) became acquainted with psychoanalytic literature during this period.

These reviews and articles were accurate and fair-minded as well as critical and speculative. For instance, in his review of *The Interpretation of Dreams* in *The Journal of Philosophy, Psychology, and Scientific Methods*, Wells (1913*a*) summarized the major concepts and the organization of the book in a balanced and concise fashion. He praised Freud's style highly, as was to be expected of an expert in German and a connoisseur of fine literature, but considered that the volume was "not very systematically put together...abounds in repetition...rambles interestingly along, more or less free association fashion" (p. 554), and briefly but sharply criticized the concept of "wish." He gave a sarcastic and devastating criticism of the translation, and was even more sharply critical of Brill's introduction:

> "No one is really qualified to use or judge Freud's psychoanalytic method," runs part of the translator's preface, "who has not thoroughly mastered his theory of the neuroses—'The Interpretation of Dreams,' 'Three Contributions to the Sexual Theory,' 'The Psychopathology of Everyday Life,' and 'Wit and Its Relation to the Unconscious,' and who has not had considerable experience in analyzing the dreams and psychopathological actions of himself and others. That there is required also a thorough training in normal and abnormal psychology goes without saying." This is at best an ungallant flight from criticism, since no one lives who has these qualifications; hyperbole may be justified in proselytizing for a faith, but in scientific matters one is better concerned with the justice of the criticism than with the competence of the critic [pp. 554–555].

The end of the review may perhaps be taken as Wells's motto: "He is the most fortunate who is not prevented by factors of personal affect from seeing and using what is advantageous in all" (p. 555).

In his articles Wells was perhaps less friendly to psychoanalysis. He was more inclined to criticize sharply what he considered to be arbitrary in the methods and claims of psychoanalysis, while simultaneously engaging in speculations not backed by either the psychoanalytic or the experimental method. In his "Critique of Impure Reason" (Wells 1912) he endeavored "to point out some special reasons why these doctrines have not had, and in their present form ought scarcely to expect, sympathetic recognition at the hands of a discriminating psychology" (p. 89). Although he did not deny either the role of symbolism in dreams or that of "the hidden tendency" in parapraxes, he concluded: "Whatever of these theories be true or false, there seem to have been but scattered attempts to submit them to the test of experiential [experimental?] conditions" (p. 92). He also took exception to the "resistances" argument, using the reverse of it on psychoanalysts to ask whether or not their theory attracted a certain kind of person, "a type of personality that would be attracted to psychoanalysis by the very prominence it gives to sexual factors...perhaps affording to the sexual feelings a not disagreeable stimulation of the safer and cheaper sort" (p. 93). But his vision was much keener than is implied by the foregoing. In "On Formulation in Psychoanalysis" (1913*b*) he wrote: "Upon the basis of a body of observational data, probably the most intimate ever focussed upon psychological questions, are constructed many theories of mental function, scarcely one of which has been assimilated to the psychology of scientific method" (p. 217). On the other hand, he asked (p. 227):

> Has due care been exercised to keep the interpretation of your splendid body of observational data within the limits of what they really showed, or is it often subordinated to impressiveness of statement, with just a tinge of what we clinically know as the "desire to astonish"? Have you never said "Freud has discovered," where he only surmised? The same looseness of formulation that, perhaps, facilitated their applicability to data of clinical observation, has unquestionably retarded their assimilation with the more rigid standards of experimental proof.

Wells felt "strongly that an ameliorated formulation will not only make it easier for every one to appreciate adequately what is already known, but will obviate many natural barriers of resistance to the correct interpreting of future observations" (p. 218). Nevertheless, if we look at his papers (1916, 1917), and even a late paper (1935), "Social Maladjustment: Adaptive Regression," in the *Handbook of Social Psychology*, which anticipates some of the concepts of psychoanalytic ego psychology, we find that Wells's massing of literary allusions from many languages (his philological background stood him in good stead here) and anthropological references left him open to the same kind of criticism that he directed at psychoanalysis.

Thus we see this perhaps most sympathetic critic of psychoanalysis caught up in difficulties similar to those of Freud and his followers. But all in all, we must conclude that his considerable role in introducing and reconciling psychoanalysis to academic psychology has largely remained unappreciated and unrecognized. I say unappreciated because, from my own observations and those of others, this wise, scholarly, insightful, most sympathetic teacher as well as critic of psychoanalysis has never been given his due. Perhaps he was handicapped by his reserve, his lack of dominating presence, his superficial "stiffness," and the low "mumbling" style of his communication. In any case, he never had the impact he should have had—more's the pity. But let me reiterate: neither his colleagues at the Psychopathic nor those at Harvard really appreciated him. He was a true teacher in the best sense.

Final Comments

What are the broader implications of the personal material I have been setting forth—broad implications despite the fact that they stem from the relatively narrow context of Worcesterian psychoanalytic developments? The major one is what I see as the limited view taken by most psychoanalytic—particularly medical psychoanalytic—historians of the factors they interpret as playing a role in the course of the history of psychoanalysis. They appear to me to be too much carried away by the obvious, direct, and literal, and insufficiently sensitive to the less direct influencing factors. Such insensitivity is reflected in unmindfulness of the inferences that flow from two fundamental Jamesian principles. One is what Thorndike called James's most significant discovery in psychology: the existence of "fringes" of mental states. The other is James's emphasis on the concept, not unrelated to the first, of "habit:" the importance of those "smallest strokes of virtue and vice," the minor repetitive experiences in our environments and in our actions which play such momentous roles in the establishment of attitudes, receptivities, responses—both automatized and nonautomatized. In a way, the distinction resembles the difference between an emphasis on the part that trauma plays in development, as opposed to the much less prominent and remarkable, but equally effective, part that habit plays in development.

Or, to be somewhat more definite, there exist in our environments a multitude of factors of an indirect, subtle kind that coalesce indistinguishably to achieve perhaps an even deeper influencing effect than that achieved by the direct, grander influences so obvious to all. Rapaport and I (Shakow and Rapaport 1964) have considered both types of factors in our monograph and pointed out the different significances of each. I daresay such factors operate in other fields of endeavor as well.

More specifically, in relation to psychoanalysis, I am pointing out what Rapaport and I considered in detail, namely, that a major part of Freud's influence has resided in his effect on conceptions rather than on concepts. Precise ideas play a direct role in influence, but sometimes an even greater role is played by other, approximate, factors. Freud's influence must be gauged by the reactions to any idea that demonstrably originated in his observations and theories, regardless of whether the idea came from original sources or, instead, from such less precise factors as secondary sources, popularizations, partially convinced persons, atmosphere, or even hearsay. In the latter circumstances, we deal with conceptions rather than concepts. Conceptions refer to the broad, less defined and less structured matrix from which theories and concepts crystallize. Concepts have definitions; conceptions make use of any term, and apply concepts in a common sense way disregarding, or even ignoring, their definitions. By and large, theories are the only terms that have a conceptual status. Terms used outside of the theory become conceptions, as they were before the theory gave them definitions as concepts. Thus, as far as psychoanalysis is concerned, what becomes accepted is Freud's view of man and his pioneering in new areas for psychological study. Slowly the realization has come that it was Freud who awakened interest in human nature, in infancy and childhood, in the irrational in man; that he is the fountainhead of dynamic psychology in general, and of psychology's present-day conceptions of motivation and of the unconscious in particular. Although there are many striking exceptions, it is for the most part his conception of these fields of study and his observations in them, not his concepts and theories about them, that have been accepted. When the theory itself is referred to, it is usually transformed into some "common sense" version or is taken at the level of its clinical referents.

What has occurred then has been increasing acceptance without proportionate growth of conversance; acceptance of Freud's conception of man but not of the means by which he derived it; in fact, an influence that was not accompanied by true understanding. But, generally, this is what we have to live with, and in most cases it appears sufficient to affect our culture. And this is in general what characterized the Worcester-Clark scene I have described.

It is in such a broad context that I wish to point up the reminiscences I have presented, leaving aside the more obviously direct influences. The importance of the nonmedical, in the Clark and Worcester scenes, as elsewhere in the development of psychoanalysis, cannot be minimized. Willoughby and his impact on Clark students and on the state hospital, Zinn and Róheim, Dollard, Boisen and his group, Jellinek, the psychology group—these are some of the nonmedical influences that played a great role in keeping psychoanalysis prominent. The importance of the teachers of the nonmedical students, so many of whom became teachers themselves: Hill with social workers, theologs, and occupational therapists, Willoughby in his teaching of psychologists and ministers, the Psychology Department personnel and its training of so many clinical psychologists and clinical teachers; the place of lay psychoanalysts in the analysis of prominent theoreticians and researchers; the influence of highly respected persons in their remote specialties, such as Jellinek (compare in this context, William Morton Wheeler and A.G. Tansley), whose acceptance of psychoanalysis gave it a positive aura; the place of receptive, even if psychoanalytically uncommitted, administrators like Bryan, who provided facilities for the analytically experienced, and educational opportunities for those who sought training—these, as well as such contributions from the medical group, all made up some of the indirect influences that resulted in making the Worcester area an important source for the spread of psychoanalytic ideas.

Thus it is not only the practitioners who received training of a direct-line institute kind along Freudian lines who contributed to the spread of psychoanalytic ideas. In fact, the question may be raised whether there is truly such a thing as a univocal Freudian product. Thirty-five years ago Glover circulated his well-known questionnaire on psychoanalytic technique to twenty-nine practicing English analysts, twenty-five of whom replied. As if anything were needed to convince the observer that psychoanalytic practice and theory indeed require a large umbrella to cover even the anointed! So many approximations to central Freudian notions in theory and practice seem acceptable. Over the years, despite so much effort on the part of the *echt*, the umbrella has necessarily had to become even larger. And in this parlous period when psychoanalysis is under such constant criticism and struggling with so many fundamental problems, particularly as to its contribution as a scientific movement, is such facing up to reality so lamentable?

References

Alexander, F., and T.M. French (1946). *Psychoanalytic therapy: Principles and application.* New York: Ronald Press.

Angyal, A. (1941). *Foundations for a science of personality.* New York: Commonwealth Fund.

——— (1965). *Neurosis and Treatment.* New York: Wiley.

Anthony, E.J. (1973) review of "Autism and Childhood Psychosis," by Frances Tustin. *Psychotherapy and Social Science Review, 7,* 14–21.

Bacon, S.D. (1963). "E.M. Jellinek, 1890–1963," *Quarterly Journal of Studies on Alcohol, 24,* 587–590.

Balint, M. (1954). "Obituary of Géza Róheim," *International Journal of Psycho-Analysis, 35,* 434–436.

Billinsky, J.M. (1969). "Jung and Freud (The end of a romance)," *Andover Newton Quarterly, 10* (November), 39–43.

Boring, E.G. (1950). *A history of experimental psychology.* 2nd ed.; New York: Appleton-Century-Crofts.

Bryan, W.A. (1936). *Administrative psychiatry.* New York: Norton.

Dollard, J. (1934). "The psychotic person seen culturally," *American Journal of Sociology, 39,* 637–648.

Eissler, K.R. (1971). *Talent and genius.* New York: Quadrangle.

Harrington, M.A. (1915). "The psychic factors in mental disorder," *American Journal of Insanity, 71,* 691–732.

——— (1934). *Wish-hunting in the unconscious.* New York: Macmillan.

Hendrick, I., ed. (1961). *The birth of an institute.* Freeport, Maine: Bond Wheelright.

Huston, P.E., D. Shakow, and M.H. Erickson (1934). "A Study of hypnotically induced complexes by means of the Luria technique," *Journal of General Psychology, 11,* 65–97.

Jellinek, E.M. (1912). "A saru eredete [On the origin of footwear]," listed in Géza Róheim review in *Bericht über die Fortschritte der Psychoanalyse 1914–1919.* Vienna: International Psychoanalytische Verlag.

Klein, M. (1932). *The psycho-analysis of children.* New York: Norton.

LaBarre, W. (1966). "Géza Róheim (1891–1953): Psychoanalysis and anthropology," in F. Alexander, S. Eisenstein, and M. Grotjahn, eds., *Psychoanalytic pioneers.* New York: Basic Books.

Malamud, W. (1935). *Outlines of general psychopathology.* New York: Norton.

McDougall, W. (1923). *Outline of psychology.* New York: Scribner.

——— (1926). *Outline of abnormal psychology.* New York: Scribner.

Meyer, A. (1951). *Collected papers of Adolf Meyer*, vol. II, *Psychiatry*. Baltimore: Johns Hopkins Press.

Münsterberger, W., and B. Domhoff (1968). "Géza Róheim," in D.L. Sills, ed., *International encyclopedia of the social sciences*, vol. 13, p. 543. New York: Macmillan and Free Press.

Putnam, T.J. (1931). "Boston Society of Psychiatry and Neurology," *Journal of Nervous and Mental Disease, 74*, 64–67.

Rosenzweig, S. (1942). "The photoscope as an objective device for evaluating sexual interest," *Psychosomatic Medicine, 4*, 150–158.

——— (1943*a*). "An experimental study of 'repression' with special reference to need-persistive and ego-defensive reactions to frustration," *Journal of Experimental Psychology, 32*, 64–74.

——— (1943*b*). "Sibling death as a psychological experience with special reference to schizophrenia," *Psychoanalytic Review, 30*, 177–186.

——— (1944). "An outline of frustration theory," in J. McV. Hunt, ed., *Personality and the behavior disorders*, vol. I, chap. 11, pp. 379–388. New York: Ronald Press.

——— and H. Freeman (1942). "A 'blind test' of sex-hormone potency in schizophrenic patients," *Psychosomatic Medicine, 4*, 159–165.

——— and D. Shakow (1937*a*). "Mirror behavior in schizophrenic and normal individuals," *Journal of Nervous and Mental Disease, 86*, 166–174.

——— (1937*b*). "Play technique in schizophrenia and other psychoses. I. Rationale," *American Journal of Orthopsychiatry, 7*, 32–35.

Ross, D. (1972). *G. Stanley Hall: The psychologist as prophet*. Chicago: University of Chicago Press.

Shakow, D. (1940). "One psychologist as analysand," *Journal of Abnormal and Social Psychology, 35*, 198–211.

——— (1972). "The Worcester State Hospital research on schizophrenia (1927–1946)," *Journal of Abnormal Psychology, 80*, 67–110.

——— and D. Rapaport (1964). *The influence of Freud on American psychology. Psychological Issues, No. 13*. New York: International Universities Press.

——— and S. Rosenzweig (1937). "Play technique in schizophrenia and other psychoses. II. An experimental study of schizophrenic constructions with play materials," *American Journal of Orthopsychiatry, 7*, 36–47.

——— (1940). "The use of the tautophone ('verbal summator') as an auditory apperceptive test for the study of personality," *Character and Personality, 8*, 216–226.

——— S. Rosenzweig, and L. Hollander (1966). "Auditory apperceptive reactions to the tautophone by schizophrenic and normal subjects," *Journal of Nervous and Mental Disease, 143*, 1–15.

Spitz, R. (1953). "Obituary of Géza Róheim," *Psychoanalytic Quarterly, 22*, 324–327.

Terman, L.M. (1932). "Lewis M. Terman: Trails to psychology," in C. Murchison, ed.,

A history of psychology in autobiography, vol. II. Worcester, Mass.: Clark University Press.

Wells, F.L. (1912). "Critique of impure reason," *Journal of Abnormal Psychology, 7*, 89–93.

——— (1913*a*). Book review: "S. Freud, *The Interpretation of Dreams*,"' *Journal of Philosophy, Psychology, and Scientific Methods, 10*, 551–555.

——— (1913*b*). "On formulation in psychoanalysis," *Journal of Abnormal Psychology, 8*, 217–227.

——— (1916). "Mental regression: Its conception and types," *Psychiatric Bulletin*, N.Y. State Hospital, *1*, 445–492.

——— (1917). "A summary of material on the topical community of primitive and pathological symbols. ('Archeopathic symbols')," *Psychoanalytic Review, 4*, 47–63.

——— (1935). "Social maladjustments: Adaptive regression," in C. Murchison, ed., *A handbook of social psychology*. Worcester, Mass.: Clark University Press.

Willoughby, R.R. (1929). "An adaptive aspect of dreams," *Journal of Abnormal and Social Psychology, 24*, 104–107.

——— (1931). "The efficiency of short psychoanalyses," *Journal of Abnormal and Social Psychology, 26*, 125–130.

——— (1932). "A scale of emotional maturity," *Journal of Social Psychology, 3*, 3–36.

——— (1933*a*). Book review: "M. Klein, 'The psycho-analysis of children,'" *Journal of Social Psychology, 4*, 257–261.

——— (1933*b*). "A note on a child's dream," *Journal of Genetic Psychology, 42*, 224–228.

——— (1935). "Magic and cognate phenomena: An hypothesis," in C. Murchison, ed., *A handbook of social psychology*. Worcester, Mass.: Clark University Press.

——— (1940). "Some articulations between psychoanalysis and the rest of psychology," *Journal of Abnormal and Social Psychology, 35*, 45–55.

Zinn, E.F. (1924). "History, purposes and policy of NRC committee on sex problems," *Mental Hygiene, 8*, 94–105.

Pierre Janet
and His American Friends

H.F. ELLENBERGER

Few among the major pioneers of the psychological sciences have been as much neglected by medical history as Pierre Janet. One of the enigmas of science is why fame is bestowed upon certain men, and not upon others. There is a common belief that posterity automatically restores the balance, granting fame to those who deserve it, in the measure to which they deserve it, and letting the others fall into oblivion. Nothing is further from the truth. We know practically nothing of the mysterious powers that raise certain men to full glory and dim the memory of others, and that create positive or negative legends.

It is perhaps characteristic that among the Greeks, Clio, the muse of history, was the daughter of Mnemosyne, the goddess of memory, in contrast with Lesmosyne, the goddess of oblivion, and that the Greek word for truth, *aletheia*, etymologically defines truth not so much as the contrary of lie and error as the contrary of forgetfulness. From this perspective truth is what we manage to rescue from the abyss of oblivion.

As for Pierre Janet, it is as though fame had played a strange game with him. As a young professor of philosophy who pioneered in psychopathological research, he started on a brilliant career. When in 1889, at the age of thirty, he published his book *Psychological Automatism*, his contemporaries had the feeling that a star of the first magnitude had risen in the firmament of psychology. This impression was confirmed by his subsequent research and contributions on subconscious fixed ideas, multiple personalities, psychological strength and weakness, the function of reality, the psychological analysis of hysteria and psychasthenia, and his treatise on *Psychological Healing*, a book of 1,100 pages, filled with numerous and impressive case histories.

For some mysterious reason, however, after 1920 Janet's fame seemed to decline slowly in his own country. More and more, he became identified with the stereotype of the promoter of a purely descriptive and static psychiatry. This happened just at the time when he was shifting from psychological analysis to psychological synthesis and was beginning to build a new behavioral system of mighty amplitude and profound originality. Comparatively few people seem to have been aware of this new development in Janet's work. His unfinished book, *Psychology of Belief*, on which he had been working for years, remained unpublished. His papers and vast correspondence were destroyed. His unique collection of rare psychological books was scattered. The only extant recording of his voice seems to have disappeared. He had never been filmed, nor has anyone established a Janet Archives. This is why it is so difficult to reconstruct the history of Pierre Janet. There remain, however, his writings, a few data from archives, and testimonies from those who had known him in later years. With these sparse data, and with information received from his two daughters, I shall attempt to rescue from oblivion a few glimpses of Pierre Janet and his relations with his American friends.

Pierre Janet was born in Paris in 1859, and there he died in 1947, having been thoroughly Parisian in manner, spirit, and speech. He was the nephew of Paul Janet, a noted philosopher, but, following the example of his teacher Théodule Ribot, he strove to found a new psychology on the scientific basis of experiment and clinical observation. Janet joined Charcot's staff at the Salpêtrière not so much as a pupil, but rather as an experienced collaborator. In 1902, he was appointed professor of experimental psychology at the Collège de France. His life is thus mainly the story of his work, interspersed with a few journeys in Europe and overseas, and enriched by many contacts with prominent scientists. Pierre Janet had many opportunities of making American friends during his American journeys and among the visitors he received from overseas. It would not be an exaggeration to say that in Continental Europe few scientists remained in such close contact with America as Pierre Janet.

Janet had received the usual academic education of his time, with strong emphasis on Latin, Greek, and philosophy. His main inspiration came from the philosopher Maine de Biran. For Descartes's principle "I think, therefore I am," Maine de Biran had substituted "I will, therefore I am," and this new principle became the starting point of Janet's concrete, pragmatic psychology. There was from the start a sort of preestablished affinity between Janet's perspective and American philosophical thinking. Janet divided psychology into two processes: analysis and synthesis. Psychological analysis consisted of identifying the basic elements of psychic life, without, however, following the classical division into intellect, affectivity, and will. He distinguished general levels of awareness: subconscious and conscious, and a hierarchy of tendencies.

His research in psychological analysis started in 1886, the same year in which he first came in contact with the Anglo-Saxon scientific world. The twenty-two year old professor of philosophy in Le Havre experimented with suggestion at a distance. These experiments were witnessed by visitors from Paris, and by a delegation of the British Society for Psychical Research.

Janet's first encounter with American psychologists seems to have occurred in 1889. He had just brilliantly defended his thesis *Psychological Automatism*. This was the year of the great Universal Exposition, organized in Paris by the French government to celebrate the centenary of the French Revolution. To emphasize the cultural value of this event, the government had decided that an uninterrupted succession of scientific congresses would take place during the exposition, a true innovation at that time. Thus it happened that the First International Congress of Psychology was held in Paris from August 6 to 10, with 160 registered participants. There were four sections. The first one was under the chairmanship of William James. In the third section, devoted to problems of hallucination, both William James and Pierre Janet participated in the discussion. Overlapping with that congress, the First International Congress of Hypnotism took place from August 8 to 12. Here, too, we note among the participants the names of William James and Pierre Janet. In the following year appeared James's long-expected *Principles of Psychology*, containing accounts of Janet's first experiments.

The Second International Congress of Psychology took place in London in 1892. Janet read a paper which included the story of a famous patient, Mme. D., whose "subconscious dreams" he investigated with the threefold approach of hypnosis, automatic writing, and "automatic talking," that is, letting the patient talk at random about anything that occurred to her. Among the speakers is listed the name of another American who was to become a lifelong friend of Janet, James Mark Baldwin.

The Third International Congress of Psychology took place in Munich in 1896, and gave the participants the impression of a gigantic meeting. There were, indeed, no fewer than 450 registered participants, and 176 papers were read in four languages. Janet read a paper on the therapeutic rapport between the therapist and the patient. Among the American participants were William James, James Mark Baldwin, Stanley Hall, and Edward Titchener.

The Fourth International Congress of Psychology was held in Paris from August 20 to 25, 1900, on the grounds of the new great Universal Exposition. Pierre Janet was general secretary. Americans who attended included William James, James Mark Baldwin, Stanley Hall, Titchener,

George T. Ladd, Hugo Münsterberg, and Morton Prince, who read a sensational paper on the genesis and development of the personalities of Miss Beauchamp, and who was to become another lifelong friend of Janet.

Also in 1900, an International Psychological Institute was founded in Paris. Pierre Janet was appointed general secretary, and one of the members of the International Committee was William James.

From that time on, Pierre Janet's reputation was firmly established in the United States. His textbook on hysteria was translated into English under the title of *The Mental State of Hystericals*, and was considered a classic. No wonder that Janet received an invitation to participate in the International Congress of Arts and Science that had been organized at the 1904 Universal Exposition of Saint Louis, Missouri—his first journey to the United States, which he considered one of the highlights of his life.

According to family tradition, Janet realized that he really had to learn English for such an occasion. In the neighborhood lived a lady teacher of English. Janet asked her to give lessons to him and his wife. The teacher's method was to have them translate into English an old-fashioned novel by Bernardin de Saint-Pierre, *Paul et Virginie*. It was a touching love story, supposed to take place on Reunion Island, and the author, who was a good botanist, had complacently described the magnificent trees and flowers of that tropical island. Janet's great hobby was botany, so he enjoyed the lessons, but when he came to America, he and Mrs. Janet found to their dismay that they were unable to understand anything or to make themselves understood, in spite of their extensive familiarity with exotic botany. Nonetheless, both of them thoroughly enjoyed their trip.

Janet read his paper, "The Relations of Abnormal Psychology," on September 24, 1904, in the section of abnormal psychology of the Congress. The chairman of the section was Edward Cowles, the secretary was Adolf Meyer, and the two speakers were Pierre Janet and Morton Prince.

Janet's itinerary on this trip included visits to the Rocky Mountains, Yellowstone Park, Niagara Falls, Montreal, Quebec City, and the Saint Lawrence River. On his way back to Paris, he read a paper, "The Psycholeptic Crises," by invitation before the Boston Society of Psychiatry and Neurology on October 20. As was his custom, he wrote his family long letters that he illustrated with his own drawings, especially of trees and flowers that he saw on his travels. Janet was enthusiastic about America; he treasured a scrapbook with pictures he had collected. He liked to tell the story of how he met a bear in Yellowstone Park who had devoured a tourist on the previous day!

Two years later, in 1906, came Janet's second invitation to America, to give a series of lectures on hysteria, from October 15 to the end of November, at Harvard University. These lectures were subsequently published directly in English, under the title *The Major Symptoms of Hysteria*. This time, Janet's knowledge of English had notably improved. However, according to family legend, it once happened that coming back from one of his lectures, he overheard somebody saying: "This Janet says quite interesting things, but what a terrible accent!"

Evidences of his growing popularity are to be found in American periodicals of that period. When Morton Prince founded the *Journal of Abnormal Psychology*, he made it a point to request the collaboration of as many prominent men as possible, and the saying goes that Freud entirely disapproved of the idea, whereas Janet liked it very much. As a result, in the first issue of the journal, in April 1906, the leading article was a contribution "On the Pathogenesis of Some Impulses" by Pierre Janet. Almost at the same time, one of the founders of the American Society for Psychical Research, James H. Hyslop, wrote to Janet asking him to express his opinion on psychical research. Janet answered with a twenty-page letter which was published in the first volume of the society's journal; he showed himself keenly interested and extremely cautious about parapsychology, and did not forget to point out that from his own personal experience the most difficult and original part of the project would be, he felt, to secure the necessary funds.

It is noted in the first volume of the society's journal for 1907 that Pierre Janet was one of the main speakers at the International Congress of Psychiatry in Amsterdam; among the participants was a well-known American figure, James Jackson Putnam.

The year 1909 is famous in the annals of psychiatry on account of the celebration that was held at Worcester, Massachusetts, for the twentieth anniversary of the founding of Clark University. Overshadowed by that event was Janet's reading of a report on the subconscious (a term he had himself created) at the International Congress of Psychology in Geneva. His concern was to distinguish the subconscious, a clinical concept, from the unconscious, a philosophical concept; however, he was misunderstood as having denied his previous concept of the subconscious.

In spite of this, when Münsterberg edited a collective work on *Subconscious Phenomena* in 1910, one of the five contributions was by Janet, along with that of Morton Prince. It was the time when psychiatric opinion in America was wavering between the ideas of Freud and those of Janet. In 1910, a publication edited by W.B. Parker was issued serially under the title *Psychotherapy*. It contained a contribution by A.A. Brill on Freud's psychoanalysis and a discussion by Richard C. Cabot on the "Varieties of Psychotherapy." Of all existing methods, Cabot gave preference to Janet's therapy, which he ranked before those of Dejérine, Freud, and Jung.

The last public confrontation between Janet's "psychological analysis" and Freud's "psychoanalysis" occurred during the 17th International Congress of Medicine in London in August 1913. One of the discussions was on psychoanalysis, which was criticized by Janet and defended by Jung. Among the discussants of Janet's report were three Americans: Isador Coriat stood in favor of Freud, Walsh in favor of Janet, while T.A. Williams expressed a balanced opinion. One year later, World War I broke out, and international scientific relations were greatly affected.

When the war was over, many things changed. Janet's great book on psychotherapy, whose publication had been delayed on account of the war, was printed in 1919, an English translation appeared in 1925 under the title *Psychological Healing*. Although a few chapters of this book seemed out of date, Janet's prestige remained high. In 1921, he was invited to participate in the festivities organized for the centenary of the Bloomingdale Hospital. It was his third journey to the United States. Janet read his paper on "The Relation of the Neuroses to the Psychoses" and participated in no fewer than five congresses—two in Boston, two in Atlantic City, and one in Niagara Falls. In Boston, he read a paper on "Psychasthenic Delusions," and again, one of the discussants was Adolf Meyer.

In 1925, Janet was sent by the French government as an exchange professor to Mexico. On his way back, he again toured the United States and delivered lectures at Princeton, Pennsylvania, and Columbia universities.

Janet's fifth trip to America took place in 1927. A symposium was held at Wittenberg College, Springfield, Ohio, from October 19 to 23, to celebrate the inauguration of their new psychological laboratories. An impressive list of celebrities, from both Europe and America, was invited. Janet, who received an honorary doctorate there, embarked on one of his favorite topics, "The Fear of Action." Among the other speakers was his old friend Morton Prince.

Janet's last journey to the United States followed an invitation to the tercentenary of Harvard University in 1936. The seventy-seven year old man met there many of his old friends and former visitors from America. His head was full of new ideas and new projects. Ernest Harms, one of his former students, reports that Janet embarrassed him by asking whether he had read his latest book. "When I denied this, he came back: 'You have to keep up with me, since I still plan to write ten more books.'" He also visited Saratoga Springs, Poughkeepsie, Baltimore, and Washington. In Boston he talked on "Psychological Strength and Weakness in Mental Diseases." This was Janet's swan song as far as America was concerned.

But the story of Janet's relations with America is, of course, not limited to an account of his travels and his encounters with Americans at international congresses. If Janet exerted a deep influence on several American psychological and psychiatric circles, he himself was strongly inspired by American contacts. A perusal of Janet's works shows that he drew from American sources in several periods of his life. During the period when he was mainly concerned with psychological analysis—that is, with the exploration of the subconscious, the study of hysteria, and multiple personalities— he frequently referred to Weir Mitchell, William James, and Morton Prince. In his studies of psychological strength and weakness, he referred to James's *Energies of Man* and to the theories of George Beard.

Janet's great treatise *Psychological Healing* is filled with reference to American sources, such as Parker's *Psychotherapy*, a publication infrequently quoted by European authors. Janet's book also contains an historical section with substantial accounts of Christian Science, Mind Cure, and similar movements; it is obvious that he gathered this information during his stays in America.

In the period when he began to elaborate his powerful construction of a psychological synthesis—that is, his theory of the hierarchy of functions, and his system of enlarged behaviorism, Janet drew very much from two Americans, Josiah Royce and especially James Mark Baldwin. The term *socius*, which he liked, was borrowed from Baldwin. There are great similarities between Janet's concept of schizophrenia and that of Adolf Meyer, whom he had met on various occasions in America and Europe, and Janet quoted him in that regard. Another remarkable parallel can be shown between Janet's theories of personality and those of George Herbert Mead; however, there is no evidence that these two men knew about each other.

Janet acquired many friends among the people he met in America or who visited him from abroad. It is greatly to be regretted that his correspondence with many of them has been lost. Janet was the kind of man who was extremely careful in checking the accuracy of facts. Thus, he wrote to Weir Mitchell in order to clarify the story of his father's famous case of multiple personality. That patient had been known in France as "Mary Reynolds" and as "La Dame de McNish." French authors told these stories as concerning two different patients, but Janet found from Weir Mitchell's answer that in fact the two case histories concerned the same person. (In another instance Janet learned through a letter from William James about his impressions of the San Francisco earthquake.)

Among the many people who visited Janet, three Americans left a vivid impression in the minds of his daughters. One was Morton Prince, whom they remembered propped in the middle of the ladder in their father's library, singing the "Marseillaise." As to James Mark Baldwin, who also spent several years in Paris and was a frequent visitor at the Rue de Varenne, Janet said, "We talked so much with each other that I don't have to read his books." There was also Macfie Campbell, who had been Janet's host during one of his visits to Cambridge, Massachusetts.

It should not be overlooked that several among Janet's American visitors and friends significantly contributed to our knowledge about his personality and work. Janet loathed any kind of publicity; he never granted interviews to journalists, and hated to talk about his private life. The only autobiographical account we have of him he wrote in answer to a request by Carl Murchison for his *History of Psychology in Autobiographies*. Another American, Elton Mayo, first pointed out the great value of Janet's theories with respect to industrial psychology. Percival Bailey of Chicago was one of the best informed people about Janet's psychology, and wrote excellent accounts of his work that were published in American journals. During the academic year 1921–22, Janet gave a series of lectures at the Collège de France on the psychology of religion. A visitor from America, the Rev. Walter M. Horton of New York, a distinguished theologian and historian of religion, was in the audience. He took detailed notes and upon his return to America published a substantial English digest of these lectures. Janet never fulfilled his intention of publishing a book on the psychology of religion, but thanks to Horton this very important part of Janet's thinking was rescued from oblivion.

It is appropriate to conclude with a few impressions of Janet as related by one of his American friends—a Boston physician, Harry Kozol, who worked with him for some months in Paris in 1929.

> Janet had numerous English-speaking patients, including Americans, and after a kindly but penetrating interrogation of the young psychology

student before him he issued an invitation to assist him in dealing with these patients. It was eagerly accepted.

Janet dwelt and practiced in an opulent apartment located at 54 rue de Varenne in the elegantly ancient St. Germain section of Paris. The Janet apartment was on the second or third floor of the gray stone building. His consulting room was rather small but elegantly furnished with an antique desk, a small satin-covered divan, and two or three small satin-covered chairs. Much of the room was covered with well-filled bookcases. The draperies on the windows were of heavy brocade. All in all it was exactly what one would have expected under the circumstances.

In physical appearance Janet was quite short—perhaps 5 feet 5 inches in height. He had an impressive beard and wore pince-nez. He must have been quite slim the better part of his life, but was now beginning to put some weight about his girth.

What sort of person was he? One word would best describe his manner: staccato. His was a truly staccato personality. But he appeared to be comfortable with himself and not tense or accelerated. He was precise in his questions and in his diction. He tended to make short, sharp chopping gestures with his extended hand in order to emphasize his points. He took his histories and kept his records in longhand. In questioning a patient he was strictly matter of fact and made no attempt to put his patient particularly at ease or to ingratiate himself. He never hurried a patient and he was meticulously thorough in eliciting descriptions of the patient's complaints, but he made every moment count and tolerated no digressions or any unnecessary amplifications. He wrote rapidly and in a very small hand. Had he been arbitrary one might have accused him of being a martinet, but in fact he was very kind and impressed his patients as being so by the intensity and concentration that he devoted to their problems. He spoke English quite well but encouraged his patients—and his young English-speaking assistants—to speak French. He was particularly kind to my young wife, urging her to come to the office with me when we were going to discuss some cases and encouraging her to speak French.

Janet was a man of prodigious energy and productivity. He had a subtle sense of humor, which was betrayed only by the twinkle in his eye.

I must make what Janet called an "acte de terminaison." Information about the relation of Janet to his American contemporaries is still rather scanty, and I hope that amid the historical material unearthed by present-day American researchers, further—and perhaps more substantial—data will emerge. It is also my hope that the personal and scientific relations between Europe and North America will remain as fruitful in the future as they were in the past between Pierre Janet and his American friends.

References

Pierre Janet, "The Relations of Abnormal Psychology," *International Congress of Arts and Science, Universal Exposition*, St. Louis, 1904. vol. 5, Boston 1906, pp. 737–753.

———, *The Major Symptoms of Hysteria* (New York and London: Macmillan, 1907).

———, "On the Pathogenesis of Some Impulsions," *Journal of Abnormal Psychology, 1* (1906–1907), 1–17.

———, *Journal of the American Society for Psychical Research, 1* (1907), 346–351, letter.

———, "La Psycho-Analyse," *17th International Congress of Medicine*, London 1919, Section XII; I, p. 13–64, II, 51–55.

———, "Le centenaire de l'Hôpital Bloomingdale," *Annales Médico-Psychologiques*, lle série, 79e année (1921), II, 467–474.

———, "The Relation of the Neuroses to the Psychoses," In: *A Psychiatric Milestone: Bloomingdale Hospital Centenary, 1821–1921*. (Society of the New York Hospital, New York, 1921), pp. 115–146.

———, *Psychological Healing: A Historical and Clinical Study*. (New York, Macmillan, 1925), 2 vols.

———, Autobiography in Carl Murchison, ed., *A History of Psychology in Autobiography* (Worcester, Mass.: Clark University Press, 1930), vol. 1, pp. 123–133.

———, "Psychological Strength and Weakness in Mental Diseases," in *Harvard Tercentenary Publications: Factors Determining Behavior* (Cambridge, Mass.: Harvard University Press, 1937), pp. 64–106.

Hugo Münsterberg, et al., eds., *Subconscious Phenomena* (Boston: Richard G. Badger, 1910).

W.B. Parker, ed., *Psychotherapy: A Course of Reading in Sound Psychology, Sound Medicine, and Sound Religion* (New York: Centre Publishing Co., 1909), 3 vols.

Martin L. Reymont, ed., "Fear of Action as an Essential Element in the Sentiment of Melancholia," *The Wittenberg Symposium: "Feelings and Emotions"* (Worcester, Mass.: Clark University Press, 1928).

Elton Mayo, *Some Notes on the Psychology of Pierre Janet* (Cambridge, Mass.: Harvard University Press, 1948).

Percival Bailey, "The Psychology of Human Conduct: A Review," *American Journal of Psychiatry, 8* (1928), 209–234.

Walter M. Horton, "The Origin and Psychological Function of Religion According to Pierre Janet," *American Journal of Psychology, 35* (1924), 16–52.

Dr. Ernst Harms, personal letter.

Dr. Harry Kozol, personal letter.

DISCUSSION

Otto Marx, presiding

EDNA HEIDBREDER: This sense of gratitude toward James comes from the fact that he was dissatisfied with the psychology of his own day and took measures to correct the situation. If there was an official psychology at that time, it was that of Wundt, which had been imported to the United States, and of course James was a vigorous critic of it. On the other hand, I think it is characteristic of James that he was not willing to sweep his criticism under the rug. He took it seriously, and discussed it in *The Principles of Psychology*, which was one reason *The Principles of Psychology* was as influential as it was. Throughout it he took up the standard topics, gave the standard views on the subjects, and then gave his own views, which were often very different indeed.

Not only was *The Principles of Psychology* a great success in its own day, it has remained so ever since. On any list of great books that I have looked over, there are two on psychology that appear regularly: William James's *Principles of Psychology* and Sigmund Freud's *Interpretation of Dreams*. I think that James's book is so well written and such a pleasure to read that even today it gives a sense of what was going on in psychology at the time James finished it in 1890. I think it might also be said that, for all his delightful wildness, James was a conscientious author. One cannot read the *Principles of Psychology*, especially the footnotes, without realizing this. Academic psychologists must be grateful to James for the freshening of psychology.

ROBERT I. WATSON SR.: Although William James put his heart and soul into *The Principles*, it was not necessarily the sort of book that could be used as a text. Hence he prepared "James," the briefer course, which for many years was best known as "Jimmy."

Professor Aaron has pointed out the tepid aspects of turn-of-the-century Boston. It seems, as he has indicated, somewhat incongruous that these other, scientific interests emerged. William James was an intellectual adventurer. He moved from topic to topic, but for this reason he could not follow through on some of his ideas. We have heard about his relation to the unconscious, and about the variety of ways in which he was related to many seminal movements. I would suggest, however, that he perhaps never thoroughly understood the work of Freud, and that much of James's work related to his interest in subliminal phenomena.

BENJAMIN RIGGS: James was not altogether out of touch with the unconscious in dreams. He dreamed that he had had a rhyme come through his head: "Hoggamus Higgamus men are polygamous; Higgamus Hoggamus women monogamous."

I believe it was also he who invented the comparison between the tender-minded and tough-minded. If that is the case, there is an interesting parallel in modern psychological concepts of ego strength and ego weakness in terms of adaptational flexibility to meet stress, and some of his discussion of the functions of the tender-minded were really quite close to our adaptational concepts of ego function.

SANBOURNE BOCKOVEN: William James had a direct effect on psychiatry through Elmer Ernest Southard, who worked closely with him and took his philosophical seminars for some time. As the first medical director of the Boston Psychopathic Hospital, Southard and those who followed exercised considerable influence on American psychiatry, I think all traceable to William James.

BARBARA ROSS: I think James's work on volition, on the inner control of the individual at various times—individual differences in the ability to cope under different circumstances—comes out best in *Varieties of Religious Experience*, which was published twelve years after *The Principles*. In *Varieties of Religious Experience*, it seems to me, he incorporated a clear understanding of what had been and what was going on in psychology, in medicine, in psychiatry, in neurology, in mental healing, and whatever else was related to the entire movement at the time. I feel that he had an understanding of the theories, of the methods, of the discoveries; and furthermore, he related all the information within a broader perspective than others who were more concerned with their own specific directions and supporting data. James coordinated and synthesized information from all directions. I certainly agree that he and Freud had much more in common than I alluded to in my paper, and that will, volition, and attention were extremely important to James.

I would like to respond to Dr. Marx's earlier comment that James is not to be found in the two psychological journals.[1] We must not forget that different factions at various times have tended to contribute to and to read certain journals and not others; this has been and still is a problem in cross communication. James was concerned with getting information to the American public as well as to professionals. Many of his articles did appear in *The Nation*, the *Atlantic Monthly*, and other major periodicals read by a diverse audience. However, most of his work, in fact, was published in psychological journals, which leads me to believe that he was trying to reach primarily psychologists. Nevertheless, when he felt the need, as he often did, he addressed neurologists and others through various and appropriate media.

OTTO MARX: Dr. Ellenberger in his interview in *Psychology Today* referred to both Freud and Jung as having undergone what he termed creative illness.[2] I know from reading *Varieties of Religious Experience* that James himself apparently had some similar difficulties. I wonder if you could comment on the nature of his personal anguish.

BARBARA ROSS: James wrote a letter that one of his greatest problems was that he had his ups and downs, but every time he was on a down, so to speak, he made those feelings known. About 1893 he experienced what he referred to as a depression, which was serious enough that he actually went to a mind curer. In another letter, he said that he had eighteen sittings with the mind curer and that he believed it was quite possible that the mind curer had a great deal to do with his recovery. James was very emotional, especially during the earlier part of his life; he was trying to find his way and, as the son of a millionaire, was able to float around a bit more and take more time perhaps than others. He wanted very much to be an artist and his letters contain a number of excellent drawings, yet his father discouraged him, feeling that William was meant to be among the scientific. The entire James family was a rather hypochondriacal group. Henry had his problems; his sister Alice, it is said, was a lesbian, and died quite young in England, where she was living with a woman friend. But William, being the so-called veritable storm bird, certainly experienced a number of depressions, and, as he said, it made him much more sympathetic to morbid feelings. He knew well that such feelings existed and that they ought to be dealt with on what he considered to be a functional or practical level. It was characteristic of James not to talk much about what he could not experience himself.

An excellent dissertation is available in the Harvard library on Renouvier's influence on James.[3] Besides Renouvier, Lotze may have been another powerful force in James's thinking. When, two years before he died, James was asked who were the most influential people that he could remember, Richard Hodgson was one and I believe the other was

Renouvier. Bergson of course was important—James supported his point of view and encouraged Putnam and others to do the same.

EDNA HEIDBREDER: I think there is a certain similarity between James and Hall in that both of them were decidedly dissatisfied with the state of American psychology, though of course in different ways. I have the feeling that both men were enormously influential through direct contact with their students.

I should like to ask Professor Ross whether the rumors that one hears about Hall's seminars at Clark were true, that is, that in them he branched out into psychoanalysis much more than was customary at the time in graduate seminars.

DOROTHY ROSS: In later years he had a large number of his students working on psychoanalytic topics, and since the seminars were organized around work that his students were doing and papers that they were presenting, I think that such rumors were probably true. In either 1912 or 1913 he wrote White or Jelliffe, I forget which one at the moment, that he had formed a Freud Club—he called it a dream club among his students, since they were discussing their dreams. Edwin Boring, who was a more experimentally oriented psychologist, remembered that there was so much Freud on campus that the experimental psychologists were totally disgusted.

It is also interesting that these two men were the only ones who were ever elected twice to the presidency of the American Psychological Association, and both of them were mavericks. I think that says a good deal about the men and also about the American Psychological Association.

ARCHANGELO D'AMORE: It should not pass without notice that Hall was also president of the American Psychoanalytic Association, contrary to the roster of the association, which shows William A. White as president in 1918. In White's correspondence files, which I have been examining, I have found correspondence with Emerson and Hall that reveals that Hall was the only nonphysician president of the American Psychoanalytic Association and the notice for the 1918 meeting in Atlantic City indicated that Hall was going to deliver the presidential address, but it did not give the subject. In a letter to White, Hall expressed his regrets that he had been ill and unable to give the presidential address, but that it would have been on the subject of hate; from Professor Ross's talk, I now realize why he would have chosen that subject.

BRUCE TUCKER: Professor Ross, I wonder if you would comment on Hall's role as an editor, both of journals and in the larger context of the development of psychoanalytic thought. You said that he was on the outside of developments in Boston; do you think that in some way his role as an editor affected his influence on the movement?

DOROTHY ROSS: He was very influential as an editor. During the early part of the 1890s, the *Journal of American Psychology*, which he founded in 1887, was the only journal in psychology available. It was, however, the difficulties that various people were having with Hall as editor that encouraged them to form the rival *Psychological Review*. Hall's journal was never a provincial organ for Clark; he co-edited it with Titchener and it became an important journal in publishing a lot of early work that is of significance to psychoanalysis. For example, Hall had his students doing studies of dreams of early childhood development, some of which Freud himself quoted, and they were all published in the *American Journal of Psychology* and therefore had a wide audience.

KENOST: We recently held an Oscar Pfister Symposium in Zurich, and I had the opportunity to read quite extensively in Pfister's work. His psychoanalytic method book is dedicated to Stanley Hall, whom he called one of the outstanding founders of the experimental psychology of religion. How far is he recognized as such in America and how much did he influence Freud in this field?

DOROTHY ROSS: This always remained an important topic of interest for Hall. He had a number of students working in the field, and in fact at one point founded a journal of religious psychology, though it was not able to sustain itself for many years. But again his work in that field was genetically oriented; a number of his students began to investigate, as he had done earlier, the subject of conversions among adolescents, and he brought together a lot of data on this subject. His work also had a fairly wide influence among theologians, especially his whole psychotherapeutic approach, which probably led to some of the developmental work on psychological, or pastoral, counseling in this country.

BARBARA ROSS: I think perhaps Hall's interest in religious conversion might have come from his old teacher William James who talked about religion in a functional kind of way, saying that it was something like what experimental laboratory science had been for him when he was younger; it was there when he needed it. He implied that religion is something that in adolescence might help to get over difficult times.

ROBERT I. WATSON SR.: The founding of the *American Journal of Psychology* in a sense was all a mistake. Hall was granted a sum of money by a totally unknown donor in Baltimore who was not really interested in psychology but thought that he was helping to found a phrenological journal; that particular form of activity was often called psychological research.

EVEOLEEN REXFORD: I would like to mention the tremendous influence that Hall had, not only in this community but in the country in general, in the founding and development of the child guidance movement and child psychiatry. The child study associations to which Hall gave so much attention for a number of years were extremely important in disseminating ideas of child development and in making more popular the notion that perhaps one can do something about children's troubles and ought to try to develop institutions to carry on this particular work. All of us interested in adolescence as a field of study could spend a great deal of time in Hall's monumental work, and although there are many points with which a number of us would not agree today, still practically every problem that we are busy with, whether psychological, social, or intellectual, received a great deal of attention in that work.

LILLIAN SALTMAN: In the Hall correspondence at Clark there is a very touching letter, dated 1910, from Dr. Hall to Dr. Healy, about his searching for a social worker who was also trained in psychology who would be able to help him in his work with children.

References

[1] See Otto M. Marx, "American Psychiatry Without William James," *Bulletin of the History of Medicine, 1* (1968), 52–61. The two journals that Marx checked for references to James's *Principles of Psychology* (1890) were the *American Journal of Insanity* and the *Journal of Nervous and Mental Diseases*. Writes Marx, "we are left with the conspicuous absence of William James's name from the journals of neurology and psychiatry."

[2] Jacques Mousseau, "Freud in Perspective, a Conversation with Henri F. Ellenberger," *Psychology Today*, March 1973, pp. 50–60. See also, Henri F. Ellenberger, *Psychoanalytic Review, 55* (1964), 442–456, and Ellenberger, *The Discovery of the Unconscious* (New York: Basic Books, 1970), pp. 447–448, 672–673, 889–891.

[3] "The Philosophy of Charles Renouvier and its Influence on William James" is a dissertation submitted in partial fulfillment of the requirement for the degree of doctor of philosophy, department of philosophy and psychology, Harvard College, by Wilbur Harry Long, June 1, 1925.

HENRY FOX: My remarks are particularly related to the papers on William James by Professor Barbara Ross and on the Worcester State Hospital by Professor David Shakow. Since I majored in philosophy during the late twenties, I was particularly interested in the contributions of William James, and I chose to obtain medical training at the Johns Hopkins Medical School because of what I had heard about Adolf Meyer, the professor of psychiatry. I have been vividly aware of how these two men prepared the way for me and for so many others to respond with deep personal conviction to the discoveries of Freud.

In May 1966, one hundred years after the birth of Adolf Meyer, Theodore Lidz gave the Adolf Meyer lecture at the annual meeting of the American Psychiatric Association at which I was one of the invited discussants and Dr. Lawrence S. Kubie was the moderator. Lidz had stated that "in contrast to other countries, American psychiatry had achieved a genetic-dynamic approach prior to the impact of psychoanalysis. The way had been prepared by Meyer and his teachings." Lidz also stated that Meyer "insisted that the patients' life experiences were pertinent to etiology and provided guides to treatment and that interest in the physiological must fit into study of the total pattern of a person's current behavior and its biographical origins—a genetic-dynamic approach. He understood that human behavior can only be comprehended properly through study of its integration at the symbolic level—the psychobiological orientation that overcame the mind-brain parallelism. He combatted the 'neurologizing' of psychiatry."[1]

During the discussion of this paper by Lidz, I made some remarks on current trends in psychobiology and psychoanalysis. I pointed out that both Meyer and Freud began as neuropathologists and that both were greatly influenced by the neurological model of the nervous system as hierarchic and integrative (Hughlings Jackson and Sir Charles Sherrington). Meyer used this as the background for his concept of psychobiological functions as "mentally integrated." As David Rapaport has pointed out, inhibition at lower levels by higher ones served Freud as a model for the conceptualization of conflict.[2]

Both Meyer and Freud had an unusual capacity for grasping the pattern to which details belong. Although both moved away from a primarily neurological base, they continued to be greatly interested in the biological setting for psychobiological events.

From my own experience of training in psychiatry under Adolf Meyer and then as a psychoanalyst, it has not seemed to me that the essential contributions of psychobiology and psychoanalysis conflict. Although it is true that Meyer objected to what he considered a premature conceptual systematization as presented by some of the psychoanalysts who came to this country, later developments in ego psychology (particularly the work of people like Hartmann, Kris, Loewenstein,[3] Kubie,[4] and Rapaport) have emphasized observable patterns of adaptation, and Freud himself, of course, constantly revised his concepts right to the end of his life. Although both Meyer and Freud had to counteract the strong tendency of the times to consider hereditary factors as fixed and unmodifiable, nowadays psychobiology and psychoanalysis seem to be moving along easily in an atmosphere represented by a concept of the continuous interaction of the experiential and the innate.

In spite of these important similarities, which greatly helped to create an outlook favorable to Freud and to psychoanalysis, my memories concerning Meyer as a teacher are that he did not really understand or make us aware of the leading psychoanalytic concepts concerning the patient's transference to the physician and the physician's countertransference that were so clearly described by Ralph Greenson.[5] On the basis of personal discussions with Meyer, Theodore Lidz concluded that he "did not properly grasp the nature of the transference relationship, either as a therapeutic lever, or as a means of focussing biographical data." Lidz reported that Meyer had difficulty seeing why his personality study or the distributive analysis that he taught, which were aimed primarily at providing intellectual insight, were not adequate.

While I was a member of Meyer's staff, he discouraged me from undertaking a psychoanalysis, so that I postponed it until almost the age of forty, which undoubtedly reflected my personal transference to him. He was intrinsic to my own development as a psychiatrist.

After graduating from a progressive school that had been much influenced by the ideas of John Dewey, I went to Harvard College, where, as I have stated, I became primarily interested in the writings of William James. As C.H. Faust described it, aspects of Dewey's views "were seized upon by the progressive movement in education which stressed the student-centered rather than the subject-centered school, education through activity rather than formal learning, and vocational or occupational education rather than the mastery of traditional subjects."[6] Faust added that the philosophy on which Dewey's views of education rest had been labeled pragmatism, although he himself favored the term "instrumentalism" or "experimentalism." Faust pointed out that William James's *Principles of Psychology* early stimulated Dewey's rethinking of logic and ethics by directing his attention to the practical function of ideas and concepts. Henry D. Aiken reminds us that in his *Essays in Radical Empiricism* James "presents a theory of 'pure experience' which rejects the radical bifurcation between mind and its object and hence between mind and body or matter that is the heritage of the Cartesian tradition."[7] He adds that "in destroying the dualism between mind and its object and between mind and matter James was left with the conclusion that the ultimate nature of reality is in no way distinct from that of experience itself."

Alfred Lief reported that John Dewey came to Chicago in 1894 and began a lasting intellectual companionship with Meyer (who had gone to the State Hospital at Kankakee in 1892).[8] William James had recently published his two-volume *Principles of Psychology*, and Meyer was introduced to his writings by Paul Carus, publisher of *The Monist*. As Lidz pointed out, Meyer then found himself caught up in one of the most exciting phases of American intellectual history.

Meyer's skepticism concerning the dogmatic use of diagnostic categories has for many years seemed meaningful and useful to me, and to those of us who deal with the personal responses of people in sickness or in health. The son of a Swiss Zwinglian minister and the nephew of an old-fashioned, capable family doctor, Meyer seemed to combine a good deal of each of them in his own way of life. His father's liberalism and distrust of Calvinist doctrines of exclusive salvation seemed to find expression in Meyer's eschewal of dogma in any form, even when clothed with the dignity of so-called science. And his criticism of the use of Freud's concepts of the id, the ego, and the superego in a way that ignored the complex reality of human behavior made a great impression on me. Although Freud himself was much more tentative and flexible in the use of these concepts than some of his followers, a reference, for instance, to the ego as "struggling" with the id or with the superego becomes anthropomorphic[3] and justifies the original objection made by Adolf Meyer.

Although in his own development Meyer had obviously been influenced by his father, the minister, he had become a physician like his uncle and, for a time, used to make house calls for him. This undoubtedly helped to give him a clear appreciation of what things make a difference to sick people. It is perfectly natural for a physician in a small canton, in contrast to the urban specialist, to think of people as tending to behave in a certain manner under certain conditions and to see resemblances to outstanding traits in the family tribe. He does not feel impelled to make any hard and fast distinctions between the influence of heredity and that of environment, but accepts without fatalism the fact that people have a certain make-up.

Adolf Meyer led the way to freeing our concepts of human behavior from what he often described as the "mereliness" of the physical-chemical chopping block. He emphasized that, in comparison with the lower animals, man's more highly developed nervous endowment and play of symbolism had brought new possibilities for choice, for spontaneity, and for true responsibility.[9]

Adolf Meyer provided crucial leadership for psychiatry's shift of interest from the insane asylum to the mental health of people living and working in both their family and community settings. Psychobiology as he developed it certainly has fundamental relevance for the current practice of general medicine. And the most important implication for the nonpsychiatrist is the active recognition that no matter what the complaint that brings the patient to a physician for diagnosis and treatment, the family history is never "noncontributory."

Both William James and Adolf Meyer lived in New England and trailblazed entirely new ways of thinking about human life and development. And both of them have had a profound influence on the acceptance of psychoanalysis and the development of psychotherapy and general medicine on the New England scene.

References

[1] Theodore Lidz, "Adolf Meyer and the development of American psychiatry," *American Journal of Psychiatry, 123* (1966), 320.

[2] David Rapaport, "Psychoanalysis as a Developmental Psychology," in Merton Gill, ed., *Collected Papers of David Rapaport* (New York and London: Basic Books, 1967).

[3] H. Hartmann, E. Kris, and R.M. Loewenstein, "Comments on the Formation of Psychic Structure," *Psychoanalytic Studies of the Child, 2* (1946), 16.

[4] Lawrence S. Kubie, "Some Implications for Psychoanalysis of Modern Concepts of the Organization of the Brain," *Psychoanalytic Quarterly, 22* (1953), 21–68.

[5] R.R. Greenson, ed., "The working alliance," *The Technique and Practice of Psychoanalysis* (New York: International Universities Press, 1967), I, pp. 190–209.

[6] C.H. Faust, "John Dewey," *Encyclopedia Britannica*, vol. 7, 1960, pp. 296–297.

[7] H.D. Aiken, Introduction, *Pragmatism and America's Coming of Age, Philosophy in the Twentieth Century* (New York: Harper and Row, 1971), paperback ed., vol. 1.

[8] A. Lief, ed., *The Commonsense Psychiatry of Dr. Adolf Meyer* (New York: McGraw-Hill, 1948), p. 44.

[9] Henry M. Fox, "Somatic symbolization versus psychosomatic dualism," *Psychiatry: Journal of the Biology and Pathology of Interpersonal Relations, 5* (1942), 7–13.

Illustrations

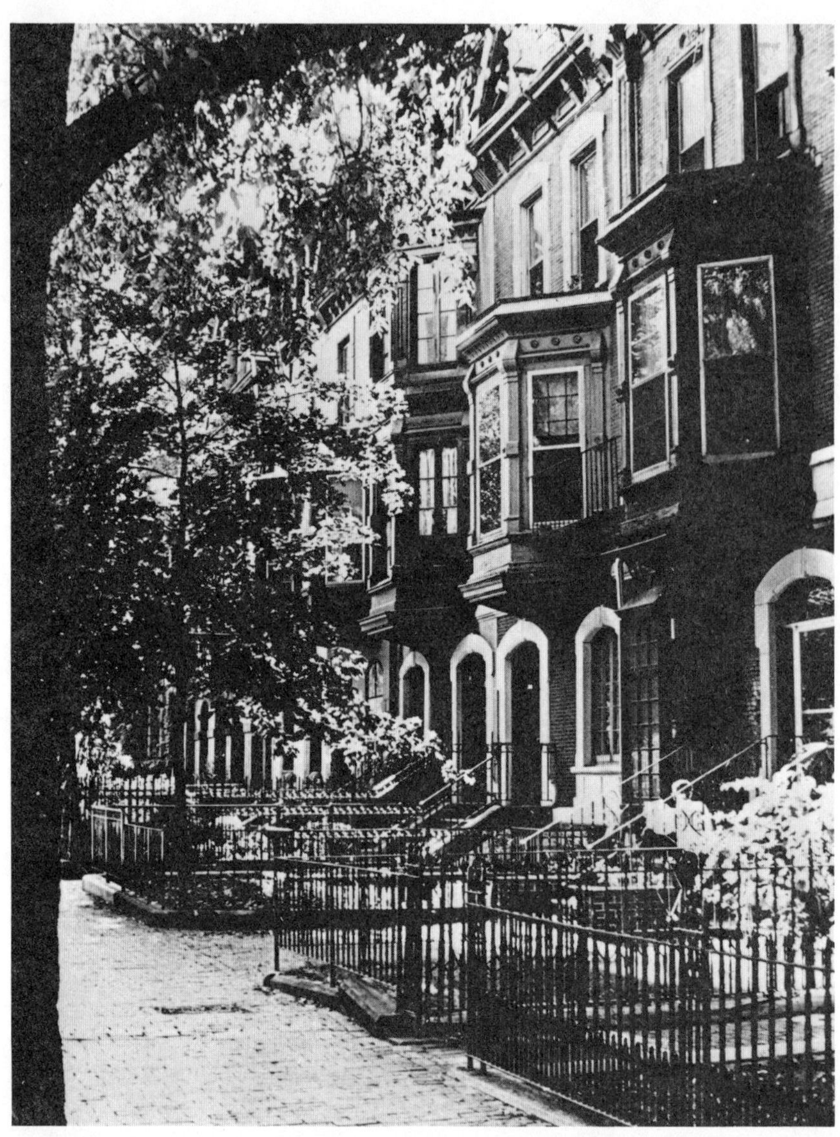

1. Marlborough Street, north side, looking west from Exeter, 1870s to 1880s. J.J. Putnam's house was at 104-6. *Public Information Office, Boston Redevelopment Authority.*

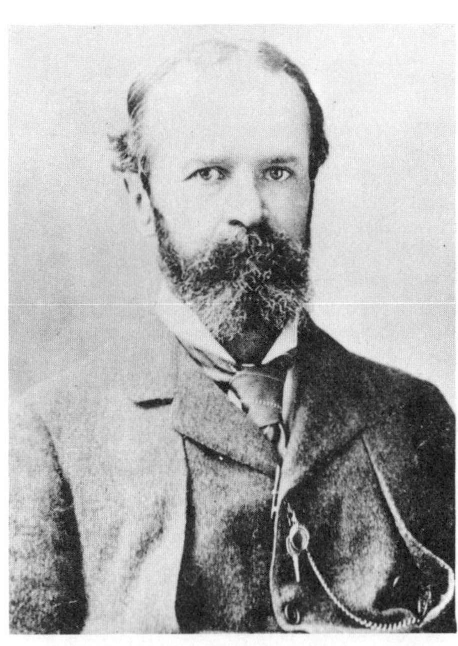

2. William James photographed for the *Boston Budget*, 1901. *Harvard University Archives.*

3. William James and Josiah Royce about 1900. *Harvard University Archives.*

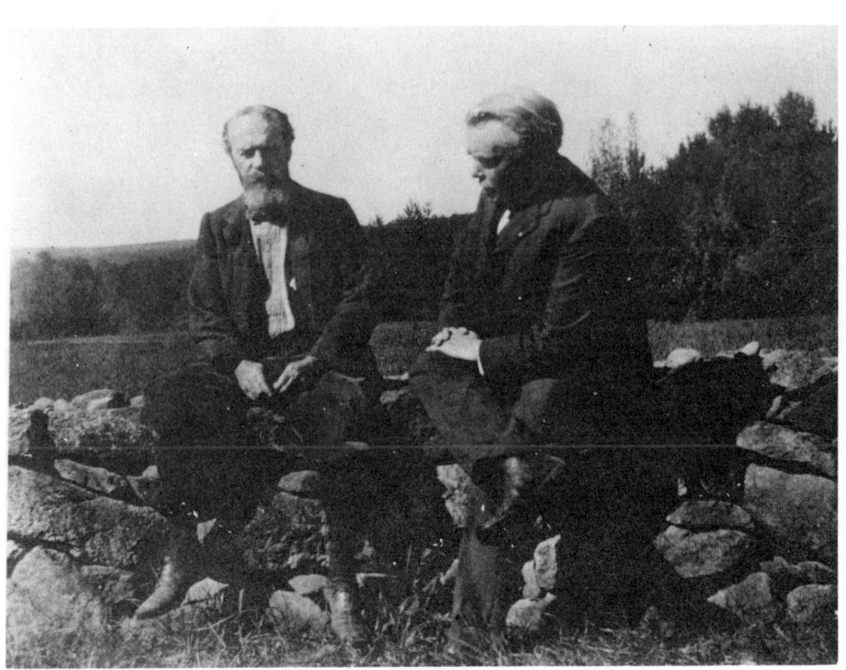

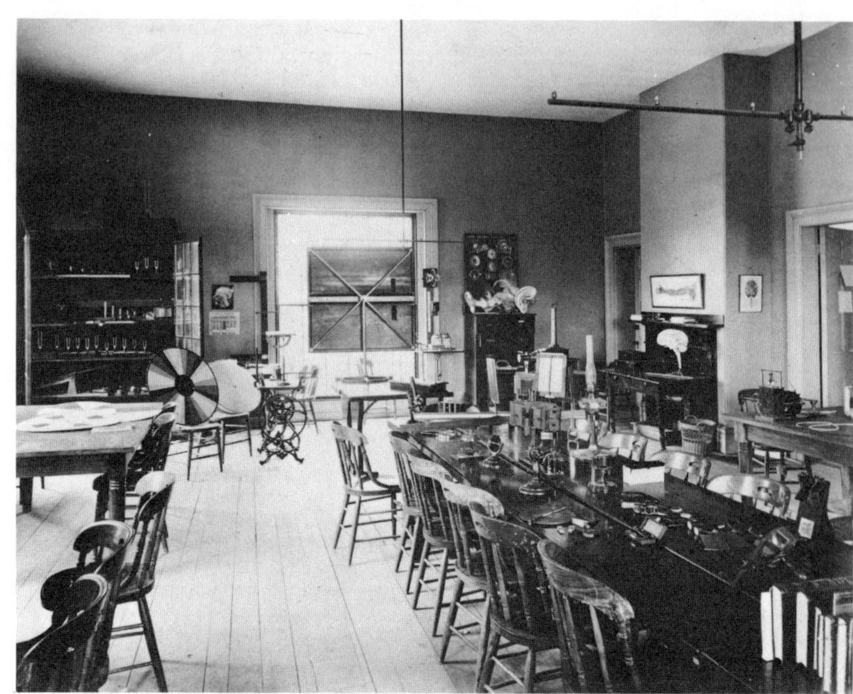

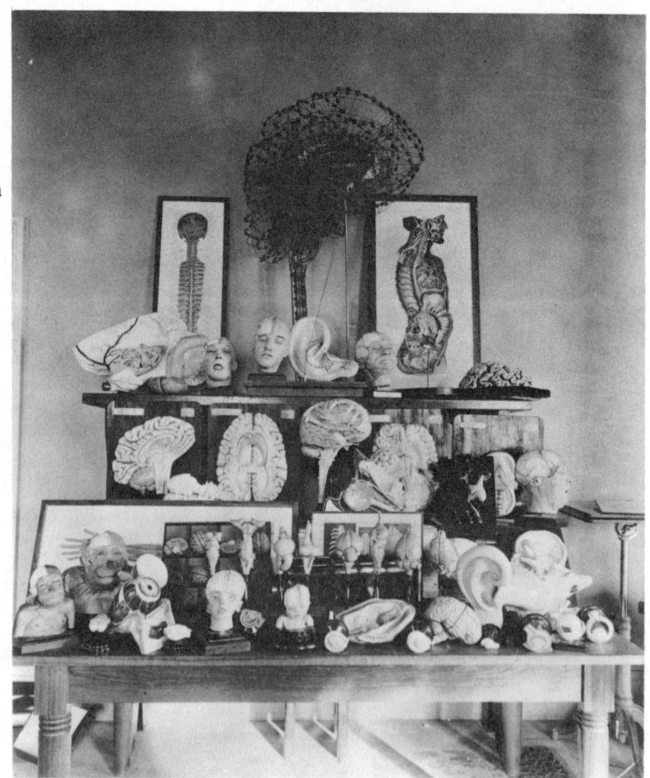

4. *a.* William James's Psychological Laboratory in Dane Hall, Harvard University. *b.* Wax specimen from James's laboratory. Both photographs were taken especially for the Harvard University exhibit at the World's Fair, Chicago, 1893. *See Herbert Nichols, "The Psychological Laboratory at Harvard,"* McClure's Magazine, *October 1893, pp. 399-409.*

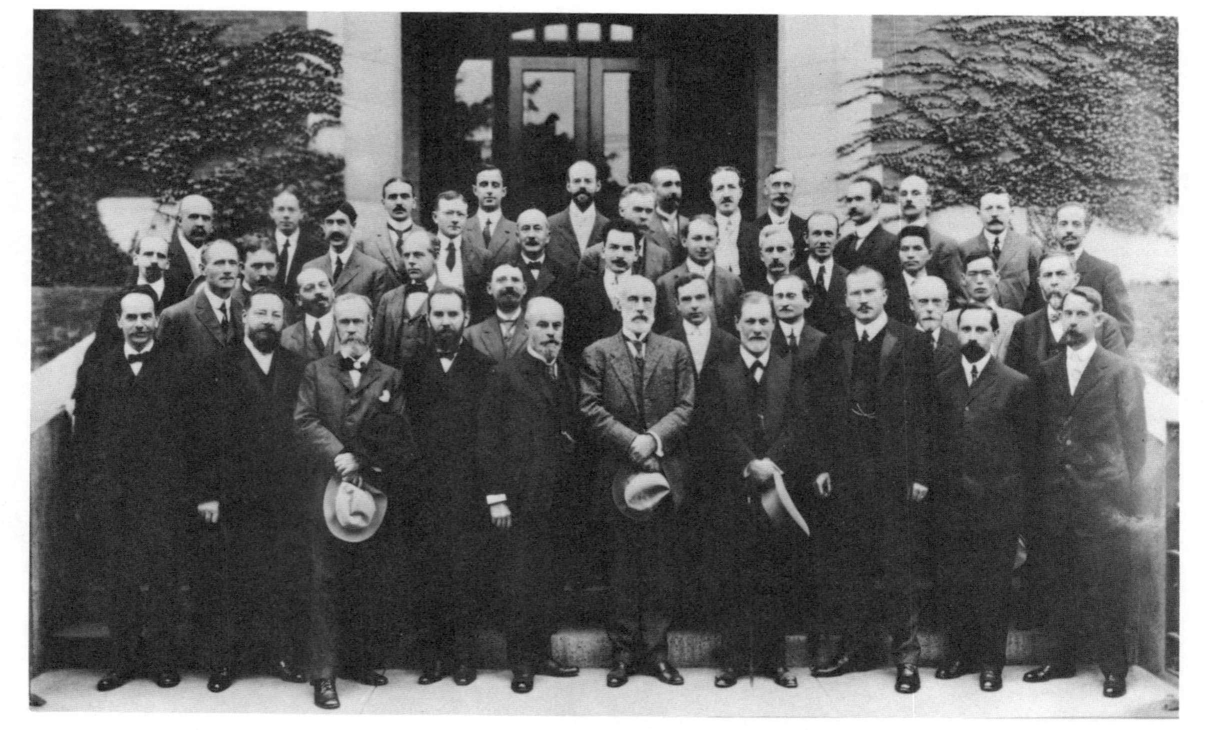

5. Psychology Conference Group, Clark University, September, 1909. *Beginning with first row, left to right:* Franz Boas, E.B. Titchener, William James, William Stern, Leo Burgerstein, G. Stanley Hall, Sigmund Freud, Carl G. Jung, Adolf Meyer, H.S. Jennings; *second row:* C.E. Seashore, Joseph Jastrow, J. McK. Cattell, E.F. Buchner, E. Katzenellenbogen, Ernest Jones, A.A. Brill, Wm. H. Burnham, A.F. Chamberlain; *third row:* Albert Schinz, J.A. Magni, B.T. Baldwin, F. Lyman Wells, G.M. Forbes, E.A. Kirkpatrick, Sandor Ferenczi, E.C. Sanford, J.P. Porter, Sakyo Kanda, Hikoso Kakise; *fourth row:* G.E. Dawson, S.P. Hayes, E.B. Holt, C.S. Berry, G.M. Whipple, Frank Drew, J.W.A. Young, L.N. Wilson, K.J. Karlson, H.H. Goddard, H.I. Klopp, S.C. Fuller. *Courtesy of Clark University.*

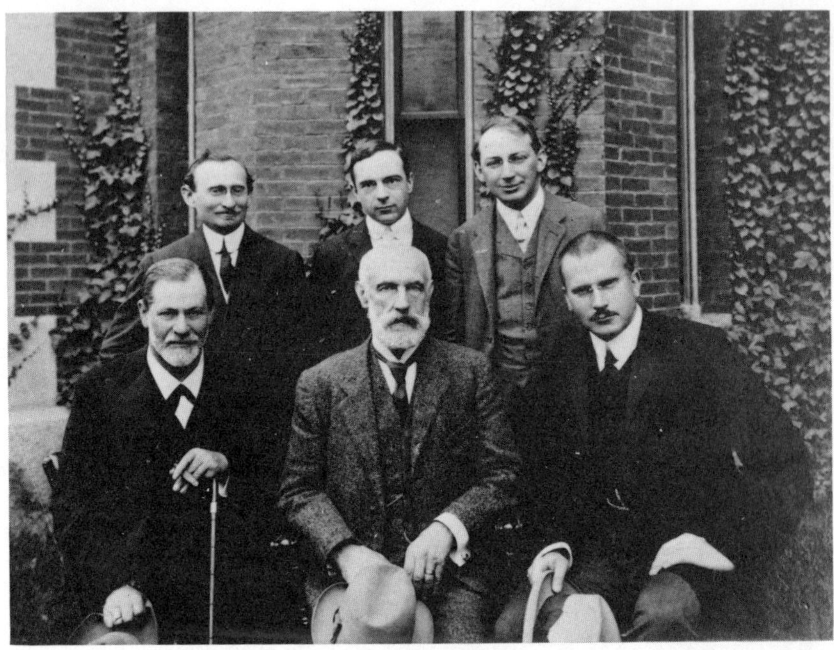

6. A small group picture at Clark, 1909. *Front row, left to right:* Sigmund Freud, G. Stanley Hall, Carl A. Jung; *back row, left to right:* A.A. Brill, Ernest Jones, Sandor Ferenczi. *Courtesy of Clark University.*

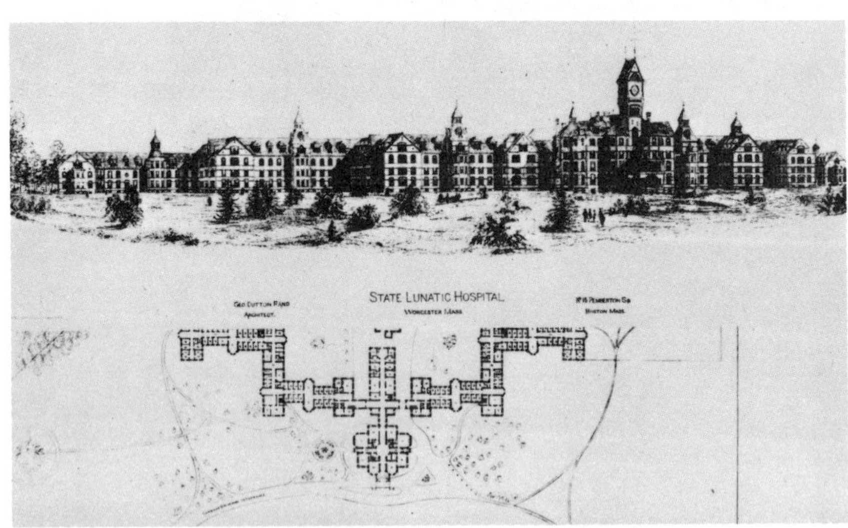

7. Worcester State Hospital. The *forty-eighth Annual Report of the Trustees of the Lunatic Hospital at Worcester for the year ending September 30, 1880.*

8. David Shakow, 1971.

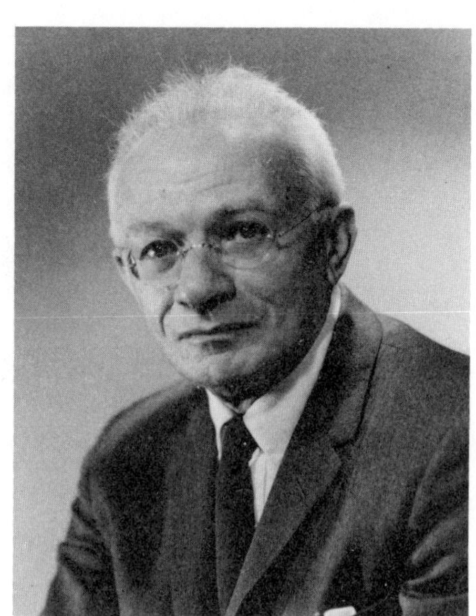

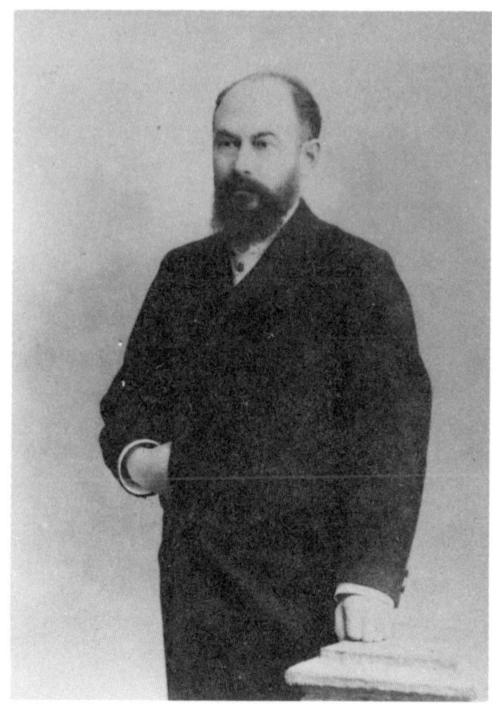

9. Pierre Janet. *Boston Medical Library Collection, Countway Library.*

Popular Psychotherapy Movements

The Mental Healing of Mary Baker Eddy

JULIUS SILBERGER, JR.

One of the lesser known relationships in the history of psychiatry and psychology is that of Mary Morse Patterson, who was later to be known as Mary Baker Eddy, the leader of Christian Science, and Phineas Parkhurst Quimby, who greatly influenced the direction of her life.

Mary Morse had been the spoiled youngest of six children, three boys and then three girls. She was invalided from the time of her earliest girlhood, well before adolescence, by a whole spectrum of variable physical symptoms, including seizures of one kind and another, muscular and skeletal aches and pains, dyspeptic, biliary, and intestinal dysfunctions, tantrums, fatigues, insomnias, nightmares, trance states, in fact all of the florid symptoms that George Beard was later to group together in the clinical state he would call neurasthenia, the *American malady*.

Mary had ruled her family with the tyranny of the weak, competing with her father, an inflexible, domineering, and litigious man, who was disposed more readily toward tyranny of *force*, but whose determination was no match for that of his infuriating, beloved youngest daughter. Her symptoms interfered with her education, for she could not attend school regularly. She never achieved the formal standards of spelling and punctuation that her sisters and brothers did. But she had at her disposal qualities of willfulness, of self-importance, of a sense of personal consequence that would carry her safely on, despite her physical idiosyncracies. And she was always able to appear to others as a significant person.

Mary's first marriage to George Washington Glover ended with the death by yellow fever of her husband of six months, leaving her six months pregnant and so helpless an invalid that the mere sound of a cart in the road outside her father's farmhouse would send her into paroxysms of pain. Her father would take her into his arms and rock her to comfort her. She never raised her son, George, who was ultimately to go off in the care of a hired girl when his mother remarried, living first nearby, for many years, and then moving off to the Midwest. Her second marriage, to Dr. Daniel Patterson, an itinerant dentist, did not occur until two years after her mother had died and her father had remarried, an event she had greeted with the most intense outrage and personal loss.[1]

At the age of forty-one, she was facing the failure of this marriage; her husband, who had always considered her a person who needed and relied upon his strength, was preparing now to leave her behind in poverty while he went to Washington to seek his fortune in the Union Army. It was 1862. Before leaving, however, Dr. Patterson wrote Phineas Quimby, who had a healing practice in Portland, Maine, asking him to heal his wife, and Mrs. Patterson herself wrote later. She was interested in other healers, too, and went first to the Vail water cure in Hill, New Hampshire, where kindly encouragement, plain living, and the admonition not to talk about her physical discomforts were not enough to relieve her of her sufferings. In August 1862 she wrote Quimby from there[2] saying that she should have gone directly to him rather than to the Vail establishment, for in the two or three months that she had been there, she had become progressively weaker. She wondered whether Quimby thought she would have the strength to make the journey to see him—whether she might be so weak when she arrived that he would not be able to help her. Perhaps it would have been better for her to go back home to Sanbornton Bridge, to die in the company of friends, but she had to make a decision soon.

It took two months more for her to get to Portland, Maine and to Quimby, but finally she arrived on October 10, 1862. Julius Dresser, one of Quimby's patients, described in his diary Mrs. Patterson's entry into their group:

> The most peculiar person I have seen of late is Mrs. Patterson, the authoress, who came last Friday, a week ago today, from Vail's water cure in Hill, N.H., where Melville, Fanny Bass and I were, and is now under Dr. Quimby, and boarding also, at Mrs. Hunter's. She was only able to get here, and no one else thought she could live to travel so far, but today she, with Mrs. Hunter and sister, Nettie and I went up into the dome of the "New City Building" up seven flights of stairs, or 182 steps. So much for Dr. Quimby's doings.[3]

As for her writing, which she took very seriously, Mrs. Patterson wrote topical poems and essays which she would send to newspapers and which were occasionally accepted. She herself soon seconded Dresser's testimonial, for she wrote a eulogy of Quimby that was published in the Portland *Courier* on November 7, which I quote at some length both as an example of her enthusiastic literary style and also because of her description of what she believed Quimby's beliefs to entail:

When our Shakespeare decided that there are more things in this world than was dreampt of in your philosophy! I cannot say of a verity that he had a foreknowledge of P.P. Qimby. And when the school Platonic anatomized the Soul and divided it into halves to be reunited by elementary attraction—and heathen philosophers averred that old Chaos in sullen silence brooded o'er the Earth until her inimitable form was hatched from the egg of Night; I would not at present decide whether the fallacy was found in their premises or conclusions, never having dated my existence before the flood...

But when by a falling apple an immutable law was discovered, we gave it the crown of Science, which is incontrovertible and capable of demonstration, hence that was wisdom and truth...Hence the following demonstration:

Three weeks since and I quitted my sick room en route for Portland. The belief in my recovery had died out of the hearts of those who were most anxious for it. With this to the Vail water cure, in Hill, New Hampshire, where mental and physical depression I first visited P.P. Quimby, and in less than one week from that time I ascended by stairway of one hundred and eighty-two steps to the dome of the City Hall, and am improving ad infinitum. To the most subtle reasoning, such a proof, coupled too as it is with numberless similar ones, demonstrates his *power* to heal. Now for a brief analysis of this power:

Is it Spiritualism: Listen to the words of wisdom. "Believe in God believe in me; or believe in me for the very work's sake!"

Now then his works are but the result of superior wisdom which can demonstrate a science not understood: hence it were a doubtful proceeding not to believe in *him* for the works' sake. Well then, he denies that his power to heal the sick is borrowed from the spirits of this or another world...

Again is it by animal magnetism that he heals the sick? Let us examine. I have employed electro-magnetism and animal magnetism, and for a brief period have felt relief from the equilibrium that I fancied was restored to an exhausted system, or by a diffusion of concentrated action, but in no instance did I get rid of a return of all my ailments, and because I had not been helped out of the error in which opinions involve us, my operator believed in disease independent of the mind, hence I could not be wiser than my teacher. But now I can see dimly at first and only as trees walking, the great principle which underlies Dr. Quimby's faith and works; and just in proportion to my right perception of truth, is my recovery. This truth which he opposes to the error of giving intelligence to matter and placing pain where it never placed itself, if received understandingly changes the currents of the system to their minimal action and the mechanism of the body goes on undisturbed. That this is a science capable of demonstration becomes clear to the minds of those patients who reason upon the process of their

> cure. The truth which he establishes in the patient cures him (although he may be wholly unconscious thereof) and the body which is full of light, is no longer in disease. At present I am too much in error to elucidate the truth, and can touch only the keynote for the master hand to make the harmony. May it be in essays instead of notes, say I. After all, this is a very *spiritual* doctrine—but the eternal years of God are with it and it must stand firm as the rock of ages. And to many a poor sufferer may it be found as by me, "the shadow of a Great Rock in a weary land."[4]

If we were to assume that such florid sentiments testified to genuine appreciation, we would be misreading Mrs. Patterson, who could be moved to enthusiasm by a multitude of causes and characters of varying importance. But her feelings for Quimby and his ideas about healing were to become the dominating influence of her life from this point on. That he would not think so much of *her* was unimportant. She needed a cause to identify herself with and a person who would not discourage the hopes she would place in him; someone she could idealize, someone who was close enough to be reassuring, but distant enough that the wear and tear of real friendship would not get in the way of her illusions.

Quimby gains his place in our story because he filled that place in Mary Patterson's life, but even if Christian Science and Mary Baker Eddy (Mrs. Patterson, divorced from Patterson in 1873, married Asa Gilbert Eddy on January 1, 1877) had never been, Quimby would deserve a vivid paragraph in the history of American medicine for his originality and influence on others, and because he was such a prototype of the ingenious, practical, and eccentric Yankee craftsman.

Phineas Parkhurst Quimby was one of seven children, born in Lebanon, New Hampshire, on February 16, 1802. His father was a blacksmith. When he was two, the family moved to Belfast, Maine, where he was to live most of the rest of his life. He had little formal schooling. His writings show a sketchy command of spelling and punctuation, worse even than Mrs. Eddy's own. His son said of him that "he was very argumentative and always wanted proof of anything, rather than an accepted opinion. Anything that could be demonstrated he was willing to accept; but he would combat what could not be proven with all his energy, rather than admit it as a truth."[5] One imagines a determined young man, in hardheaded revolt against his father's authority, making his own way in the world, and inspiring in his children a similar grudging admiration, a willingness to acknowledge, but not to emulate. However much he was to inspire certain of his patients, Quimby could never persuade his own children to choose to carry his work forward.

His first trade was that of making clocks with wooden movements. He invented a number of improvements in the manufacturing process, including, for example, a bandsaw for cutting small parts that is essentially the kind used today. His receptiveness to new technological discoveries and new ideas led him to an interest in daguerreotypy, and for a time he made a business of taking daguerreotype portraits.

In 1836 and 1837, a Frenchman named Charles Poyen began to demonstrate mesmerism in towns along the New England coast. By 1837, Poyen claimed to have introduced the practice to at least forty amateurs.[6] Like many who were to follow him, Poyen had first become interested in mesmerism as a way to relieve his own physical pains, and emphasized that aspect in his demonstration. In 1838 Quimby was witness to one of these sessions and began to experiment with the method on anyone he could persuade to volunteer. In short order he discovered an enormously suggestible young man named Lucius Burkmar. When Quimby would put him into mesmeric sleep, Burkmar would diagnose the pains of ailing people brought before him and make prescription for their relief. He even treated Quimby himself, claiming to reunite separated parts of Quimby's kidneys so that they would no longer cause him pain, and astonishing Quimby by the success of his treatment.

In Quimby's day, the fashionable notions of what influenced human behavior and therapeutics included phrenology, animal magnetism, and spiritualism. There was less of a spread then than there is now between the level of sophistication of the interested intelligent layman and that of the specialist, just as there was less of a difference between the cultural and intellectual life of a middling-small town in Maine and that "Hub of its Universe," Boston.

Thus, Quimby had greater access to the leading edge of investigation into these popular beliefs than we today would likely expect of a man of his background and education, however talented. Similarly, he expressed his ideas in the style of his age; his distinction lay not in the readiness with which he incorporated the conventional scientific attitudes of his time into his practice of mesmerism, but rather in his capacity to question the conventions and to make new and original observations that would modify his practices and his beliefs.

He was at first very much influenced by prevailing notions of phrenology and of animal magnetism. Here, for example, are some excerpts from an account of him published in a Belfast, Maine, newspaper on April 27, 1843:

> Mr. Quimby is a gentleman in size rather smaller than the medium of man, with a well proportioned and well balanced Phrenological head, and with the power of concentration surpassing anything we have ever witnessed. His eyes are black and very piercing, with rather a pleasant expression, and he possesses the power of looking at one object without even winking for a great length of time. Thus, when he commences to magnetize, he fixes his eyes upon the subject's and neither moves nor winks until he entirely accomplishes his object.
>
> We were present a few days ago when a subject [Lucius Burkmar] was under the magnetic influence, and saw some few experiments upon focal magnetism, clairvoyance, etc. When the subject was thoroughly magnetized, and the bandages placed over the eyes, Quimby placed his finger upon the organ of self-esteem and inquired whether it was not very wrong to allow slavery in this country and was answered, no, no!—that slavery was one of the best institutions in the world, and that one half of the world were just fit to be the slaves of the other. He then asked the magnetized, what he thought of himself, and was answered that he possessed all power, that he should one day be a great man, that he should be governor, and even more, that he should be President of the United States! Just as he had spoken the above, Quimby passed his hand to the organ of Reverence, and the subject instantly changed his tone and thoughts, and said, oh!, he should never be anything but a poor miserable mechanic, that he could not do anything, etc.[7]

The reporter goes on to describe clairvoyant diagnosis, with Quimby having only a lock of a patient's hair, and other manifestations of clairvoyance under trance, such as taking the subject in spirit to a place where he had never been and asking him to describe what he saw there in his mind's eye. In the newspaper account, Burkmar was taken in spirit to the laboratories of Bowdoin College, where he describes all kinds of interesting things and, at the end, thanks the reporter for having suggested a visit to such a delightful place.

Quimby was not then primarily interested in using mesmerism to heal, but he did participate in inducing anesthesia. A letter dated Belfast, April 19, 1845, from A.T. Wheelock, M.D., to the editor of the *Boston Medical and Surgical Journal*, describes an example of anesthesia by hypnotism that Quimby had induced the preceding year. A young woman who was to have a nasal polyp removed requested that she be mesmerized so that the procedure might not hurt. Quimby was called in and assisted successfully, much to the surprise of Dr. Wheelock, who had thought that he was simply humoring his patient. He wrote, "She evinced not the slightest symptom of pain, either by groaning, sighing or motion whatever, but was in all respects precisely like a dead body. I felt convinced that I might as well have amputated her arm."[8]

Among the other "successful magnetizers" mentioned in the newspaper articles of the time was one John Bovee Dods, a minister. If Quimby was not then particularly interested in healing, Dods was, and he borrowed Burkmar for a time, using him to diagnose and to prescribe medicines which Dods would then prepare and sell to the patient.

Dods articulated a physiological theory based on his enthusiasm for electricity as a life principle.[9] All normal and pathological operations of the organism were caused by electricity, he said. The apparent weightlessness of this "substance" explained how the soul could exist and yet be thought immaterial. It was composed of electricity. The movement of the blood was caused by its intrinsic electrical pulsation, he felt, the heart serving only as a regulator of the flow. Electrical influences could come from within or without. "Human magnetism" was an example of electrical influence from without, and, obeying the same laws that governed other electrical phenomena, was less effective in a moist atmosphere than in a dry, because the electrical energy could not be concentrated in a moist atmosphere. Therefore, one could not mesmerize during a thunderstorm, and mesmeric currents were more likely to be effective in a ring of people hooked up to each other by way of a series of galvanic batteries. Dods felt that he had the key to life. His enthusiasm must have been infectious.

Burkmar was full of these ideas when he returned to Quimby after a season with Dods. He was now, in the trance state, a confident healer. Diagnoses and prescriptions composed in Latin rolled off his tongue with professional self-assurance. Quimby was puzzled by the Latin, which Burkmar could recite, but with no more understanding of it than Quimby had. He must have learned it somewhere. When Burkmar would come out with one of these expensive prescriptions in Latin, Quimby said, he would mesmerize him again, and Burkmar would prescribe the simple, homely herb remedies that Quimby was more familiar with and that cost less; Quimby observed that the patients seemed to do just as well with these simples as they did with the more erudite remedies prescribed by Burkmar-Dods. He concluded that the patient's belief in the encounter was the most effective healing force. Quimby had been surprised that Burkmar had been able to make *his* pains disappear, and felt that Burkmar's explanation of reconnecting the parts of his kidneys had not made sense. Could he too have been made better by his own belief in Burkmar? It seemed so to him.

One doubt led to another. Quimby began to question the other "facts" of animal magnetism, that the trance relation between people operated by an electrical force from one upon the other, that it was dependent on meteorological conditions, and the like. He satisfied himself that he could mesmerize just as effectively in a moist atmosphere as in a dry, if only he were confident of his ability to do so. He could mesmerize in the midst of a lightning storm if he wanted to. And he began to experiment with the healing technique, eliminating the middle man, Burkmar, and treating the patient directly either by putting him in a trance and suggesting health, or by convincing the patient directly without recourse to mesmerism at all.

The notion had been that it was Burkmar who healed, not Quimby. Burkmar's capacity to heal was supposed to reside in some innate talent for clairvoyance, which could be released from subjection to everyday conventionality when he was put in a mesmeric trance. In this state, it was thought, he could see into the patient's body, thereby divine what was amiss, and prescribe accurately. It was thought that the prescription was the curative agent, but that this technique of diagnosis and prescription was more accurate than that of ordinary doctors simply because they did not have the same insight into the patient's body that Burkmar had, clairvoyant in his trance.

What Quimby did now, though, was to reject the notion that the patient was healed by the medicine. It was by belief, he said. That was the powerful agent in the encounter, the patient's belief that he was sick and that he would be cured. The healer's practice served only to verify the patient's beliefs, in the illness and in the cure.

Quimby thought that it ought to be possible to attack the notion of illness more directly. According to his incipient views, people visited illness upon themselves by their own notions of illness. It was not that the illness was imaginary; it was real enough, but it was caused by the patient's beliefs, by his mental state. Now, if only the patient's attitude toward illness could be changed, if only he could be convinced that illness was a matter of belief, then the harmony between his mental state and his body could be reestablished and the body would heal itself.

A healer, then, according to Quimby, ought to help the patient to redress his mental attitude toward illness; once that was done, the aim of healing, absence of illness, would be accomplished by the patient's own body, in conjunction with his purified mental state. That was the goal that Quimby sought in his practice.

His technique was described by his son George who had served as his secretary during the time of his most extensive practice of healing:

> Instead of putting the patient into a mesmeric sleep, Mr. Quimby would sit by him; and, after giving him a detailed account of what his troubles were, he would simply converse with him, and explain the causes of the troubles, and thus change the mind of the patient, and disabuse it of its errors and establish the truth in its place; which, if done, was the cure. He sometimes, in cases of lameness and sprains, manipulated the limbs of the patient, and often rubbed the head with his hands, wetting them with water. He said it was so hard for the patient to believe that his mere talk with him produced the cure, that he did this rubbing simply that the patient would have more confidence in him; but he always insisted that he possessed no "power" nor healing properties different from anyone else, and that his manipulations conferred no beneficial effect on the patient, although it was often the case that the patient himself thought they did. On the contrary, Mr. Quimby always denied emphatically that he used any mesmeric or mediumistic power.[10]

Quimby believed that he discerned the patient's pain without requiring that it be shown or described. When he would sit beside the patient, pains would arise in his own body, reflecting those of the patient's body. By attending to his own inner feelings, he would have a sure guide to a sense of the patient's inner feelings. Then he could describe accurately what the patient felt. This accuracy would presumably convince the patient of Quimby's authority, and the patient would be ready to receive Quimby's theory of illness. It was believed that the healer took on himself, in some part, the burden of the patient's suffering, and that once a connection to the patient had been made, one could exert an influence in spirit, at some distance, without the requirement of one's corporeal presence. Such ideas were common currency at the time; it was supposed to be a perfectly reasonable way to bridge separations—a supplement to what could be communicated by letter.

Such was the form that Quimby's beliefs and practice had taken by the time Mrs. Patterson first consulted him.

I wish now that I could tell in detail the story of Mrs. Patterson's involvement with Quimby and his ideas. She would write to him and visit him not only for the relief of her varying and ever-changing aches and pains, but also for a kind of spiritual communion. She would report to him her eager efforts to spread his beliefs by lecturing, by bearing testimony from her own case, and by trying her hand as a healer, but only as a representative of and witness to his ideas. In her healing attempts, she tended so to identify herself with the sufferers that she would take on their symptoms to a threatening degree. For example, a Miss Jarvis, a patient of Quimby's, had had to leave him at Portland and return to her home in Warren, Maine. At Miss Jarvis's request, or at her own suggestion, Mrs. Patterson accompanied her and took on the job of resident healer. She wrote to Quimby[11] describing her experiences. When Miss Jarvis, asthmatic, came near her, she would herself be set to coughing. The strain imposed other symptoms on her—insomnia, constipation. She was glad, she told Quimby, that he himself, never having been an invalid like her, was immune to such influences, for she needed him to come to her, in spirit, to cure her of her own diseases and to give her the courage to go on.

But Quimby became ill himself. He and his followers said that he had been giving so much attention to others that he could not give proper care to himself, and when he died, in early 1866, Mrs. Patterson suffered a complete physical collapse. She begged Julius Dresser, another of Quimby's patients, to take his place as her healer. Dresser declined, at least for the moment, and Mrs. Patterson withdrew, brooding and helpless, living for some years on the charity of kindly superstitious and dyspeptic ladies in small country towns.

Four years later she found a young man, Richard Kennedy, twenty-one years old, with whom she entered into an agreement that he would practice her concept of healing, at that time almost wholly derived from Quimby, while she would share his income and devote herself to her labors in the theory of illness. The long march began that would lead to Christian Science, crystallized today largely in the form in which she was to leave it forty years later, when she died.

I cannot here discuss her later denial of Quimby, or her repudiation of her attachment to him, or the other healing movements that were inspired by Quimby's influence on his patients. Two of these achieved some importance: the Mental Hygiene beliefs of Warren Evans and the New Thought Movement founded by Julius and Annetta Dresser.

Quimby had had some notion that the major messianic task of Christ was in healing the sick by encouraging beliefs harmonious with health. This later presented Mrs. Eddy with the germ of a solution to the question, if God be all good, how then can evil exist in the world? It was because, she would say, men in their incorrect relation to God suffered from the errors of mortal mind. That is, evil represented the manifestation in the world of men's ideas when they turned away from God; evil was, therefore, only an illusion, which would be dissipated when people put themselves into proper resonance with the Divine Spirit. The Bible contained the keys to this realignment, and thus to the dissipation of evil, including illness and death.

These then were some of the ideas that were in the air when more formal dynamic psychiatry began to make a place for itself in America. Like psychoanalysis, Christian Science and Mental Hygiene and New Thought derived from mesmerism, by the curious transformations of which I have given only the briefest outline. They denied the importance of the details of history and experience in one's emotional life, and tended to look outward to some authority or ideal belief for their understanding. But they did at least testify to the powerful interconnections between beliefs and body-feelings, and it is from this testimony that they have derived their authority and much of their success. That is what I hope will be the story for another time.

References

[1] See, for example, a letter she wrote to her brother George on Thanksgiving Day, 1850, in anticipation of her father's remarriage, in Robert Peel, *Mary Baker Eddy, The Years of Discovery, 1821–1875* (New York: Holt, Rinehart and Winston, 1966), p. 96, and in Ernest Sutherland Bates and John V. Dittemore, *Mary Baker Eddy, The Truth and the Tradition* (New York: Alfred A. Knopf, 1932), p. 50.

[2] The Phineas Parkhurst Quimby Papers, 1859–1866, (Washington, D.C.: Library of Congress Photoduplication Service), reel 3, frames 1382–1383. These letters are also available published in the first printing only of Horatio W. Dresser, ed., *The Quimby Manuscripts* (New York: Thomas Y. Crowell, 1921), pp. 147–148.

[3] Bates and Dittemore, *Mary Baker Eddy, The Truth and the Tradition*, p. 88.

[4] Phineas Parkhurst Quimby Papers, frames 1478–1479.

[5] George A. Quimby, "Phineas Parkhurst Quimby," *New England Magazine, 6* (1888), 267–276.

[6] Charles Poyen, *Progress of Animal Magnetism in New England* (Boston: Weeks, Jordan, 1837).

[7] Phineas Parkhurst Quimby Papers, frames 1435–1437.

[8] Quimby, frame 1427.

[9] John Bovee Dods, *The Philosophy of Electrical Psychology* (Boston: Fowlers and Wells, 1852).

[10] George A. Quimby, *Phineas Parkhurst Quimby*, p. 272.

[11] Phineas Parkhurst Quimby Papers, frames 1411–1413, letter 12 from Warren, Maine, 1864.

Medical Psychotherapy and the Emmanuel Movement in Boston 1904–1912

SANFORD GIFFORD

Introductory Remarks

The Emmanuel Movement may seem a distant episode, almost forgotten among other popular psychotherapy movements at the turn of the century. Our present reconsideration is based on its interest as a significant social phenomenon and as a mirror that reflects many of the passionate contradictions and shifting opinions in the scientific life of its time. When the few existing psychiatrists in practice were sequestered in asylums for chronic psychoses, and even fewer internists and neurologists were interested in treating office patients with everyday neuroses, the Emmanuel Movement deserves to be regarded: (1) as a radical experiment in community mental health, offering free psychotherapy to "men and women of all social classes, of any religion or none whatever"; (2) as the first application of group methods to the treatment of neuroses, directly derived from Dr. Joseph Pratt's "class method" of treating tuberculosis patients at home; and (3) as an attempt to use nonmedical therapists under medical supervision, an effort which distinguished the Emmanuel Movement from all other "mind cure" and faith healing movements, but which failed to ward off the antagonism of the medical establishment.

Besides its interest as a reflection of current scientific controversies, the Emmanuel Movement was a product of three sources that converged in the prepsychoanalytic psychotherapy of that era, based on suggestion, hypnosis, and "moral persuasion." One source was the associationist psychology of the German universities, exemplified by James and Royce, and another was derived from nineteenth century French neurology, from Charcot and Bernheim to Janet, as practiced by Prince and Putnam. A third source was the local tradition of "medical psychotherapy," advocated by Edes and Putnam in the 1890s and practiced by internists like Pratt and Richard C. Cabot. One of the inherent contradictions in the Emmanuel Movement was the fact that its founders were both well-trained clinical psychologists, with doctoral degrees from European universities, as well as clergymen in a conservative church. Apart from its use of group methods and its mass following, the Emmanuel Movement provided psychotherapy indistinguishable from that offered by the psychologists, the internists, and the "office" neurologists.

At that time, for example, William James, Josiah Royce, Hugo Münsterberg, and Boris Sidis practiced psychotherapy without evoking criticism from the medical profession. Although all but Royce happened to have degrees in medicine, they were considered clinical psychologists rather than physicians. The same kind of psychotherapy was practiced by internists like Cabot and Pratt, and also by Prince, Putnam, and others trained in neurology. Very few in any of these professional groups had had experience with chronic institutionalized psychoses.

The Emmanuel Movement seems to have been destroyed by its own popular successes, precisely because it satisfied a widespread need that was not fulfilled by the small number of other professionals who treated neuroses. And it was these patients who otherwise sought treatment in anti-scientific faith healing sects like Christian Science and New Thought, with which the Emmanuel Movement was easily confused by the public. These popular successes were publicized by a new type of journalism, and the ensuing controversies evoked opinions from all the eminent physicians and intellectual figures of that era.

The Tradition of Medical Psychotherapy

The founder of the Emmanuel Movement was Dr. Elwood Worcester, an Episcopal clergyman and Rector of the Emmanuel Church, a conservative, upper-class parish in Boston's Back Bay. His interest in mental illness derived from the prevailing currents in late nineteenth century thought which William James had called "The Mind Cure Movement" in 1902.[1] In a well-known passage in *The Varieties of Religious Experience* he suggested that the American public was unusually receptive to this movement "due to its practical fruits, and the practical character of the American people has never been better shown than by the fact that this, their own decidedly original contribution to the systematic philosophy of life, should be so intimately knit up with concrete therapeutics."

Medical psychotherapy seemed more prominent in Boston than in other American cities at that time, and contributed directly to the distinguishing features of the Emmanuel Movement. Of the four men who played some part in the Emmanuel Movement, Putnam and Coriat will be described by other members of the symposium, but the two internists,

Cabot and Pratt, were the most closely involved and require some separate attention.

Dr. Richard C. Cabot (1868–1939) came from one of those ancient, wealthy, complicated Boston families like Putnam's, with a tradition of strong interests in medicine, philosophy, and philanthropic concerns. His father was an architect, philosopher, and the biographer of Emerson; his cousin, Joseph Lee, devoted his life to social work; and his wife became a distinguished teacher and writer on psychology and ethics. Cabot was known for his medical achievements, as a gifted teacher and clinician, and the author of many textbooks on physical diagnosis and heart disease. He introduced the weekly clinico-pathological conference that has become a tradition in most teaching hospitals. He was chief of medicine at Massachusetts General Hospital from 1912 until his retirement, where Putnam had been chief of neurology and carried out the first "psychoanalytic" treatment of hysteria in 1904–06. But Cabot was unusual among physicians as a philosophy student of Josiah Royce and as the author of many popular books about ethics, psychotherapy, and religion. He was the first appointed professor of social ethics at Harvard College from 1920 to 1932, and an early advocate of prepaid medical care. In 1913, he had almost been expelled from the Massachusetts Medical Society for his radical views, and he was accused by his conservative colleagues of "publicly advertising the faults" of the general physician.

He was best known as a pioneer in the application of social work to medical care in a general hospital, for which he had sought the support of Putnam in 1905. A year later, in collaboration with Miss Ida Cannon, he published the first of many articles and books on the relation between medicine and social work.[2] Like Putnam's interest in psychotherapy, Cabot's interest in medical social work seemed to arise from an empirical dissatisfaction with therapeutic results. About the typical Massachusetts General Hospital clinic patient he wrote "I needed information about his home, about his lodgings, his work, his family, his worries, his nutrition...Facing my own failures day after day...my work came to seem almost intolerable."[3] His ethical and religious concerns, however, came from the moralistic traditions of his background, and make his once influential writings almost unreadable today, with a blend of good intentions and denatured Christianity that flavors so many products of New England Protestantism.

Joseph H. Pratt (1872–1956) had a similar lifelong interest in the influence of psychic and social factors on illness of all kinds. Educated at Yale and Johns Hopkins, he came to Boston in 1898, and after a few years in pathology he became an instructor in medicine at Harvard Medical School until 1917. He was professor of clinical medicine at Tufts Medical School from 1929 until his retirement. His interest in emotional aspects of illness evolved in the course of treating indigent tuberculosis patients who could not afford to stop working or to pay the small fee for the public sanitarium at Rutland. Although his method of home care was derived from current ideas about the importance of fresh air, he used group methods from the beginning and increasingly recognized the influence of emotional attitudes on the outcome of illness.

Pratt soon established a close cooperation with the Reverend Worcester, who came to Boston in 1904, and Pratt's first meeting using the "class method" was held at Emmanuel Church in July 1905. Perhaps characteristically, the first report of its successes appeared in the *Journal of the Outdoor Life*, although many subsequent articles were published in more conventional medical journals.[4,5] In retrospect, the class method seems naïve, undynamic, and highly moralistic, in the nonreligious sense of preaching "right living." It was also authoritarian, in demanding absolute obedience to a primitive regimen of fresh air, bed rest, and weight gain by drinking milk. Pratt, in a later paper,[6] explained his preference for the term class, rather than group treatment, because of its essential emphasis on instruction. He invariably referred to the social worker, who played a major role in leading the group, as "the friendly visitor," the traditional term in an earlier preprofessional era of social work. Nevertheless, he consistently emphasized the essential importance of the weekly group meeting, the small size of the group for encouraging close relationships, and the personal qualities of the physician and social worker in obtaining successful results.

Within a few years Pratt recognized the value of group methods in treating other conditions, and a later review article[6] refers to the use of the class method for undernourished children by W.R.P. Emerson at the Boston Dispensary in 1908, for diabetic patients by W.G. Smillie at the Peter Bent Brigham in 1914, and for weight reduction among diabetics by Mrs. Jacobson at the Massachusetts General. Pratt[7] attributed his application of group methods in the treatment of "the common neuroses" to a chance meeting with Coriat, who was emerging from the Boston Medical Library full of enthusiasm for Déjerine's book on psychotherapy. This popular book reflected the current methods of Janet and Dubois, and it was translated into English in 1913 by Jelliffe, a pioneer psychoanalyst in New York. Pratt found Déjerine's viewpoint congenial, "that the neuroses are of emotional origin and that *emotional training and re-education* are the essential elements in their treatment," which echoed his lifelong adherence to Oslerian precepts about obedience to medical rules.

For many years Pratt had applied Déjerine's methods of "emotional re-education" to individual patients, emphasizing his belief that the common neuroses should be treated by the general physician, not the psychiatrist. In 1930 he adapted his class method to the treatment of ambulatory clinic patients with neuroses as well as physical symptoms. These weekly meetings continued for over twenty years at the Boston Dispensary[7] under the apt but unfortunate name of the "Thought Control Clinic." Pratt repeatedly stated that his excellent results were not due to intellectual insight or persuasion, quoting Déjerine's remark that hysteric and neurasthenic patients were not cured "by reason or by syllogisms. They are only cured when they come to believe in you." In his individual case results he encouraged patients to talk freely about their lives and pointed out significant relationships between personal events and the onset of symptoms. But he frankly acknowledged that his method was a form of faith healing, and his weekly meetings included many ritualistic details of his tuberculosis groups: calling the roll, collecting written reports of improvement, reading testimonials aloud, and a "relaxation exercise" with closed eyes which Pratt called a mild form of hypnotic suggestion.

In doing justice to the originality of these early physicians—Cabot as a leader in establishing medical social service in the general hospital, and Pratt as a pioneer in the use of group psychotherapy—we must also acknowledge a certain naïveté and the dilute Christian morality that pervaded their attitudes toward patients. These qualities were an inescapable part of their background and historical period, and we recognize their sermonizing tone in the works of such dissimilar figures as William James, Teddy Roosevelt, and an early psychoanalyst like Jelliffe. This pervasive tone helps to explain our early response to psychoanalysis, as Burnham and Hale have shown, as an essential part of the myth and the reality of American innocence.

The derivatives of a denatured New England religiosity and the optimism of the Progressive Era, in its interaction with European experience, anti-clericalism, and scientific materialism, can be recognized in a man like Putnam, who had renounced all formal religious beliefs but remained deeply committed to certain secularized moral convictions about free will that he hoped to convert Freud and Jones into sharing. These qualities also help us to understand conflicting attitudes toward the Emmanuel Movement, which was a complex product of this interaction between religious innocence and scientific experience, at a time when the actual practices of medical psychotherapy and religious spiritual counseling were virtually indistinguishable. Pratt[7] acknowledged this when he quoted an earlier Boston physician, Dr. James Jackson, Putnam's grandfather (from "Letters to a Young Physician," 1855): "The priest had the parish for his cure, the physician the sick for his."

To remind ourselves of these pervasive qualities in popular thinking, in the United States and especially in New England, defines a major difference in attitudes toward psychotherapy before and after the first World War. When Ives Hendrick[8] was asked what psychiatric residents were taught during the 1920s about nonanalytic psychotherapy, he recalled that the first precept was to listen to the patient and suspend all moral judgments on what he had to say. When Pratt[9] still held that "the psychoneuroses are due to an initial change in the *moral* or mental state" (italics added), they represented the attitudes of two different eras.

Dr. Elwood Worcester and the Emmanuel Movement 1906–1912

The life and family background of Dr. Worcester himself will also illustrate some crosscurrents of nineteenth century America. He was born in 1864, in Massilon, Ohio, and grew up in Rochester, New York, but his father came from a New England family that contained many ministers and physicians. "Oddly enough, several of its physicians have been preachers, and more than one of its ministers has practiced medicine."[10] The most famous of these was the Rev. Thomas Worcester, who established the Swedenborgian church in Boston, and another was a physician said to have brought the stethescope to this country from his medical education in Europe. Worcester's father was an amateur geologist who made and lost several fortunes prospecting in the Ohio and Mississippi River valleys. Worcester himself was an only son, with three older sisters who teased and adored him; two later committed suicide and one drowned in the Galveston flood. Though he scarcely spoke until he was three, he recalled vivid visual and tactile memories dating from his second year. At six he had terrifying preoccupations with physical decay after the death of a favorite aunt. When he was sixteen, following his father's death and his mother's blindness and emotional prostration, he attempted to support the family by working in the New York Central freight warehouse. Here, "one dark and gloomy day in February," he had a mystical experience, in which the yellow wall suddenly seemed brightly lit and a voice spoke to him, saying "Be faithful to me and I will be faithful to you." He retained a lifelong interest in the occult, at a time when psychic phenomena were seriously investigated by respected scientists.

Worcester sought counsel about his vision with the Rev. Algernon Crapsey, a mildly heretical minister and gifted orator who emphasized the social applications of Christianity. After a year of disciplined self-study, teaching himself Greek and Latin, he won a scholarship to Columbia University. He worked his way through college, completing three years of the Episcopal Seminary in one year of prodigious study. Then he went to the University of Leipzig for a doctorate in philosophy and psychology, where he was strongly influenced by Wundt and even more so by Fechner, whom he revered as a saint and later wrote a book about. After completing his dissertation on John Locke, he became professor of philosophy, psychology, and "Christian evidences" at Lehigh University in 1890.

Except for his religious training, this background of Swedenborgianism, scientific German psychology, and an interest in the occult recalls the James family, and his admiration for Fechner recalls Freud, who derived his libido theory from Fechner's "constancy principle." During his years at Lehigh he began to read Charcot, Bernheim, and Janet, because he believed that "human nature...could be understood only through the knowledge of psychopathology." When he turned from teaching psychology to the ministry in 1896, his first parish was in Philadelphia, where he became a friend of Dr. Weir Mitchell, and he attributed the idea of the Emmanuel Movement to a remark of Dr. Mitchell's on one of their weekly walks.

When Dr. Worcester came to Boston in 1904 as Rector of Emmanuel Church, Dr. Pratt sought his help in treating tuberculosis patients by the class method. As previously described, the first meetings were held in the chapter house in 1905, and this project continued independently of the Emmanuel Movement for eighteen years. After a successful year with tuberculosis patients, Dr. Worcester decided in 1906 to form a similar class, "for the moral and psychological treatment of nervous and psychic disorders." He sought medical supervision from various prominent physicians, and his closest collaborator became Dr. Isador Coriat, a young neurologist and psychiatrist who had trained under Morton Prince and Adolf Meyer at Worcester State Hospital. His other close collaborator was his own assistant, the Rev. Samuel McComb, an Anglo-Irishman with a Ph.D. in psychology from Oxford. The first meeting began with four lectures by Drs. Putnam, Cabot, Worcester, and McComb, and the audience was informed that the two physicians and the two clergymen would be present for individual counseling the next morning. To Dr. Worcester's amazement, 198 men and women arrived, including "several hack-loads of patients from a local asylum, sent down...I suppose, to have a joke on Dr. Putnam." The initial function of the physicians was to examine each patient and refer all organic disorders to appropriate clinics. The procedure thereafter consisted of weekly group meetings, conducted jointly by one physician and one clergyman, with individual counseling as requested. Apparently this format continued unchanged for many years.

The nature of the psychotherapy is known from the writings of Dr. Worcester and many sympathetic physicians and psychologists, including a pamphlet of William James, and from the book, *Religion and Medicine*,[11] in which Worcester, McComb, and Coriat collaborated and wrote separate chapters. Sixteen of its twenty chapters are didactic lectures on "psychopathology," as the term was then used to convey preanalytic concepts of the "subconscious mind," and their content is indistinguishable from other similar popular books of that decade by Sidis,[12] Jastrow,[13] and Münsterberg.[14] Their monotony now lies in the undynamic quality of Janet's concept of hysterical dissociation. Although the subconscious mind was conceived as a dynamic force, influencing behavior without conscious awareness, its manifestations were chiefly found in hypnotic phenomena, hysterical symptoms, and the repetitious cases of amnesia and "multiple personality" reported by Janet and Flournoy in Europe and by Prince in this country. Freud's *Psychopathology of Everyday Life* is favorably mentioned in one of Coriat's chapters as "an interesting little book," but one that merely adds dreams and slips of the tongue to other evidences of unconscious activity.

These bland didactic lectures may seem a tepid broth instead of the fiery potion we imagine when we read about the enormous following and the fierce public controversies that the Emmanuel Movement inspired, during the years of its increasing popularity from 1906 to 1912. But it represented the most advanced and dynamic psychotherapeutic method then available, until Freud's Worcester lectures in 1909. (We assume that its successes depended on the personality of its leaders, the shared group experience of the weekly meetings, and the common sense wisdom of its individual counseling.)

Opposition of the Medical Establishment, 1908–1912

From the evidence of newspaper files,[15] 1909 marked the high tide of the Emmanuel Movement, and in that year two characteristic publications appeared. One was a journal, called *Psychotherapy*, subtitled *A Course of Reading in Sound Psychology, Sound Medicine and Sound Religion*, which contained many articles about the Emmanuel Movement, several about psychoanalysis by Brill and Putnam, and an introduction by Cabot, called "The American Type of Psychotherapy."[16] Cabot proclaimed, in effect, the triumph of our native contributions to the art, while acknowledging its European sources in Dubois and Déjerine. He also suggested that its advent had been retarded here by a decade, compared to Europe, because of the widespread influence of Christian Science and other faith healing cults. In Europe, he proposed, "there has been no movement among the laity, where psychotherapy has been wholly in the hands of the physicians, [and] its scientific and reasonable sides have been developed." The other publication, a small book, *Psychotherapeutics*, edited by Dr. F.H. Gerrish,[17] contained similar papers by Prince, Putnam, Sidis, and E.W. Taylor, while Ernest Jones contributed a skillful popularization of Freud, using surgical metaphors and presenting psychoanalysis as "the second stage in the evolution of psychotherapy."

In 1908 the Emmanuel Church had offered a summer school for theological students, and a similar course for Tufts medical students was announced for the fall, to be given by Dr. Morton Prince and the Rev. A.B. Shields. Prince gave a commencement day address on psychotherapy, defending its ancient traditions and scientific respectability in France over the past twenty-five years and attacking his conservative Philadelphia colleagues for calling it "a Boston fad."

As popular enthusiasm for the Emmanuel Movement increased, its successes, as well as opposition from many different quarters, were magnified by newspaper publicity. There is no doubt that Dr. Worcester was surprised and sincerely distressed by the publicity, which he endured as the price of helping large numbers of patients. Some complaints from his genteel parishioners, about crowds of indigent patients in their church, suggest that many admired his intentions but wished his meetings were conducted elsewhere. He was attacked by conservative clergymen, from within his church and from other denominations, for the emotionality of his following, as if his weekly lectures were revivalistic camp meetings, yet he was always supported by the benevolent neutrality of Archbishop Lawrence. Naturally the Emmanuel Movement was attacked by Christian Science and other antimedical faith healing sects, on the grounds that Jesus had not limited the healing function of the church to nervous and mental disorders.

The major opposition came, however, from the medical establishment, expressed with every degree of vehemence, sometimes politely acknowledging Dr. Worcester's personal integrity, sometimes expressing bitter denunciation. But the universal point of attack, underlying all shades of opinion, was the simple issue of professional status: nonphysicians were treating patients with medical illnesses, even if these illnesses were functional and not organic. The opposition of most rank-and-file physicians no longer seems surprising, knowing the conservative character of the profession then and now; even in the eighteenth century the first official acts of the Massachusetts Medical Society were to increase fees and oppose vaccination. But the attacks were disappointing to Dr. Worcester, who always believed that a real collaboration between the clergy and medicine was possible, and who never advocated psychotherapy without medical supervision. He received no support from his fellow psychologists, and his chief defenders remained the physicians—Pratt, Cabot, Coriat, and a few others who originally helped in founding the Emmanuel Movement. And they were a minority within their profession, and each, for his own reasons, gradually drifted away in later years.

Surprising, however, are the reactions of two physicians who joined the conservative medical opposition to the Emmanuel Movement, primarily over the issue of lay psychotherapy. Putnam is the first. He had initially been sympathetic to the Emmanuel Movement and had given the opening lecture at its first meeting. Without reviewing the detailed evidence in his unpublished letters and his lengthy article in the *Harvard Theological Review* of 1909,[18] there is reason to suspect that he was in some conflict about his position. He repeatedly emphasized Dr. Worcester's personal qualifications and the widespread unfulfilled need for outpatient and office psychotherapy. But his extreme distaste for the weekly group meetings, which he stopped attending, suggests that his strongest aversion was to the sensationalism of the newspaper publicity. Burnham[19] describes a similar fastidious reaction when Putnam first encountered psychoanalysis. Putnam's article is a lengthy study in ambivalence about the respective roles of minister and physician in treating mental illness. In a footnote he admits that psychologists without medical training may be allowed to treat patients because in such small numbers no question arises of "a new medical specialty." Whether Putnam was also put off by the religious auspices of the Emmanuel Movement we can only speculate.

Having renounced religion and boldly espoused psychoanalysis, his persistent need to reintroduce ethical and metaphysical issues into analysis at least suggests some unresolved conflicts.

The second physician is Freud himself, who happened to arrive in Boston for the Worcester lectures at the height of the public controversies about the Emmanuel Movement. In one of his few newspaper interviews (Boston *Transcript*, Sept. 11, 1909), he deplored psychotherapy without medical training, while acknowledging that psychotherapy was "as old as illness, and [that] we doctors could not give it up if we wanted to because...the patient has not the slightest intention of giving it up." His principal objection was more explicitly to the religious element, expressed as his distaste for the public's "weakness for everything that savors of mysteries." This objection is not unexpected, in view of his lifelong antireligious attitudes, which reappeared in his much later judgment of the Emmanuel Movement. In a 1934 reply to an inquiry from the Rev. J.G. Greene,[20] a Unitarian minister who wrote the only recent history of the Emmanuel Movement, Freud wrote: "Perhaps one should be sorry that so much energy in America has poured forth in these religious movements. But America is overrich in energy." His objection to psychotherapy by laymen is paradoxical, however, because his advocacy of lay analysis was also one of his lifelong convictions, staunchly upheld even when it threatened to split the American and European analytic groups.

The Latter Days of the Emmanuel Movement, 1912–1929

In 1909, in response to medical criticism, Dr. Worcester appointed a new medical board, including Dr. Joel E. Goldthwaite, and imposed stricter rules of supervision, so that "an internist remains throughout in charge of every case." But the establishment was not really appeased because, according to Dr. J.J. Thomas, "clergymen will still go on giving medical treatment." At any rate, the Emmanuel Movement seemed to fade from public notice after 1912, partly as a result of Dr. Worcester's decision to avoid public controversy and to refuse information to the newspapers. He and Dr. McComb quietly continued their work as before until Dr. Worcester's retirement as Rector in 1929.

Dr. Worcester's writings of this period,[21] and his autobiography of 1932,[10] are more interesting than earlier ones for their reflective tone, their vivid clinical vignettes, and his impressive therapeutic successes. He and Dr. McComb provided, in effect, what would now be called a walk-in service, group psychotherapy, individual crisis intervention, and long-term supportive relationships of considerable intensity. A woman with globus hystericus, for example, referred by a surgeon who had proposed a sham operation, was successfully treated by the brief exploration of some fairly obvious dreams as pregnancy fantasies. Many hundreds of depressed and suicidal patients sought treatment over the years, and though Dr. Worcester accepted them all, against Dr. Cabot's advice to avoid psychotic depressives, there were no deaths from suicide, an enviable record for any psychotherapist.

Another remarkable feature of these later years was Dr. Worcester's increasing admiration for Freud, and the extent to which he accepted analytic theories and assimilated them into his therapy. He had always believed in the influence of childhood experiences, but he now defended Freud's theories of childhood sexuality as "a truth of the highest value" and the interpretation of dreams for its "amazing capacity to discover law where all is chaos," precisely those aspects of analysis that Cabot and other pre-Freudian psychotherapists had found so objectionable. But he was deeply disturbed by Freud's concept of the unconscious as "a seething cauldron" of forbidden wishes, and compared it with St. Paul's "arraignment of human nature." The widespread public acceptance of the Emmanuel Movement, as Hale[22] has recently suggested, may have played some part in the popular receptiveness to Freud here in New England.

One practical outgrowth of the Emmanuel Movement deserves mention: the first use of group methods in the treatment of alcoholism. In 1911 Mr. Ernest Jacoby, a businessman and parishioner of Dr. Worcester's, organized a self-help group for alcoholics that met weekly in the basement of the church. As a separate project from the weekly Emmanuel meetings, this group eventually dissociated itself from the church and moved to other quarters. Later, another businessman and former patient of Dr. Worcester's, Mr. Courtnay Baylor, became a full-time volunteer and continued his work with alcoholics. After Dr. Worcester's retirement, Baylor incorporated a version of the Emmanuel Movement as the "Craigie Foundation," to avoid exploiting the church and to protect it from "the drawbacks of a popular movement."

References

1 William James, *The Varieties of Religious Experience* (1902) (New York: The Modern Library, 1929).

2 Richard C. Cabot, *Social Service and the Art of Healing* (New York: Moffat, Yard, 1909).

[3] ———, Remarks quoted in Biographical sketch, *American Dictionary of Biography*, vol. XXII, Supplement 2. (New York: Scribner's, 1958), p. 83.

[4] J.H. Pratt, "The Class Method of Treating Consumption in the Homes of the Poor," *Journal of the American Medical Association, 49* (1907), 755–759.

[5] ———, "Results Obtained in the Treatment of Pulmonary Tuberculosis by the Class Method," *British Medical Journal, 2* (1908), 1070–1071.

[6] ———, "The Principles of Class Treatment and their Application to Various Chronic Diseases," *Hospital Social Service, 6* (1922), 401–411.

[7] ———, "The Use of Déjerine's Methods in the Treatment of the Common Neuroses by Group Psychotherapy," *Bulletin of the New England Medical Center, 15* (1953), 9–17.

[8] Ives Hendrick, personal communication, May 1971.

[9] J.H. Pratt, "The Influence of Emotions in the Causation and Cure of Psychoneuroses," *International Clinics*, 1934.

[10] Elwood Worcester, *Life's Adventure* (New York: Scribner's, 1932).

[11] ———, Samuel McComb, and Isador H. Coriat, *Religion and Medicine. The Moral Control of Nervous Disorders* (New York: Moffat, Yard, 1908).

[12] Boris Sidis, *The Psychology of Suggestion* (New York: Appleton, 1903).

[13] Joseph Jastrow, *The Subconscious* (Boston: Houghton, Mifflin, 1905).

[14] Hugo Münsterberg, *Psychotherapy* (New York: Moffat, Yard, 1909).

[15] Isador H. Coriat, Scrapbook, 3 vols. Clippings from U.S. and Canadian newspapers, magazines, and medical journals, 1906–1943. Archives of Boston Psychoanalytic Institute and Francis A. Countway Library of Medicine, Boston.

[16] W.B. Parker, ed., *Psychotherapy, A Course of Reading in Sound Psychology, Sound Medicine and Sound Religion*, 3 vols. (New York: Centre Publishing Company, 1908–1909).

[17] F.H. Gerrish and others, *Psychotherapeutics* (Boston: Badger, 1909).

[18] J.J. Putnam, "The Service to Nervous Invalids of the Physician and of the Minister," *Harvard Theological Review, 2* (1909), 235–250.

[19] John C. Burnham, *Psychoanalysis and American Medicine, 1894–1918*, Psychological Issues, Monograph 20 (New York: International Universities Press, 1967).

[20] Sigmund Freud, unpublished letter to J.G. Greene, 1934. Translated by Ingrid B. Gifford. Archives, Countway Library of Medicine.

[21] E. Worcester and S. McComb, *Body, Mind and Spirit* (Boston: Marshall Jones, 1931).

[22] Nathan G. Hale, Jr., *James Jackson Putnam and Psychoanalysis* (Cambridge, Mass.: Harvard University Press, 1971).

Clifford W. Beers and the Mental Hygiene Movement

NORMAN DAIN

I

One of the most compelling problems in the history of psychiatry is the alternation between optimistic and pessimistic, therapeutic and custodial, environmental and hereditary, psychological and somatic attitudes, theories, and practices regarding mental disorders. How can this cyclical pattern be explained? Why have zealous men and women found it necessary to repeat, and in much the same terms, calls for reforms—reforms that have in practice benefited relatively few of the mentally disordered and that even in their limited scope have inevitably been overwhelmed by countertendencies, only to be revived again as if they were entirely new proposals? This paper, a partial summary of a more extensive statement in my forthcoming biography of Clifford W. Beers, expresses some thoughts on the subject and uses as a case study certain aspects of Beers's work in the mental hygiene movement that he started in New Haven, Connecticut, in 1908 and dominated until 1939.

A decade ago, in a study of pre-Civil War concepts of mental illness in the United States, I described the rise and then, briefly, the decline after the Civil War of the nineteenth century moral treatment or milieu therapy movement. Further research and reflection upon this period of decline and then the rise of another reform movement at the turn of the century have led me to seek to generalize beyond the specifics of a particular reform era.

The characteristics of reform efforts over the past two centuries in the United States in the mental health field are complex and have exhibited important differences. Nevertheless, essential similarities are discernible; they probably arise from common forces that determine the life cycle of modern reform movements. The central problem of mental health reform movements from their origin in the eighteenth century to today is, I believe, their inability to secure humane, therapeutic treatment for the mass of mentally disordered persons. This well-documented failure is the key to the recurrent gradual decline of reform efforts relating to patient care, the replacement of optimistic attitudes by pessimistic ones, and a tendency to blame the so-called insane for their own intractable illness, either through poor heredity or harmful life styles. With the exception of penicillin therapy for paresis, few effective somatic therapies for the major mental disorders have been discovered; the very useful tranquilizing and antidepressant drugs are not cures. Nonsomatic treatment, therefore, has remained crucial in coping with mental disorders. And from this situation arises in part the difficulty of caring effectively for the majority of institutionalized mental patients because such treatment requires a deep concern for the quality of the patients' lives.

The emotional, behavioral, and intellectual disorders called mental illness have been greatly affected by the social environment; this will invariably continue until some effective somatic therapy is developed. Sufferers from the usually long-term, often chronic mental disorders have traditionally lived in the closed social system called the hospital, mostly at public expense, and if they were "cured," they had to face the social and economic perils of having been mental patients. For two centuries, despite the efforts of physicians and lay reformers to persuade the lay public as well as the medical establishment to take a clinical view of mental disorders, and to acknowledge them as ailments amenable to rational treatment by professional personnel inside and outside the hospital, mental illness still stands in a special, vulnerable category, intimately related to social attitudes and the social structure.

Essential to the implementation of the reforms espoused by Dorothea Dix in the nineteenth century and Clifford Beers in the twentieth were changes not only in attitudes but also in the social structure and organization of society at large. To improve conditions in mental hospitals and to sustain these improvements required sympathetic support, encouragement, and pressure from the outside. Society had to provide, among other things, funds for the institutions and rewards for those who worked there, as well as external conditions that contributed to rather than negated the therapeutic practices initiated in the hospitals. In different ways, then, the community must be no less therapeutically oriented than the asylum.

In fact, however, American society has not been structured to favor therapeutic practices or even minimum humane care for the majority of mental patients in or out of mental hospitals. Federal and state governments did assume responsibility for the mentally ill, but for the most part at less than minimum expense and with limited concern. And this is true also for other persons unable to function independently in the community

—the severely physically handicapped, the retarded, the aged, the orphaned, and the extremely poverty-stricken.

The credo of individual success so proudly described by generations of commentators on the American scene encouraged the belief that the achievement of power, that is, control over one's own and especially other people's lives (usually synonymous with wealth), was the best criterion of personal value. The democratic rhetoric that spoke about the equality of man within a profit-motivated society led in practice to the view that everyone must compete for wealth and power, so that the inequality of status that increasingly characterized American society became a valid measure of inherent worth. More than in most Western societies, in the United States the possession of material riches gave men and women an aura of success and the respect, consideration, and, in times of illness, the concern of their community. The powerless, usually the poor, were held personally responsible for their condition and as such merited perhaps pity but not esteem. Medical services were distributed on the same basis as all other services and goods: the upper classes, who could pay, were treated relatively well, while the lower classes usually received what they could command or pay for—indifference and neglect, if not actual mistreatment.

During periods of reform, efforts were made to modify the hostile, negative, or uncaring attitudes toward the lower classes. Human nature was described as perfectible—possessing something of the divine—and morally innocent—the product of forces beyond the individual's control, yet essentially malleable. All that was needed to eliminate most of mankind's ills was to shape a favorable environment. In the case of mental illness, reformers believed that they could create the proper circumstances both in and out of the hospital without going much beyond educating the public or the politicians, who were to supply the funds. Explain the real nature of mental disorders and the conditions that would restore patients to sanity, and in time public men, on their own or because of popular pressure, would act appropriately to attain these ends. That a profit-oriented society, dedicated to amassing wealth and power and viewing government as handmaiden to this process, might find these goals not always compatible with a deep concern for the needs of people who did not have power was not generally recognized. From this perspective, the great stress upon somatic therapies during periods with a pessimistic outlook on mental disturbances can be seen in part as an effort to break out of a dilemma that seemed unresolvable in sociological terms, rather than simply as a concession to despair and the avoidance of social problems, as

I and others have contended.

Reform movements were in a predicament of which their participants tended to be unaware. On the one hand, their leaders argued that all mental patients must be treated not according to their class position, status, wealth, education, or any other criterion that was usually applied to the insane. Rather, the simple fact of their being children of God, or belonging to the human race and being in need, would justify doing whatever was necessary to provide humane care and, if possible, a cure. On the other hand, without actually admitting it, reformers did recognize that such an appeal was too out of joint to receive serious attention by any but a few people. They therefore sought to influence the taxpaying public and tax-spending legislators. It was well known that the public was hostile to the poor, who were considered somehow responsible for their mental affliction and who must not benefit from this condition by being treated too well. So, the public was told, it would be cheaper in the long run to cure instead of simply to care for patients indefinitely, but that did not mean that living conditions in hospitals needed to be out of keeping with the socioeconomic status of the patients: the poor, unaccustomed to much comfort, needed only modest accommodations.

That society would actually benefit financially if it provided therapeutic treatment was not self-evident; as far as the public was concerned it did not prove less expensive to practice therapy rather than custody, especially since early nineteenth century psychiatrists grossly underestimated the proportion of the population that would be institutionalized. The states were forced to build not one but several hospitals each, and until 1950 it seemed that the number of hospitalized mental patients was determined largely by the available facilities, a condition that did not incline the states to support the even more expensive system that therapeutic treatment would have entailed. Given the existing social and political structure, only unrelenting pressure from reformers, other powerful individuals, and an organized, mobilized, and concerned public could persuade legislators to spend the large amounts of money necessary to change the institutional setting for mental patients and provide, in addition, adequate aftercare services for those who returned to their community.

But this kind of pressure was not maintained, and in the case of Clifford Beers's mental health movement, though the organizational vehicle survived, it abandoned Beers's early goals with respect to the lower classes, that is, the investigation of conditions in state hospitals, recommendations for reforms and efforts to have them carried out. The movement turned, instead, to more indirect approaches that organized services to the middle and upper classes and to concern with prevention of mental disorders in ways most useful to the upper classes too.

II

Clifford Beers's commitment to the mental health movement derived from his own experiences. He was a member of a New Haven middle-class family of five sons, all of whom developed psychological or neurological disorders. One died young of a probable brain tumor that precipitated epileptic-like seizures, and the other four, including Clifford, died in mental hospitals, two of them by suicide. Clifford Beers described himself as suffering from childhood anxieties, periods of depression during adolescence, and, while a student at Yale's Sheffield Scientific School, severe anxiety and tension brought on, he thought, by the trauma of caring for his "epileptic" brother. At the same time he managed to complete all his schooling, lead an active social life, and gain the respect and affection of his friends for his lively personality, clever wit, and extracurricular accomplishments. His goal being to succeed in the business world, he secured work in New York City and seemed to everyone to be a promising young businessman. But his career was cut short in 1900, when, tormented by depression and delusions, he attempted suicide. For the next three years he was a patient at three Connecticut mental hospitals—first a proprietary institution, Stamford Hall; then the well-known and respected Hartford Retreat (now the Institute of Living); and finally the state hospital at Middletown. At the retreat he passed from a depressed, deluded, hallucinatory state to high mania, from which he slowly recovered at the state hospital, to the point where he was released in September 1903, but with a poor prognosis for the future.

Though Beers reserved his most vitriolic criticisms for the physicians at the Hartford Retreat, it was there that he first formulated his scheme for reform, albeit in grandiose terms. He began his active reform campaign at the Connecticut state asylum after some bitter, brutal experiences in the violent ward. He managed to send a letter to the governor of Connecticut, with whom he had distant political connections, and who was the person ultimately responsible for conditions at the state hospital. Beers thought he could bring political pressure to initiate an investigation of alleged brutalities and nontherapeutic policies at mental hospitals. The governor did respond, indirectly, and some changes for the better occurred at the state hospital, but not enough to satisfy Beers, who decided to bide his time until he would be in a better position to accomplish more, first in Connecticut and then in other states.

Shortly after his discharge, Beers's former New York employers rehired him, thus providing him with a model for appropriate, empathetic behavior of employers toward former mental patients and for aggressive, self-confident behavior of the latter in seeking jobs. But he soon became elated again, enough to require a stay at the Hartford Retreat for a month, after which he went back to his job. At the retreat and afterward, he worked on his reform schemes, evolving a two-pronged approach. First, he would inform the public in an autobiographical account about conditions in mental hospitals and offer his recommendations for changes. Second, through his autobiography and personal contacts, he would try to interest influential and wealthy persons in founding an organization that would work to make mental hospitals humane and therapeutic, to educate the public about mental illness as part of a plan to promote preventive measures, and to help former patients reenter the "normal" world.

Beers carried out his plans. He wrote his autobiography, which he sent in 1906 to William James, who read it with interest and approval. This encouragement enabled Beers to win further financial assistance from friends and relatives and the time off from his work necessary to prepare the manuscript for publication. James thereafter and until his death in 1910 became Beers's most loyal supporter. He recommended Beers to his own publisher and wrote a flattering preface to the book. To Beers's numerous requests, often of a burdensome nature—editing, letter writing, and pleading his cause—James said no only in a very few instances where he felt inadequate to the task. In poor health and refusing almost all other appeals for assistance, James volunteered to write to John D. Rockefeller in behalf of the organization that Beers founded and even sent $1,000 of his own money to help Beers out of financial difficulties incurred in financing the new mental hygiene movement. James played an as yet untold and important role in that organization and in the life of Beers, whom he found enormously appealing and felt it a privilege to help.

In 1908 Longmans, Green published Beers's book, *A Mind That Found Itself*, which created a sensation and made Beers famous. (It still sells about a thousand copies a year.) That same year Beers founded the Connecticut Society for Mental Hygiene, and in 1909, with the active support of James, Adolf Meyer, William Welch, Jane Addams, Julia Lathrop, and a host of academicians, physicians, and university presidents, he formally established the National Committee for Mental Hygiene. Two years later, at Welch's suggestion, the steel magnate and philanthropist Henry Phipps donated $50,000 to the committee, which enabled it to employ Dr. Thomas W. Salmon as director of special studies and to start a series of investigations of state hospitals all over the country. Eventually this activity petered out, to be replaced by popular educational campaigns, preventive services like child guidance clinics, research into schizophrenia and other mental disorders, and professional training in psychiatry.

These newer programs were valuable; they influenced the field of psychiatry, helped numerous persons, and anticipated the functions of the National Institute of Mental Health. But they also represented a turning away from a direct concern with hospitalized patients and hospital conditions, a trend that, with a few notable exceptions, could also be seen in the growing psychiatric-psychoanalytic establishment in the United States. The beneficiaries of the changed goals tended to be educated, middle- and upper-class persons who responded to educational campaigns and could take advantage of psychiatric services on a private basis. Even when the committee's new projects were planned to serve a broad range of people, such as the child guidance clinics, considered to be a key preventive program for society as a whole, the original design was thwarted: when the focus shifted from coordinating community placement services for children to provide in-house treatment by professionals at the clinics, the clientele gradually became largely middle class.

Beers was involved in all the struggles within the national committee about its direction, and served as idea man, gadfly, fund raiser, and, in the view of some committee members, overall pest. All the successive medical directors of the committee recognized that it was peculiarly Beers's organization and that he always had the last word, albeit he would take advice when it suited his purposes. By the 1920s he began to give a good deal of his energies to creating an international mental health movement and in 1930 succeeded in founding an International Committee for Mental Hygiene and financing a spectacular international meeting in Washington, D.C., attended by over 3,500 delegates from fifty-two countries. He was receiving increasing public recognition; among his many awards was the red ribbon of the Légion d'Honneur, and numerous newspaper and magazine articles described his work. He remained deeply involved with the national committee, especially as principal fund raiser, and it may be that the difficulty in finding donors during the late depression years of the 1930s contributed to his falling victim to severe melancholia in 1939, almost forty years after his first attack. This time he went to Butler Hospital in Rhode Island, where he died in 1943.

As for the national committee, it remained in existence until it merged in 1950 into the National Association for Mental Health. In 1949 the federal government, in establishing the National Institute of Mental Health, realized an early dream of Beers's that the resources of the national government should be applied to psychiatric research and treatment. Yet the plight of the institutionalized insane had not changed much from the time he had first described it in 1908. Again the public was shocked by revelations of abuses and neglect, this time by various writers, including Albert Deutsch, who had earlier written a classic history of mental illness in the United States with Beers's support and under the sponsorship of the National Foundation for Mental Hygiene, a funding organization established by Beers to support the work of the national committee. And in 1961 the Joint Commission on Mental Illness and Health, appointed by federal law, addressed itself to the question, "Why Has Care of the Mentally Ill Lagged?"

III

The nature of the society in which they lived and their acceptance of its social-political structure and its ideology created problems and contradictions for reformers like Clifford Beers and forced them to make certain choices that seemed practical, but that contributed to vitiating their original goals. Beers's failure to significantly relieve the boredom, brutality, and neglect suffered by mental patients—miseries that he knew so well—was predictable if not inevitable.

To found and then activate the mental hygiene movement Beers needed the support of influential people: medical men, especially psychiatrists, and wealthy individuals and the foundations they were creating during the early years of the twentieth century. This approach was natural to Beers, in his social and political outlook a conventional middle-class American, business minded and success oriented. Psychologically, moreover, he was drawn to successful men of affairs as authority figures whose approval enhanced his own self-image. And at a time when social services and medical research were still largely privately sponsored and political activists were not interested in mental illness, to whom else could he turn? The cause of the mentally ill had no existing power base from which it could press for change; the mentally ill themselves were singularly powerless and their friends difficult to organize. Even if Beers had wanted to work among them, the special nature of mental illness, with all the concomittant stigma, misunderstanding, prejudice, and fear, would at that time probably have precluded his making much headway without first developing a program of popular education. (His own family, so supportive during his illness, had tried to deter him from publishing his autobiography.) No doubt any such efforts would most certainly have met strong opposition from hospital superintendents.

Given conditions at the time and his own proclivities, Beers had to go to the medico-socio-economic establishment for help. But his dependence on them eventually diverted his movement from its early objective of changing hospital conditions and ameliorating the everyday lives of the masses of hospital patients. It had to go in directions that would satisfy the two overlapping groups that were crucial to its existence: reform-minded psychiatrists and men and women who had money to give. The psychiatrists wanted to make sure that the movement's activities were medically sanctioned and did not threaten their position; the wealthy and powerful, having limited interest in the mentally ill themselves, found research, specialized psychiatric clinics, and psychiatric training more attractive to finance than investigations of state hospitals.

At the outset, the nature of the national committee was determined by the outcome of a sharp conflict between Beers and the highly respected, influential, and strong-minded Dr. Adolf Meyer, appointed in 1908 to head the new Phipps Psychiatric Clinic in Baltimore. Beers considered Meyer central to establishing both the Connecticut and national organizations, and until their relationship broke off in 1910 Meyer controlled the policy of the national committee and forced Beers to accept modifications in his position on many issues.

Beers had wanted a national society, controlled by laymen accountable to a paying membership, that would appeal for funds to the public as well as to rich philanthropists. Meyer's conception was a small committee, funded privately and without a general membership; both national and state organizations were to be placed in the hands of hospital psychiatrists. Without this guarantee, written into the constitution of the Connecticut society, state hospital psychiatrists would not join; on the national committee Meyer declared that he would determine policy or resign, a common attitude of hospital physicians toward the mental health movement. Meyer insisted further that Beers must adopt the view that the culprits in the abominable hospital situation were not the physicians but the general public, which did not provide adequate financial and moral support for the state hospitals. Beers's own experience had taught him otherwise, that physicians as well as attendants, though themselves perhaps victims of the system, could not be exculpated from blame. But to win over the medical profession, the foundations, and the rich he needed Meyer's help and approval. Everyone wanted to know what Meyer thought.

After a struggle, Beers reluctantly gave in on all these issues. He could only hope that in time, with Meyer and other psychiatric leaders on his side, psychiatrists disinclined to change would see the light, but he would have to refrain from openly criticizing them. Nor must he or his movement question any of the basic assumptions held by psychiatrists, perhaps the most important of which was that the hospital as an institution and as then conceived was compatible with therapeutic and humane care—a challengeable assumption. Medical staffs received their rewards from society, albeit often paltry ones, not for conducting therapeutic institutions, but because they removed from sight masses of poor people and did so at the least possible cost to the taxpayer. Understaffed, overcrowded, bureaucratic, and with inadequate facilities of every type, especially for recreation and occupation and most of all for creating warm human relations between staff and patient, the giant state hospitals had become predominantly concerned with custody. In effect, the needs of staff and patients diverged because society did not value the recovery of poor patients enough to create and maintain therapeutic institutions and to give status and appropriate salaries to those who worked in them. The original goal of service tended to be obfuscated through bureaucratic constraints and the professional concerns of the staff. This kind of analysis, with which Beers would have agreed, had to wait more than half a century to become respectable.

The great foundations that the national committee was able to persuade to give millions to the cause were not unconcerned with hospital conditions, but they took the position that the national committee should act as an innovator for state and federal governments through investigations, studies, demonstration projects, and recommendations. If such work proved valuable, then the committee would surrender it for others to carry on; if no other agency was willing, then eventually the committee, always short of funds, must take a businessman's view and redirect its efforts, which was what was gradually done. Actually, in certain respects, the federal government did pick up the torch, but inadequately, so that with the demise of the National Committee no one was there to push consistently for improvements in hospital care. Private corporate hospitals catering to the well-to-do benefited most, for they had the resources, human and material, to take advantage of new proposals.

And even, as Beers noted, at the time when foundations supported investigations of state hospital conditions, the lives of the majority of the inmates changed little. There was never enough money to conduct more than a few investigations, and in those cases the only weapons the national committee wielded were exposure and education. Where conditions improved, backsliding was common. The committee lacked the resources to check on institutions and press them to maintain proper therapeutic and custodial practices. It could rely only upon affiliated state societies for mental hygiene, in most states an inadequate force, to effect and sustain significant changes in hospitals.

In 1924 one foundation official advised that an endowment would almost surely be forthcoming if the committee reduced its staff and thereby cut expenses by dropping many activities, and associated itself with a university, where the focus would be on research. Moves were made by the committee toward university affiliation, but Beers strongly opposed any contraction of activity, and the proposal was dropped. The foundations were not opposed to helping mental patients, but to do so was difficult short of being able to count on widespread support from state governments. And such support was not forthcoming, either before or during the depression of the 1930s. At the same time the committee was in financial difficulty, so that foundation officials thought it only sensible for it to retrench. Besides, as Meyer had much earlier stressed, research might produce a breakthrough in therapy that would enable the national committee to be more successful in the future; otherwise, not much progress could be expected unless state and federal governments changed their attitudes, something the national committee was only in the earliest stages of effecting before the 1940s.

In addition, the foundations were unsympathetic to those who forcefully challenged established authority, as discovered by Dr. Salmon, whose salary as the national committee's medical director was, after the first few years, paid by the Rockefeller Foundation. He always believed, with good reason, that the foundation dismissed him as a consultant because of his bitter dispute with government officials in charge of mentally disturbed veterans of the first World War; in his zealous concern for these men Salmon had exceeded decorum. Much less would the foundations or wealthy individuals be prepared to support a movement that would engage in vigorous political lobbying for legislation or funds for psychiatric care or that might raise philosophical issues.

The committee was not developed as an organization with any political clout. Beers's modest efforts in Connecticut to have investigatory legislation passed were not repeated because of Meyer's strong disapproval, echoed by state hospital physicians who would not join an organization that engaged in political action potentially embarrassing to them. Such opposition aside, Beers naïvely thought that all he had to do was to educate people to the true needs of mental patients and responses would be forthcoming, not only from wealthy persons but from the general public, which would demand action. Then an organized force capable of exerting pressure on hospitals could be built. It would be, in his view, in the best interests of almost the entire society, with the possible exception of hospital physicians, to eliminate abuses in mental hospitals and develop an effective program of prevention of mental illness. That people might balk at paying higher taxes to support such activities he could not at first believe. Nor did he ever see any possible inherent problems in trying to reform hospital conditions throughout the country for all patients through winning the support of rich men and women, established institutions, and the psychiatric profession.

Himself the most famous self-confessed former mental patient ever, Beers always studiously avoided seeking the active participation of his natural constituency—former patients, relatives, and their friends. Although at the beginning, in 1909, it would probably have been impossible to form such an alliance, the situation changed some twenty or so years later, no doubt partly because of the educational campaigns of the national committee and the state societies. There is evidence that by the 1930s—a time of mass social and political activity—former patients were being organized. Such groups could do what reformers could not and would not do: devote themselves to the needs of the nonaffluent majority with a sustained emotional commitment and remain on the scene even after reformers were tired or no longer influential.

In 1937 friends and relatives and former patients, their fears notwithstanding, organized an association at the Illinois Psychiatric Institute under Dr. A.A. Low's direction that is still functioning: Recovery, Inc. They published a journal, *Lost and Found*, from 1938 to 1941; won legislative changes; developed a form of group therapy; and provided members with social services, companionship, and jobs. Low communicated with the Illinois mental health society, but evidently not with Beers, who does not seem to have known anything about Recovery. When he did hear about such work he was not encouraging. In 1931, a former Presbyterian minister turned psychiatrist, Dr. L. Cody Marsh of the Worcester, Massachusetts State Hospital, asked Beers to organize a group of his former patients under national committee auspices or to finance such a group. Beers refused to do either as not being in the former patients' best interests. Besides his disapproval of such activities, Beers probably did not want the competition; he always regarded the mental health movement as his alone.

It is tempting to speculate that it might have been too threatening psychologically for Beers to be clearly associated with other former mental patients; he preferred the company of "successful" men and women, and regarded power much as the powerful did—not simply as a means of fulfilling one's potentialities, but as desirable for the control it could give over others' lives. It endowed its possessors with an appeal that Beers found irresistible, and that discouraged him from maintaining the kind of active sympathy for the mass of mental patients that was necessary if he were to keep their interests always uppermost. Indeed, Beers so identified the concerns of his cause with those of the wealthy classes that he opposed Franklin Roosevelt, who he believed wanted to tax the rich, who might then reduce their contributions to the national committee. His life spent associating with wealthy capitalists, trying to wheedle money from them, and dependent upon their generosity for his living, Beers never pondered the relation of mental disorder to the social system that they dominated.

Early in his career Beers acknowledged his conservative social outlook. In March 1908 he received a description of a proposed book, "The Call of the Insane," blaming the unjust social system for the way the insane were treated, and was asked to be a joint author. Beers took "decided exception" to the claim that "abuses are inherent in this damnable capitalistic system [and that therefore one] need not expect any radical reforms" therefrom. Instead, the author was supposed to do as Beers had done in writing his autobiography, when he had followed Meyer's advice to take a moderate and even understated position in order to win acceptance for his work.

From whom this social critic would receive approval and for what kind of work Beers did not discuss. These were questions he did not ask; he believed and continued to believe, despite his admitted failure with hospital patients, that everything was possible within the existing social structure. When a few correspondents accused him of abandoning the mental patient Beers felt hurt—he recognized the truth of the charge. He did not, however, know what to do and could only hope that in the future, perhaps after another fifty years, conditions would improve. The public needed more time to be educated by the national committee.

Some fifty years have passed, and the problems remain. But I do not wish to end on a negative note. We in the present are not necessarily doomed to repeat the past. Simply to be aware of what happened to previous reform efforts is to change the situation, and people today are asking questions largely ignored by past reformers. We may hope that the age of innocence is over.

The Settlement Movement and Medical Social Service

EUNICE F. ALLAN

Current clinical social work practice in New England derives from the convergence of two major themes. In Boston, as in other large urban centers, one theme centers on the external or environmental factors of individuals and families in distress. One resource in society's attempt to alleviate some of the stress was the settlement house, which flourished in the late nineteenth and early twentieth centuries. Familiar to all are Hull House in Chicago, the Henry Street Settlement in New York, the more local Elizabeth Peabody House, which used to be around the corner from the Massachusetts General Hospital on Charles Street, the Boston South End House, and the Rutland Corner House. Smaller cities later developed similar kinds of institutions, and all had certain characteristics that are of interest to us for their historical meaning.

The neighborhood house served several purposes. The name itself pointed to the location of a service that was accessible specifically to the neighborhood population. Initially it was to serve recreational purposes for a wide age range, with opportunities for young children, latency-age children, adolescents, young mothers, and ultimately fathers. The emphasis was on the family, and the unit for help was the group rather than the individual. There were physical facilities for athletic activities, cooking classes for girls, sewing classes for mothers, shop for boys, and the like. However, the most striking thing about all of the groups is that they tended to intervene in the sociological problems of the time through essentially educational methods. In the late nineteenth and early twentieth centuries, ethnic problems of European immigrants were a source of social strain. As an attempt to help resolve this strain, the settlement houses, in addition to instruction in skills, offered lessons in English and in preparation for citizenship. Most important was sensitivity to the immigrant's need to retain some of his own feelings of the value of his country of origin while simultaneously helping him adapt to current American life.

One of the common problems that each generation claims as

uniquely its own is the generation gap. Settlement-house workers knew well the generation gap. First-generation young people experienced enormous conflict because American society was much more permissive than the one in which their parents had been reared. Thus, these neighborhood houses identified many kinds of problems that continue to plague us today. Working at a time that preceded the formulated wisdom of Erik Erikson, they nonetheless paid strict attention to age-appropriate tasks. This they did on the basis of practical wisdom and a capacity to make observations of current reality. The cumulative experience of the settlement houses contributed a body of sociological knowledge to the new and growing field of social work.

The settlement houses were begun and primarily staffed by people who were essentially social reformers in their attitudes. The early settlement-house workers were doers who believed in action as the solution to what they saw as problems of reality in a disturbed social environment. They were closely allied to the early charity societies, out of which the more familiar family and children's agencies of recent times have developed. Their concern was with environmental difficulties and with observations of social differences and poverty. They were not, however, without their intellectuals. Current students in social work are always surprised when reading Mary Richmond to find her a lady of considerable intelligence who scientifically ordered the kinds of knowledge that were available to give guidance to the early social workers.

This body of essentially sociological observation that characterized the early period of social work, predating interest in the individual, represents one strand from which developed modern casework. Lacking was the body of knowledge that helped to explain individual behavior, for the settlement house preceded dynamic psychiatry.

The second theme influencing modern social work practice has developed by the clinical route. It began in the early part of the twentieth century. Much of it originated in New England, and more specifically in Boston. Someone has made reference to the scientific interest in the individual patient as a phenomenon of the teaching hospitals in Boston in the 1920s and 1930s. From this interest derived medical social work as well as psychiatric social work. There was, however, a very important difference, which has continued to be important. As early as 1906 in the social service department established by Dr. Richard C. Cabot at the Massachusetts General Hospital there appeared Miss Ida Cannon, one of the first medical social workers.

The need for medical social workers derived from changes in the practice of medicine. Even in urban areas doctors historically had been neighborhood physicians who knew their patients well, were acquainted with their physical illnesses and family relationships, and held themselves responsible for dealing with the total patient. However, teaching hospitals in modern urban universities became the focal point for a different kind of medical practice. It became impossible for an urban physician with teaching responsibilities in clinics serving primarily a large poor population to know very much about his patients; thus the role of the medical social worker was developed to fill that gap. That origin left its mark on the practice of the medical social worker. From the beginning there was a clear-cut distinction between the responsibilities of the physician and those of the medical social worker. These, plus the nurse, the occupational therapist, and others, came to be called the "team." The struggle for authority that sometimes characterizes the "team" has very often been blamed on the hierarchy of the hospital and the personality of the physicians, who tend to be martinets disinclined to share responsibility. The fact is that the struggle has had some basis in reality, for there were very real differences in the bodies of knowledge applied by the physician and the medical social worker. The physician knew how to deal with the physical aspects of illness, whereas the medical social worker contributed an understanding of social influence on illness and recovery. But the medical doctor having the life-saving knowledge emerged the leader. In spite of the greater flexibility currently existing within medical social service departments, this distribution of authority continues to obtain.

The development of psychiatric social work has been somewhat different, and the differences are important in explaining its current status. In about 1907, the first social service department was established at the Boston Psychopathic Hospital, jointly created by Dr. Elmer E. Southard and Miss Mary Jarrett. Mary Jarrett was a lady of great intelligence and enormous organizing ability. She and Dr. Southard developed an elaborate in-service training program which taught what psychiatrists knew about mental illness. As in medical practice and medical social work, the physician was the holder and transmitter of knowledge about mental illness while the social worker was educated about family relationships and the impact of external reality. Although the division of responsibility was similar, the demarcation was never as clear-cut and as rigid as in other areas of social work, for there was from the beginning a greater overlap in the body of knowledge that was shared by psychiatrists and psychiatric social workers, both fledgling specialists.

Miss Jarrett and Dr. Southard gave serious thought to the elaboration of a more formal training program in response to the increasing demand for psychiatric social service because of the increasing number of soldiers, returning to civilian life from the first World War, who were suffering from neurasthenia. Eventually such interest led to the establishment of the Smith College School for Social Work, the first school specifically designed for the training of social workers to work with psychologically ill patients. It ran for eight months the first year; at the end of that year it was extended to fourteen months, and it subsequently grew into a two-and-one-half year program. However, the essential point is that from the beginning a major part of the dynamic theory taught during the summer was done by psychiatrists and psychoanalysts. In those days, when transportation was difficult, analysts lived in Northampton during the summer sessions, where they were very much a part of the academic life.

Other older schools of social work arose in the context of charity organizations. They emphasized external social causes of malfunctioning, and later added psychological theory to practical experience, specifically for a subspecialty—psychiatric social work. The training of the psychiatric social worker dealt mainly with theoretical preparation, which was supplemented by supervised practice in many different settings, largely in psychiatric training centers. In those early years, state hospitals attracted some analytically trained men and thus extensive use was made of them to train social workers. Students were also trained in family and children's agencies as well as in child guidance centers.

In New England, where much of psychiatric social work developed, there was a substantial overlap in the theory of personality development offered the young psychiatric social worker and that offered psychiatrists and analysts. The overlap was not in terms of depth or of range but in substance and in point of view. In this benign climate the psychiatric social worker was free to develop her own characteristic ways of combining the old knowledge of social factors with new psychological insights in psychosocial treatment. It was a rich and fruitful period for a new young profession.

Psychiatric centers were not the only educational resource for social workers. The family agencies, having been relieved of the necessity of looking after the financial needs of the poor during the depression years, were ready to turn their attention to a study of the personalities of people who seemed unable to manage their lives. The question these agencies addressed was whether poverty or physical illness were imposed upon people from external sources, or whether inner psychological factors propelled them into uncomfortable life situations and rendered them unable to get out of such situations of their own accord. In looking for answers, social workers turned to analytic consultants for help, and on a regular basis, many family agencies employed consultants to work on particularly troublesome cases. Consultants were helpful in two areas: (1) in clarifying personality structure and providing a basis for prediction as to treatability, and (2) in enhancing an awareness of the benefits inherent in the use of a therapeutic relationship. Such an awareness merged with an increasingly sophisticated understanding of the influence of social forces to form a better-integrated body of knowledge.

Formal evidence of these changes was exhibited in the development of the professional association of psychiatric social workers, which started in 1920 as a club of social workers, was formalized as the New England Association of Psychiatric Social Workers, and ultimately became a chapter in the American Association of Psychiatric Social Workers. Up until 1939 a constant focal point of the meetings was an attempt to determine who did and who did not meet the definition of a psychiatric social worker; this served a useful purpose in encouraging and monitoring professional standards. The American Association of Psychiatric Social Workers eventually was absorbed into the National Association of Social Workers, and actively encouraged the inclusion of psychoanalytic theory in the training of all social workers.

During the last decade psychiatric social work seemed to disappear as a potent influence, only to be revived fairly recently with the establishment of a new professional Association of Clinical Social Workers. However, underlying the struggle within the professional association was the more critical issue of what kind of knowledge is needed by social workers who intervene in important ways and at crucial times in the human relations of people who are having difficulty in social functioning. This question of knowledge appeared more important than the corollary one of whether the social worker should function in a hospital with a psychiatrist or in a family agency that does not have a psychiatrist on its staff.

Regardless of the setting, the model for help became the weekly or biweekly interview, during which the psychiatric social worker explored the client's life experience with the hope of finding the psychological determinants accounting for the stress. It was questioned to what extent these explorations really led to any marked changes in the client's personality or life situation.

Some of the research did indicate that the explorations were not as productive of change as the amount of time and money invested would suggest. Nonetheless, there was no doubt that the effort succeeded in establishing a body of knowledge for a professional group, even though much of it was in the nature of clinical research with inadequate formulation of method and goal. The profession was criticized for having lost sight of the social in social casework. The caseworker was taken to task for an exclusive interest in exploring the client's inner life. It was quite true that during an interlude of twenty years the more highly trained psychiatric social worker directed a great deal of attention to the microscopic exploration of the inner life. But that period represented an essential detour and the knowledge so derived has been reconnected with people's social and environmental difficulties. The ultimate reconvergence of these two bodies of knowledge and experience is of overriding import.

Much of the learning from psychoanalytic theory took place in Boston. During the 1930s and 1940s, the Boston Psychoanalytic Institute through its educational committee offered seminars primarily for social workers on aspects of psychoanalytic theory. Many young social workers undertook personal psychoanalysis as analysands of analysts in training; such a plan met the training needs of the Psychoanalytic Institute and made it economically feasible for social workers to pursue an experience that was both therapeutic and educational.

Equipped with such experience, social workers were able to address their separate tasks and to adapt theory to the purposes of social work treatment. Early in 1940 Miss Annette M. Garrett made two very impressive attempts to formulate the theoretical material on transference and to adapt it to understanding the nature of therapeutic relationships. Her effort pointed up sharply that in issues of treatment each profession must make its own adaptation to its own treatment goals. More recently, greater attention to the structural theory has provided insight into how experiences in real life become incorporated into the developing personality. Thus the link between inner and outer life has been identified and the modern social worker has more reliable clues for helping a client find new direction in life.

This change in social work practice has come about since the earlier period of which I have spoken; still it is useful to know that the current concepts are being developed by those who were trained to understand the libidinal theory that preceded ego psychological theory.

Social workers as psychotherapists have been more generally accepted by analysts perhaps because of their original working relationship. In the 1930s, when many European-trained analysts were coming to Boston, they were not received very warmly by American medicine or American psychiatry. However, they were eagerly welcomed by social workers who were looking for just the explanatory ideas that analytic theory provided, and from this amiable past there has continued a warm and mutually supportive relationship between the dynamically trained clinical social worker and the analyst. Oddly enough, the struggle for acceptance of the social worker as psychotherapist has come from within our profession, in which the nondynamically trained workers have taken a much more critical stand toward what they regard as an ingrown preoccupation of the clinical social workers with psychotherapy for middle-class neurotics. It is an unwarranted charge, for all professional workers in a psychiatric clinic know well that the patients are not middle-class neurotics. Rather they are largely character-disordered, borderline patients who require treatment based on comprehension of the inner and outer life. That comprehension is germane to the social worker's task in the medical, psychiatric, school, or court clinics or the myriad settings in which he fulfills his role as facilitator of more rewarding functioning.

DISCUSSION

Jeanne Brand, presiding

J. SANBOURNE BOCKOVEN: There are remarkable parallels between the life of Mary Baker Eddy and the life of Dorothea Lynde Dix. She was also born in a small New England town, had the same kind of hypochondriacal story, and was a great leader in reforming the care of the mentally ill. Likewise, she had an interesting relationship with William Ellery Channing. Louisa May Alcott was another of these dynamic women coming out of New England who made such an impression, and who deserve study. It is also worth noting that the physicians of the mental hospitals in Massachusetts and the rest of New England were taking phrenology and magnetism seriously. Pliny Earle, superintendent of the Northampton State Hospital, has written a charming account of his own conflicts, between his aggressive instincts and his reverence and generosity, in almost psychodynamic-sounding language. But this was very much the content of the moral treatment era, too, which greatly influenced the care of the mentally ill based on psychological ills rather than purely physical ills.

NATHAN HALE: My impression of the Emmanuel Movement is that it was not a mass movement, but was largely confined to the Episcopal and Protestant churches, which automatically rules it out as a mass social phenomenon in what was at that point a largely Irish-Catholic city. There are two other points that I think are important and that mark a real distinction between American and European practices. The first is that one reason why the Emmanuel Movement was so viciously attacked by the medical profession was that the medical profession in America was extraordinarily weak at just this moment. In 1910 the Flexner report was about to be published, describing the low quality of American medical education. Harvard University was trying to strengthen its medical school; its sumptuous new buildings were opened in 1906. As the medical profession was striving for status, the threat to its professional role posed by outsiders such as priests and clergymen was something that could not be countenanced and was fought bitterly. The second reason that underlaid the distinction between Europe and America and ultimately had something to do with the reception of psychoanalysis was that all of these cults, as Richard Weiss said in his interesting book, *The American Myth of*

Success, were oriented toward mobility. People flocked to mind curers; the mind cure literature was full of onwards and upwards, develop yourself, make the most of yourself, heal yourself, and rise in social status. This is still a uniquely American phenomenon. In contrast to Europe, America had a precarious medical profession with a large and important interest in upward mobility.

SANFORD GIFFORD: Social workers beginning to do psychotherapy at this time did not provoke the violent antagonism from the medical profession; neither did the clinical psychologists, as I pointed out. Perhaps the medical profession was more threatened by professionally trained people like clergymen than by social workers or clinical psychologists, who were thought of as dealing with small numbers of people only.

LILLIAN SALTMAN: In its early years, psychiatric social work was in search of a theory for understanding what Mary Richmond called "character lodging." Throughout the history of psychiatric social work there is an emphasis on character, especially on faulty character. Poverty was seen as due to faulty character; somehow it was involved in the issue. "Friendly visitors," mentioned earlier by Dr. Gifford, were volunteers, women from the middle and upper classes, who served as therapists in a sense. Marian Cabot Putnam had worked with her husband for many years in the associated charities of Boston; this is the Family Service of today. At the national conference of social workers in 1887 she described friendly visiting as seeing and knowing people in their homes and trying by means of personal influence and practical suggestion to improve their condition. "Many persons agree," she noted, "in thinking that this is a good method for helping the poorest and most ignorant classes. Other persons believe that conditions under which people live, homes, schools, recreation, must be improved." Both kinds of work, she thought, are needed. Mrs. Putnam wrote, "There must be some force to help turn people to good account and that force must come from the people themselves. The visitor by sympathy, knowledge, and affection may find himself or his advice may be given and taken, where his coming brings happiness and hope and a new desire to live rightly."

The friendly visiting movement actually reached its high point in Boston. Zilpha D. Smith, who was a pioneer social worker and a supervisor to Mrs. Cabot, developed friendly visiting and started a training program in 1891. This was the beginning, in one sense, of the professional training of social workers. She started a study class—agents in training—

and then the problem arose how to train other people when you yourself are not trained. She answered this problem by beginning with the individual character of the worker, by reading, by study and reflection, and by practical experience. These friendly visitors went into the homes, and then returned to a bureaucratic agency structure for what we know today as a case conference, presided over by a paid agent, the social worker of today, who directed this work; the emphasis was always on character.

The work of the Charity Organization Society was carried into the Massachusetts General Hospital—the work that Richard Cabot and Dr. James Jackson Putnam originated with two social workers in their department in 1907. They trained their own workers because there were no trained workers available for patients suffering from neurasthenia. They called their work heart-to-heart talks, to help patients with faulty character. They worked under a physician's direction in the outpatient clinic, the beginning of what we know as the team concept of doctor and social worker. They established "a friendly relationship for helping the patient and used methods of explanation, reeducation, encouragement, and suggestion." It was from these beginnings, mostly in Boston, that the movement later taken over by Mary Richmond in her social diagnosis, the professionalization of social work, led to the search for more theory to better understand personality and character.

Illustrations

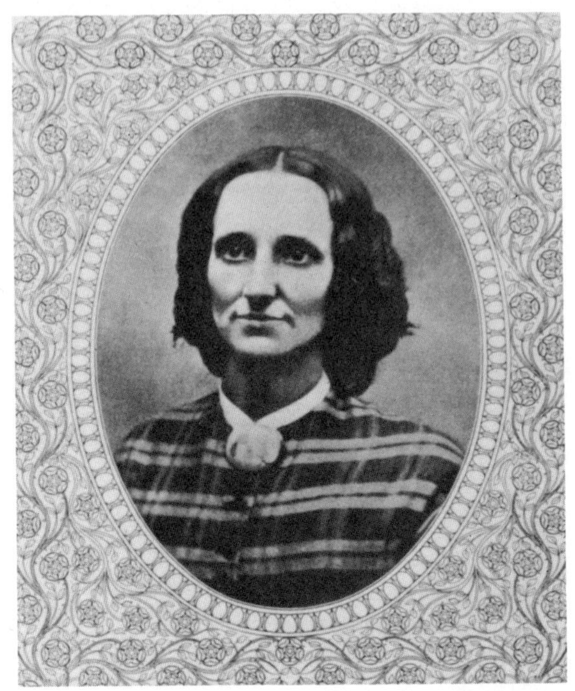

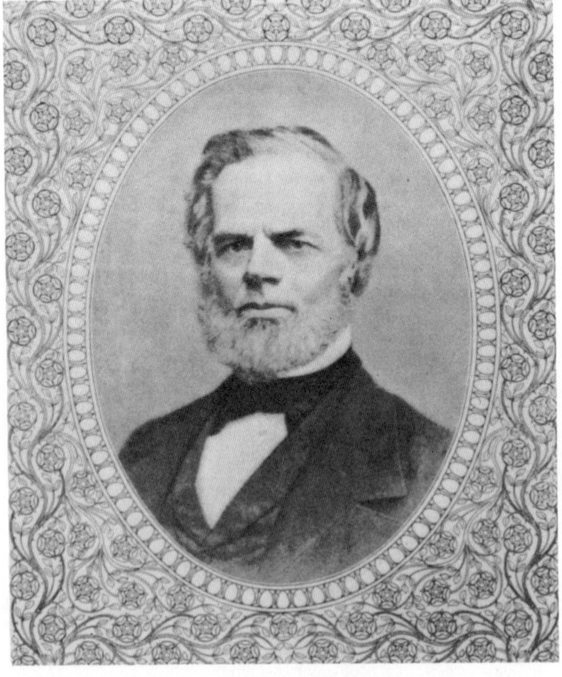

10. *a.* Mary Baker G. Eddy, from a tintype given to Mrs. Sarah G. Crosby in the summer of 1864. At this time she was being treated by P.P. Quimby, the mental healer of Portland. She was then Mrs. Daniel Patterson.
b. Phineas Parkhurst Quimby, from a photograph lent by the family. By 1859 he had developed a philosophy of life and disease, which he called "Science of Health," the "Science of Christ," and "Christian Science." *From* McClure's Maga- zine, *February 1907, pp. 342-343.*

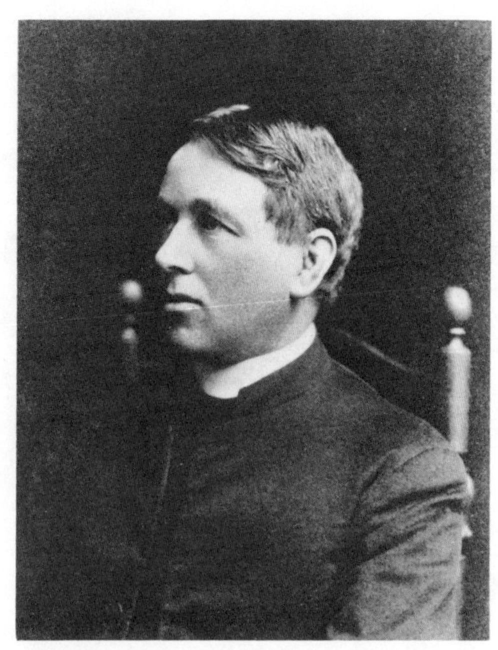

11. Rev. Elwood Worcester in 1904, founder of the Emmanuel Movement and pioneer in group psychotherapy. *Courtesy of Harley Holden, registrar-historiographer. Protestant Episcopal Diocese of Massachusetts.*

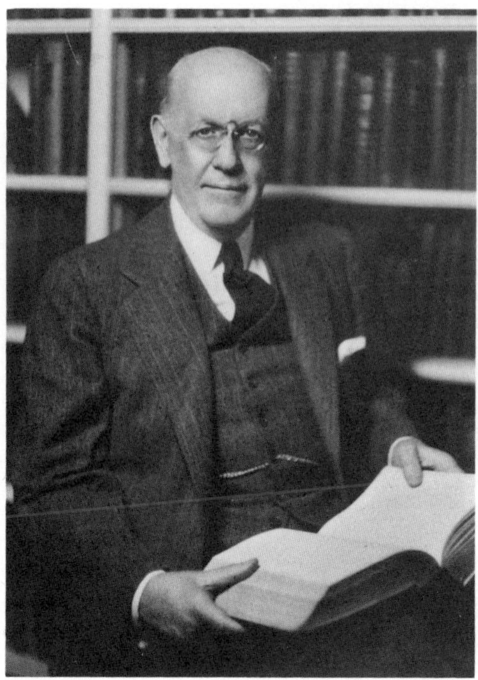

12. Joseph Henry Pratt, medical psychotherapist and pioneer in group therapy. *Boston Medical Library Collection, Countway Library.*

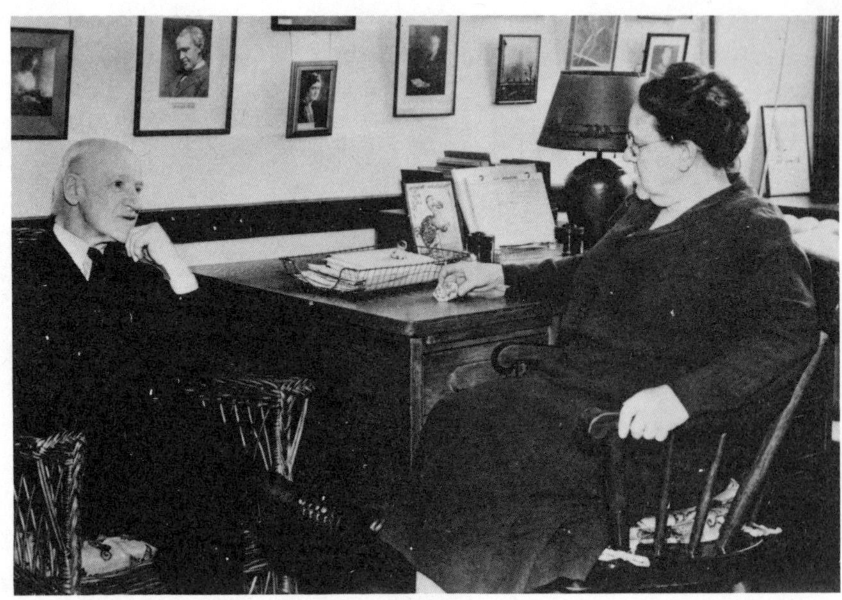

13. Pioneers in medical social service Miss Ida M. Cannon and Dr. Richard C. Cabot, 1938. *News Office, Massachusetts General Hospital.*

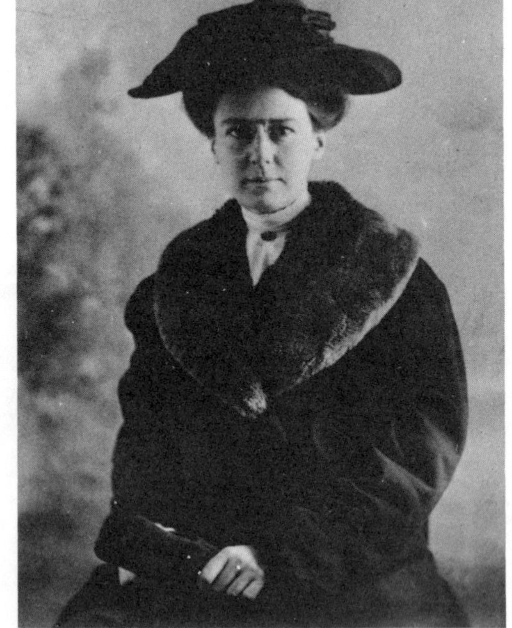

14. Mary C. Jarrett, 1905. Miss Jarrett was appointed by Southard in 1913 as the Boston Psychopathic Hospital's first director of social service, a position she held until 1918. *Greenblatt Collection, Countway Library.*

"The Age of Putnam"

James Jackson Putnam and Boston Neurology: 1877–1918

NATHAN G. HALE, JR.

Major changes took place in the years when James Jackson Putnam lived in Boston. He was born in 1846, became Harvard's first professor of diseases of the nervous system in 1874, and was a founder of the American Psychopathological Association in 1910 and of the American Psychoanalytic Association in 1911. He died in Boston in 1918.

The changes were these: from rest, diet, and electricity to the analysis of dreams, sexuality, and the unconscious; from George M. Beard's flamboyant faith in the effect of the mind on the body to Walter D. Cannon's subtle theories of interaction; from the idealism of Josiah Royce and the pragmatism of William James to the skeptical materialism of Bertrand Russell; from Harvard as a boys' clerical finishing school to Harvard as a serious university; from Boston as a Yankee stronghold to Boston as an Irish, cosmopolitan community; from Civil War to World War.

Some of these drastic shifts can be attributed to the rise of American neurology and within it the transition from a somatic to a psychological style of diagnosis and treatment. More generally, a change occurred in American culture from the Protestant piety of Putnam's youth to the scientific skepticism he deplored in his old age, particularly that of his new friend, Sigmund Freud.

What kind of personality witnessed these great realignments? Putnam was mild, determined yet diffident, committed to professional ideals, sensitive to collegial opinions yet of an extraordinary integrity. I like to think of him, impeccably dressed in tie and knickerbockers, striding along Adirondack trails with William James, or dragging Freud off on a walk the moment he arrived in Putnam's camp, to Freud's astonishment and momentary discomfort. Or to imagine him, sitting in the twilight of his study on Marlborough Street in the winter of 1911, listening to the great novelist, Henry James, describing his myriad nervous complaints and the failure of other physicians to cure his neurasthenia and obesity. Did Putnam, by then a convert, respectfully ask James for his dreams?

Or his associations? We shall never know. But James wrote him an orotund letter of gratitude a year later, in his famous final style, observing that Putnam had saved from near disaster his American trip to bury his brother William and describing his self-recovery achieved by long meditations on what he saw in his lengthy peregrinations through the streets of London.[1]

Putnam's role in the professional life of Boston, when that life was one of the most lively and influential in America, constitutes his most enduring contribution. In this role, Putnam transmitted the latest European professional and scientific advances to what was still a dependent scientific province, built local institutions to encompass those advances in a functioning reality, and approached both the ideas and the institutions with a sense of philosophical responsibility, blended from naïveté and sophistication.

Exposed to the militant scientists of the great era of European neurology—to Freud's teacher, Meynert, in Vienna, to Hughlings Jackson in London, to Charcot in Paris—Putnam returned home determined to redirect the rather complacent gentlemanly atmosphere of Boston medicine toward the hard discipline of specialization. In Vienna, as he wrote his mother, he had seen different specialists working in hospital outpatient clinics *every day*.[2] And so, armed with galvanic batteries, he set out to do likewise under the stairs of the old Bulfinch building of the Massachusetts General Hospital. He set up one of the first, if not the very first, neurological outpatient services in the United States in 1872. Through its doors passed middle- and working-class, native and foreign born patients—painters, plumbers, shoe-factory workers, housewives, school teachers, firemen. Their illnesses provided the material for his first papers on lead and arsenic poisoning, which demonstrated the need for stringent public health regulations, and on the traumatic neuroses that pointed to the need for psychological explanations. It was during the 1870s that Putnam, equipped with his own translations of Meynert's monographs, repeated some of the European experiments in brain localization with his close friends, William James and Henry Bowditch. He read all the new books and journals, particularly the German and Austrian ones.

Serious about general principles, Putnam exchanged his Unitarian piety for the equally ardent piety of science, chiefly in the evolutionary dispensation of Herbert Spencer. It was Putnam's hard German experimental outlook that prompted him to deny the claims of George Beard, in 1876, that the mind alone could create health or disease, the neurological equivalent of the views of Mrs. Mary Baker Eddy. Putnam countered Beard by insisting that, because the emotions could not be quantified, data about them must perforce be unscientific. For years he insisted on meticulous experiment and carefully accumulated data in the young profession of neurology, and this perhaps preserved him from some of the enthusiasm of his Boston friends for the seductive promise of parapsychology, from mediums and mind reading.

Yet Putnam retreated from the extreme materialistic position, and this coincided with a major shift in American neurology from a somatic toward a psychological style. In this movement he was a moving force, although not its leader, a role enthusiastically played by Morton Prince, ten years younger and considerably more ebullient. Nevertheless Putnam helped to institutionalize psychotherapy. He gave the new methods extensive application at the Massachusetts General Hospital, and he helped Prince found the *Journal of Abnormal Psychology*, remaining a major contributor.

The reasons for this great change of style in American neurology and psychiatry cannot be dealt with at length here. Part of the impetus came from defeated expectations—the absence of somatic evidence to support overextended somatic hypotheses—and from therapeutic discouragement. A new rationale and a more sanguine outlook came from new psychological data, from the European and American rediscovery of the unconscious—the rich and subtle work of Freud's immediate predecessors, particularly Charcot and Janet. Indeed, it was Putnam who brought Janet to the Lowell Institute in 1904 and to Harvard in 1906.

Boston provided a notably receptive environment for these new developments on the frontier of medical psychology for several reasons—the competition of mind cure practitioners, a long idealist tradition, the presence at Harvard of an authentic American psychological genius, perhaps the only we have had, William James, and a lesser but highly accomplished philosopher, Josiah Royce. These men exchanged ideas with their medical friends, particularly with Putnam. By 1908 he was insisting that the immediate data of consciousness—speech and gesture—were as revealing as the anatomy of the brain.

The records of Putnam's inpatient service at the Massachusetts General indicates the richness and variety of pre-Freudian therapy. Morton Prince was attempting to uncover the history of emotional symptoms by automatic writing. By 1905 Putnam was investigating patients' dreams, particularly nightmares, perhaps searching for the kinds of frightening traumas that interested the psychopathologist Boris Sidis. Most of these patients presented a myriad of presumably physical symptoms—peculiar bodily sensations, twitches, paralyses, the globus hystericus, and the like—which were meticulously investigated and described. Invariably they were treated by hydrotherapy and Zander exercises, plain talks with Dr. Putnam, and suggestion and hypnosis.[3]

Sexual complaints of patients had been important to Putnam from the beginning of his neurological career. He had been called on to treat impotence, sexual neurasthenia, and other disorders. He had never been a partisan of extreme Victorian notions of reticence or of that Victorian seminal economics which presumed that the sexual secretions, if saved, would pay preferred dividends in high endeavor and upward mobility. The records of the Massachusetts General show a complex tangle of directly sexual symptoms and unexplained, obscure psychological struggles. Take the case of a twenty-two year old worker in a shoe factory, diagnosed psychasthenic by Dr. Putnam in 1906. She complained of odd feelings in the vagina as well as a sense of the top of her head being pulled. She made great efforts to control the "proxysms," as she called them. "I do say that I feel sure no strong man would find it harder to control than I—he would not. As for a girl, she could not. All these efforts, trying to be cheerful when I suffer great depression, and trying to control my nerves are killing me."[4]

The ubiquity of such problems no doubt helped to prepare Putnam for his final contribution, his role as a catalyst of the American psychoanalytic movement and its first pillar in Boston. He tried Freud's method on his inpatient ward around 1905, with misgivings as well as with mixed results. His conversion to Freudian theory was the result of his contacts with Ernest Jones and Freud himself during and after the Clark conference. What prompted it we shall probably never fully know, though some aspects of it are clear. Putnam had an ingrained sympathy for beleaguered, unpopular causes and for forthright stands. The very opposition to psychoanalysis, once Freud's integrity had been demonstrated, increased his zeal. Putnam's repeated public stands on behalf of psychoanalysis, his lucid presentation of its advantages over previous therapies, its augmentation of his detailed knowledge of his patients, its radical hopes for cases that others considered relatively hopeless—all these smoothed the path for Freud's medical reception in the United States. Not until William Alanson White carefully broached the topic to American psychiatrists some four years later did another eminent American endorse psychoanalysis.

Putnam by no means convinced the Boston psychotherapists of the superiority of Freud's methods. Quite the contrary. The Boston school continued using Janet's and Prince's techniques into the 1930s, especially at the Boston Psychopathic Hospital and at the Austen Riggs.

Nevertheless, as he had with neurology and psychotherapy, and now with psychoanalysis, Putnam attempted to provide it with an institutional base. He lectured to students at Harvard Medical School on the subject after his formal retirement. At the clamorous insistence of Freud and Ernest Jones, he participated in the founding of the American Psychoanalytic Association, serving as its first president. Equally important, he saw that the method was applied at the Massachusetts General Hospital.

Putnam secured the appointment of Louville Eugene Emerson as staff psychologist in 1911. A student of William James, Emerson had been working at the new psychopathic hospital in Ann Arbor. Some of his cases are remarkable, including the cure of a double classical hysterical paralysis. A domestic, aged nineteen, developed severe contractures of both legs. Forced extension had failed, although her condition had been temporarily relieved when she had been blessed by a priest. Finally, the case notes read, "persistent psychoanalysis by Dr. Emerson throughout her stay here (which lasted about a month) revealed facts and dreams which were evidently the cause of the origin of the paralyses. He was able to overcome the paralyses and spasms, but with recurrence of same several times. Patient left hospital, in apparently cured condition to be treated in OPD."[6] Here was a major attempt, at a major institution, to institutionalize the use of psychoanalysis as a therapeutic tool.

Putnam attempted to reform psychoanalysis itself. From the beginning he was aware of what psychoanalysts seldom acknowledged then—the tough, recalcitrant case that did not conform to a model of inner conflict and self-possession. There were willful patients, hedonistically uninterested in socialization or sublimation or in giving up their symptoms. Cool and callous patients, Putnam called them, with devilish resistances. They needed, he thought, a sense of purpose, which the analyst must share.

Putnam reserved his doubts about the method for Freud and his analytic colleagues. It was the obverse of his outwardly enthusiastic professional role. He was one of the first analysts to see the problem of values as it relates to the symptoms of patients, and to foresee the need for some concept of the self that included development not based on conflict alone, much the kind of concept that Heinz Hartmann supplied thirty years later.

Putnam also was aware of something that has made psychoanalysis peculiarly vulnerable—its identification with a rationalist, materialistic, deterministic view of the world. It is precisely by proponents of a quite different view, what might be called romantic mysticism, that psychoanalysis is now heavily attacked.

What Putnam hoped to do, beginning with Freud himself, was to sensitize the analytic profession to its own large underlying ethical and philosophical assumptions. He failed, of course, although Freud was prodded by some of his insistence on ethics to examine the problem of conscience and of what he later called the superego.

Putnam's impact on the professional life of his native city was exercised from positions of eminence, both at the Massachusetts General Hospital and at Harvard Medical School. In the institutionalization of three major departures—the specialties of neurology, psychotherapy, and, finally, psychoanalysis—he played a role that was often decisive. Probably without him, psychoanalysis would not have found a respectable home in Boston in his lifetime.

References

[1] Henry James to James Jackson Putnam, January 4, 1912, Francis A. Countway Library of Medicine, Boston.

[2] Nathan G. Hale, Jr., ed., *James Jackson Putnam and Psychoanalysis* (Cambridge, Mass.: Harvard University Press, 1971), p. 9.

[3] Massachusetts General Hospital, Ward G, Records, I (October 1, 1903, to December 8, 1905), II (December 9, 1905, to March 6, 1908).

[4] Case of KG, Massachusetts General Hospital, Ward G, Records, II (February 12, 1906).

[5] Oscar J. Raeder, "Hypnosis and Allied Forms of Suggestion in Practical Psychotherapy," *American Journal of Psychiatry*, 13 (1933), 69–76; Horace K. Richardson, "Psychotherapeutics at Stockbridge," *ibid.*, 45–56.

[6] Case of EAC, Massachusetts General Hospital, Ward G, Records, III (January 1, 1912).

Morton Prince and Psychopathology

OTTO M. MARX

Eight months before his death on August 31, 1929, Morton Prince briefly reviewed the growth of the field of abnormal psychology and the role he had played in it. He recalled the indifference with which the early work had been met and the resistance which had hampered its development, a situation changed by Freud. Aided by public opinion which demanded that the medical profession answer the questions asked about the role of the mind in producing physical ill health, Freud had done what no one else had succeeded in doing: he made the medical profession and the psychologists take notice. In the field of abnormal psychology, psychoanalytic methods, observation, and doctrines soon displaced or obscured all other theories. Those who were not identified with Freudian psychology were "left submerged like clams buried in the sands at low water." Among them was Morton Prince and the "Boston school."[1]

In an earlier study of Morton Prince and *The Dissociation of a Personality* of 1906, I demonstrated his importance as a publicist, as a man who called upon medicine to address itself to issues and questions for which psychoanalysis soon afterwards seemed to provide the answers.[2] In this paper I will focus on Prince's work in psychopathology and offer a critical evaluation of his contribution from a historian's perspective.

But first some historically relevant background.[3] Morton Prince was born in 1854. When he died seventy-five years later, in 1929, he was an international figure. A prominent Bostonian active in civic affairs, as well as local and national politics, Morton Prince was one of the foremost neurologists in this country. As an undergraduate at Harvard, he received the Boylston Prize for his essay on *The Nature of Mind and Human Automatism*.[4] He visited the Salpêtrière in the early 1880s and inspired by Charcot and his work on hysteria, Prince turned to neurology and psychotherapeutics. He closely followed Pierre Janet in theory and approach. In 1890 his first local presentation on hypnosis was discussed by William James and Josiah Royce;[5] numerous papers followed. In 1906 *The Dissociation of a Personality* won him popular acclaim. He was invited to lecture at many universities here and abroad. At Tufts, where he was professor of diseases of the nervous system, his lectures, given from 1902 to 1912, were the first systematic presentation of psychopathology in the United States. They provided the basis for the *Unconscious* (1914), which also became a well-known text.[6] He actively worked for American participation in World War I and was personally involved in the war effort. But perhaps of greatest significance was that he founded and supported the *Journal of Abnormal Psychology* (1906), and served as its editor for many years. He organized the American Psychopathological Clinic at Harvard, which he hoped would be his monument. Prince was one of the unusual few who constantly worked for a closer collaboration between medicine and psychology, psychiatry, neurology, and psychopathology. He tried to reconcile the differences among these disciplines and effectively fought against the animosity that separated their adherents and worked to the detriment of all.[7]

To that end he espoused a "scientific psychopathology," whose history had been brief. Janet's work on hysteria had marked its beginnings. Taking off from Charcot's suggestion that certain hysterical phenomena were caused by ideas, Janet developed his theories of hysteria based on the concept of dissociation of consciousness. Experimental use of hypnosis and clinical explorations verified the theory. Prince repeated, amplified, and extended Janet's clinical and experimental work.[8]

As Henry A. Murray pointed out, the clinical approach was the hallmark of Prince's effort. Unlike other psychopathologists Prince did not continue research in biological science or neuropathology. He was also unusual in looking toward psychology for a theoretical framework. But despite his extensive observations, he did not develop a systematized theory.[9] In the preface to the *Unconscious*, subtitled *The Fundamentals of Human Personality, Normal and Abnormal*, his stated purpose was to lay a broad foundation upon which others could build without developing "any particular school of psychological theory."[10]

What was the model of the human mind which Prince proposed and which he claimed to have constructed on the solid foundation of the inductive method? The reality of a subconscious psychological life and the theory of memory as the basic mental process were the two cornerstones of Prince's theory of personality. Personality and character were made up of accumulated memory traces—physiological residues—which regardless of their unconscious, coconscious, or conscious psychological character were the elements composing the individual's psychological functions. Prejudices, beliefs, impulses, and dreams were the products of memory traces laid down in the brain.[11] According to Prince, some neuroses could be best understood in terms of a reawakening of past memories and a reexperiencing of these memories along with all of their unconscious and coconscious emotional concomitants.

Prince presented evidence to show that experience which never entered consciousness was nevertheless conserved, and he differentiated three levels of memorization.[12] Memory could be purely physiological as in the case of motor skills, psychophysiological as exemplified by thoughts linked to physiological changes, or purely mental. In all three cases the establishment of a memory trace was accompanied by a physiological change in the brain, which Prince called the neurogram.[13] A memory trace was itself a compound unit able to form affective complexes with other memory traces. A complex of memories could operate as a subconsciously functioning system and in some cases such systems functioning autonomously could lead to the establishment of separately functioning dissociated personalities. All psychological processes occurring outside the individual's own sphere of awareness Prince considered subconscious. In the subconscious sphere he differentiated between *coconscious* and *unconscious processes*. Unfortunately he slightly confounded his classification by calling the content of the coconscious sphere subconscious ideas. He reserved the term unconscious for neurophysiological processes that affected the mind, but were not part of it, being largely determined by the anatomical and physiological "prearrangements" inherent in the brain.

Whenever the equilibrium of the mind was unstable as in cases of sudden religious conversion, dreams, hysteria, or in spiritualistic mediums, the experiences of inner life "burst forth in mental and bodily manifestations of an unusual character." Unlike Freud, Prince felt it was premature to speak of "the exact mechanism" or decide to what extent "subconscious processes play their part"[14] under such circumstances. Why the mind was disturbed; by what mechanism; and finally, what particular subconscious processes were causal, remained to be worked out.

The psychoanalytic school had their own answers to these questions, but Prince found them unacceptable, feeling that the available data did not warrant such a commitment. He preferred a more tentative approach that explored the more general area of the role played by meaning. Prince did not believe that an idea or a memory of itself posed a problem to the patient, rather it was a question of its hidden meaning to the individual concerned. Meaning could never be derived from the application of a generally valid principle or scheme as Freud proposed, but had to be worked out for each case.

The psychotherapeutic process entailed three steps. First came the exploration of the subconscious for memories and the search for their meaning to the particular person. Memories acquired a particular meaning because of the setting in which they were acquired or because of the associations which they aroused. Following this it was important to isolate the memories and to see them for what they were apart from their particular settings. Finally the therapist suggested ideas and attributes to provide a new and less disturbing setting and hence a more desirable meaning for the previously harmful or painful thoughts.

In Prince's opinion therapeutic suggestion was substantially the same as education. Both depended upon the "implantation" of ideational complexes "organized" (or reinforced) "by repetition, by the impulsive force of their affective tones, or both." It was not lost on Prince that "Under ordinary conditions...*social suggestion* acts like therapeutic suggestion. But the suggestions of everyday life are so subtle and insidious that they are scarcely consciously recognized."[15]

These are but a few brief samples of Prince's thinking which seem to me typical of his work. There is little in the way of explicit theory or systematization; his writing never strayed far from his clinical examples and his approach always remained practical. Despite his stated recognition of the separation of basic from applied science, and from clinical discipline, and his recognition of the need for distinguishing facts from interpretations, he himself frequently failed in keeping these distinctions too clear.

These and other criticisms are not new and were leveled at Prince and at psychopathology at the time. William S. Taylor, professor of psychology at Smith College, wrote a small book entitled *Morton Prince and Abnormal Psychology* in 1928, and Henry A. Murray, Prince's successor at the Harvard Psychology Clinic, has offered several well-balanced overall critiques of Prince's work.[7,9] Their main points have already been stated, so that we may now supplement the psychologists' view with an evaluation of Morton Prince and psychopathology from a historical perspective.

The fact that Prince lived in Boston, his contact with James and Royce, or the visit to Charcot, each may have been decisive in his professional development. His personal qualities may also have played an important role in the way in which his work was received. His role as a teacher, lecturer, and practitioner may have to be taken into consideration. And it may well be that he exerted the greatest influence as editor of the journal he founded. But these factors should be discussed in the proper context of social, psycho-historical, or other as yet undefined historical specialties.

From the perspective of the history of science, Prince's role in the development of psychopathology as a branch of science was first discussed by Bernard Hart, a London psychiatrist, on the occasion of Prince's seventieth birthday in 1924.[16] Hart wrote that the science of psychopathology began with Janet's definition of dissociation as the first truly scientific concept. Suggestion was a somewhat vaguer but equally important idea. Hart then drew an analogy between this first phase in psychopathology as a science and the history of astronomy. He suggested that the stage in the development of psychopathology in which these concepts were elaborated—and during which Morton Prince made his contributions—was comparable to the history of astronomy at the time of Kepler.[16]

Newton and the law of gravity explained the motion of planets in ellipses around the sun. The corresponding advance in psychopathology was due to Freud. "His work marked the essential point of transition from the arid days of the academic psychology with its meticulous introspective description of mental processes, to the vigorous conceptual and dynamic method of attack which characterizes all growing science." Unfortunately discussion of the historical development of the field all too frequently remains stuck at this point.

Hart's claim has become common knowledge and everyone has heard it expressed in one form or another. Few it seems have been willing to read on and try to contend with Hart's criticism of Freudian thought. It is so much easier to celebrate the beginnings of psychological science with Freud and to relegate Janet and Prince to a prescientific age or to the era of another paradigm. Paradoxically this point of view creates many more difficulties than it solves, the least of which being that all three were contemporaries.

A notable exception to this peremptory attitude is the work of Henri Ellenberger, which provides a much more just assessment of the contributions of others to the field.[17] Although the broadly conceived approach of Ellenberger takes all possible angles into consideration, it cannot take us beyond the fact that Freud did succeed in outshining all his contemporaries in the field. It therefore seems appropriate to choose a much narrower perspective from which we can evaluate Morton Prince's position in the development of psychopathology; one which goes beyond the definition of Prince as a lesser figure in comparison with Freud.

Here the comparison of Freud to Newton is indirectly helpful. In the intervening half-century since Hart devised his astronomy-psychopathology analogy, historians of science have proposed various new conceptualizations of Newton's role in the development of physics. It is therefore no longer just a matter of accepting or rejecting the comparison of Freud to Newton, as the role of Newton in the history of science can be defined in various ways depending on one's allegiance to one of several views of the development of physics. To what extent an analogy between the history of physical and behavioral science is at all permissible will have to be discussed in a much broader context. For the moment I would like to present a point of view from the philosophy of science that appears promising and that I would like to apply in a preliminary way to my evaluation of Morton Prince's psychopathology.

Imre Lakatos recently proposed that we view the history of the physical sciences in terms of research programs.[18] A research program consists of a hard core of scientific findings, a positive method of defining new problems, and a better method for explaining the discoveries of others. A program is progressive as long as it predicts novel facts with some success. It may stagnate, another research program may become active for some time, and then another may take over. But at no time is a research program abolished or replaced. While we may have to modify Lakatos's concept of the history of science when we deal with developments in the social sciences, his scheme allows us to go beyond the traditional unilinear view of historical development. It permits us to evaluate the work of contemporaries whose work was resumed later or subsequently ignored. We are relieved of the task of setting absolute standards for the assessment of a particular approach in scientific endeavor. Importance is no longer linked to the "correctness" of specific theoretical formulations. The fruitfulness of the total research program is considered of much greater importance than the validity of one particular theory. Moreover, we can examine an individual's contribution in terms of its potential for development without regard for originality, influence, immediate failure, or success.

Looking at the work of Prince from this standpoint, which is perhaps best characterized as a broad and somewhat simplistic interpretation of Lakatos, several points become clear. Prince's work did not constitute a research program. Although Lakatos raises some serious questions about Freud's work as a research program, there is no doubt that he came much closer, for he provided a cluster of theories and hypotheses that have continued to generate a wealth of data. (The question of predictability, which is central to Lakatos's point of view regarding a research program, has to be left open pending a closer examination.) Furthermore, it becomes clear that the most important shortcoming of Prince's approach was the exclusion of himself from the investigative process and the absence of a theoretical structure that would give rise to other questions. Perhaps, unlike physical science, social science demands that we question traditional personal values and relationships, for its findings tend to reflect the investigator's experience of his own self. If this is so we cannot establish a link between Prince and his work. Being so much a part of his period and of his society was not an asset when it came to his work; it led him to accept his own role as a matter of course.

On the other hand his suggestion that psychopathology would have to be intimately related to scientific psychology was undoubtedly fruitful. But he did not work this concept out in its theoretical detail. He failed to provide the theoretical framework for what he accomplished in practice as an organizer, and as the editor of his journal.

You may share now some of my concerns regarding the extreme difficulties inherent in historical evaluation. But as Lakatos pointed out, our concept of the development of science is more than a philosophical query or an academic concern. Our view of the progress of science determines the research we pursue or support. In view of that much uncertainty regarding the development of science, we are perhaps best advised to actively support a great variety of endeavors including the work of people whose most cherished beliefs we do not necessarily share. In short, we may want to adopt an attitude and outlook similar to that which governed the lifework of Morton Prince.

References

[1] Nathan G. Hale, Jr., ed., Introduction, *Psychotherapy and Multiple Personality: Selected Essays* by Morton Prince (Cambridge, Mass.: Harvard University Press, 1975), pp. 1–18.

[2] Otto M. Marx, "Morton Prince and the Dissociation of a Personality," *Journal of the History of the Behavioral Sciences, 6* (1970), 120–130.

[3] Merrill Moore, Editorial, *Journal of Abnormal Social Psychology, 24* (1929), 249–250; Moore, "Morton Prince, M.D. (1854–1929)," *Journal of Nervous and Mental Diseases, 87* (1938), 701; Henry A. Murray, "Morton Prince, Sketch of his Life and Work," *Journal of Abnormal Social Psychology, 52* (1956), 291–295.

[4] Morton Prince, *The Nature of Mind and Human Automatism* (Philadelphia: Lippincott, 1885).

[5] *Boston Medical and Surgical Journal, 122*, (1890), 463, 475, 493. See also footnote 10 in Marx, "Morton Prince and the Dissociation of a Personality," *Journal of the History of the Behavioral Sciences, 6* (1970), 120–130.

[6] *The Unconscious* (New York: Macmillan, 1914).

[7] William S. Taylor, *Morton Prince and Abnormal Psychology* (New York: Appleton, 1928).

[8] Pierre Janet, *The Mental State of Hystericals*, translated by C.R. Corson (New York: Putnam, 1901). Janet, *The Major Symptoms of Hysteria* (New York: Macmillan, 1907).

[9] Murray, "Morton Prince, Sketch of his Life and Work," *Journal of Abnormal Social Psychology, 52* (1956), 291–295. See also reference 2.

[10] Prince, *The Unconscious* (New York: Macmillan, 1914), introduction.

[11] *Ibid.*, p. 1–14.

[12] *Ibid.*, p. 37.

[13] *Ibid.*, p. 131.

[14] *Ibid.*, p. 262.

[15] *Ibid.*, p. 289.

[16] B. Hart, "The Development of Psychopathology as a Branch of Science," in *Problems of Personality*, C.M. Campbell, ed. (New York: Harcourt, Brace, 1925), p. 231 ff. especially p. 237. Hart gave a more detailed exposition of his views in his Goulstonian Lectures held before the Royal College of Physicians in March 1926 and published in B. Hart, *Psychopathology and Its Place in Medicine* (New York: Macmillan, 1927), pp. 67–78.

[17] Henri F. Ellenberger, *The Discovery of the Unconscious* (New York: Basic Books, 1970).

[18] Imre Lakatos, "Falsification and the Methodology of Scientific Research Programmes," in *Criticism and the Growth of Knowledge*, I. Lakatos and A. Musgrave, eds. (Cambridge, England: Cambridge University Press, 1970), pp. 91–195. Imre Lakatos, "History of Science and its Rational Reconstructions," *Boston Studies in the Philosophy of Science, 8* (1971), 91–136.

Isador H. Coriat: The Making of an American Psychoanalyst

BARBARA SICHERMAN

Isador H. Coriat occupies a secure place in the history of American Psychoanalysis as "one of the leading standard bearers of the first generation."[1] As a practitioner of psychoanalysis from 1913 until his death in 1943, he thus provided a link between two generations of analysts: the pioneers, largely self-educated like himself, and the younger, European-trained men and women who helped establish psychoanalysis on a secure professional basis in the United States.

A scholarly man, Coriat wrote on such varied topics as primitive myth, the mental symptoms of paresis, anal-erotic character traits, Lady Macbeth, and medical history. He was not a major theorist; with the exception of his work on stammering and one or two late papers, his writing is facile to the point of glibness. Freud's insights into the more problematic aspects of the individual's relation to society largely eluded him.

Yet Coriat is interesting to the social historian as much for his limitations as for his achievements. For it is as a barometer of the progress of psychoanalysis that his career is most revealing. Coriat was initially the prototype of the young laboratory scientist who, dissatisfied with traditional explanations of mental and nervous disorders, found in psychoanalysis a superior theory and therapy. A study of his career helps to reveal why psychodynamic explanations ultimately seemed more promising to men of his generation than hereditary and purely somatic interpretations. The stark optimism of his early work exemplified the approach of first-generation American analysts which Freud found so disturbing. In later years, Coriat's understanding of psychoanalysis deepened, but so did his insistence on orthodoxy. His own development thus paralleled the transformation of American psychoanalysis from a loosely structured movement of individuals, some of whom expected psychoanalysis to bring about radical changes in individuals and society, to a professional discipline.

Environmental and personal considerations were important in Coriat's emergence as a psychopathologist and psychoanalyst. His residence in Boston, and his contact with the city's leading psychopathologists, fostered a receptivity to experimentation with new therapeutic techniques that led him first to the Emmanuel Movement and ultimately to psychoanalysis. Little is known about Coriat's personal life, as a colleague of many years noted with surprise at the time of his death.[2] But his marked success in Boston at an early age, his associations with the city's medical and social elite, and his rise from the slums of Boston to the presidency of the American Psychoanalytic Association could not have been matters of indifference to him.

Isador Henry Coriat was born in Philadelphia in 1875. His father was a Jewish immigrant from Morocco who arrived in the United States in 1867. Harry (or Hyram) Coriat was a member of Sephardic congregations in Philadelphia and Boston, to which the family soon moved when Isador was still a boy. Although described by his son as a manufacturer, city directories list the senior Coriat's occupation as "fancy goods," "Turkish goods," and "peddler."[3] Isador attended Boston public schools and graduated from Tufts College Medical School in 1900. Because it required no college courses for admission, Tufts attracted the sons and daughters of poorer New England families. It had recently introduced a four-year medical curriculum and modest opportunities for clinical training at Boston City Hospital and the Boston Dispensary.[4]

Between 1900 and 1905 Coriat was a resident at Worcester State Hospital, for the first two years under the supervision of Adolf Meyer, the hospital's pathologist. Although A.A. Brill suggested that Coriat's entry into hospital work was a decision "not to devote himself to organic medicine,"[5] this was not the case. Psychiatric research in state hospitals during the 1890s and early 1900s—what there was of it—was largely a matter of neuroanatomy, neuropathology, and biochemistry. Meyer wrote some important papers criticizing contemporary psychiatric trends, but his own research at Worcester was in neuroanatomy and neuropathology.[6]

Coriat proved the most prolific of the residents of that period. He published at least eleven articles based on his Worcester research, most of them on biochemistry. He studied abnormalities in the urine in various psychoses, chemical findings in the cerebrospinal fluid and central nervous system, and the chemistry of nerve degeneration. These studies demonstrated a continuing interest in chemistry; while still a student at Tufts, Coriat had been coauthor of *A Laboratory Manual for Clinical and Physiological Chemistry and Toxicology*.[7] By the end of his stay at Worcester, he had begun to investigate psychological conditions such as reduplicative paramnesia and mental disturbances in alcoholic neuritis. He also established contact with G. Stanley Hall at Clark University, and presented a paper there on the relationship between adolescence and dementia praecox.[8]

Meyer impressed Coriat, and undoubtedly stimulated his interest in psychiatric problems. A.A. Brill, a close professional friend of Coriat's, claimed that he "often spoke feelingly of these years, leaving no doubt that, like so many others, he was deeply influenced by Dr. Meyer."[9] In his papers on hysteria and dementia praecox between 1910 and 1914, Coriat adopted Meyer's psychobiological outlook and, long after Meyer had become critical of psychoanalysis, praised the work of his former mentor.

Worcester then was an exciting place for a young, scientific physician, for Meyer communicated his own exacting standards and enthusiasm for research to the residents. From him, Coriat would also have learned to gather complete case histories and to attempt to correlate physiological and anatomical findings with clinical data. These simple and obvious points constituted major innovations in American psychiatric hospitals and were perhaps Meyer's most lasting contributions to psychiatry at Worcester.

In May 1905, Coriat wrote Meyer, then in New York, that he wished to stay on in hospital work, but that advancement at Worcester was blocked "in the matter of psychiatry or chemistry." He added: "I would not be further advanced here, as far as position is concerned, in 5 years from now, than I am today."[10] This was a serious consideration, since the preceding year he had married Etta Dann, the daughter of a Boston rabbi. Thus at the age of thirty, he left Worcester for Boston and private practice.

The move to Boston changed the direction of Coriat's life. Between 1905, when he began work in the neurological service of Boston City Hospital, and 1913, when he espoused psychoanalysis, Coriat moved far from the worlds of the state hospital and biochemical research that had initially attracted him. In Boston he met the renowned physicians and psychologists who practiced psychopathological research in America. His connections with Morton Prince at Boston City Hospital, with James Jackson Putnam and others in the psychopathology study group that met at Prince's, and his philosophical studies with William James at Harvard provided the context for his developing interests. The innovative therapies and joint ventures with laymen tolerated by Boston's medical elite, then pressed by the rapid growth of Christian Science in their city, also encouraged the young man to experiment. Had he practiced in the city of his birth, still dominated by the conservative neurological outlook of S. Weir Mitchell, it is unlikely that he would have become such an enthusiastic psychotherapist or endorsed the controversial Emmanuel and psychoanalytic movements.

Most important, Coriat came under the influence of Morton Prince, physician for nervous disorders at Boston City Hospital and then at the peak of his career as a psychopathologist. Prince exerted a dynamic influence on younger physicians. A versatile and genial man, Prince was something of a showman. A student at Tufts about this time recalled Prince's first presentation in which he dramatically cured a young woman of hysteria by using a tuning fork and suggestion.[11] The year Coriat arrived, Prince published *The Dissociation of a Personality*, a sensational case study of a woman with multiple personalities. Written for a popular audience, the book received widespread, and sometimes critical, attention. It did much to dramatize the exciting new trends in psychopathology for an eager public.

Besides the impact of Prince's personality and the inherent fascination of his experimental research—Coriat described psychopathology as the "fairyland of science"[12]—Prince proved quite helpful to Coriat, then at a critical stage of his career. He sent him interesting referrals, made him a collaborating editor of the *Journal of Abnormal Psychology*, founded in 1906, and wrote an article on psychotherapy with him the following year. In a 1907 article, Coriat thanked Prince "for his continued help, suggestions and inspiration," and three years later dedicated to him his first book on psychopathology.[13]

Under Prince's influence, Coriat published several experimental and clinical studies on amnesia, followed by papers on hallucinations, hysteria, and sleep. Adopting Prince's conceptual framework, he focused on the subconscious, which he defined "as an independent consciousness, coexistent with the healthy consciousness but detached from it."[14] He regarded amnesia, for example, as a submerged patch of memories in the subconscious of the patient, but could not explain why a particular group of memories split off in this fashion.

Coriat hoped to develop precise methods of identifying and treating psychopathological states. He measured pulse rates and psychogalvanic reactions, both modifications of Jung's association tests. He also utilized various forms of psychotherapy, including hypnosis, suggestion, "analysis" (defined as inquiry into the origin of the mental state), and reeducation. For Coriat, as for Prince, psychotherapy was a matter of resynthesizing the dissociated states with the normal personality. Both men hoped to find a "rational basis" for psychotherapy, to counteract ill-conceived fads. Coriat noted the variety of techniques at the therapist's disposal: "substitution, suppression, inhibition, elimination" in some cases; "confession" in others. The difficulties in systematizing such diverse techniques, which depended on the "individuality of the physician," could scarcely be overestimated.[15]

It may have been Coriat's interest in psychotherapy—then all the rage in Boston—that attracted him to the Emmanuel Movement. The health clinic for functional nervous disorders, established at Emmanuel Church in 1906, was a cooperative venture of physicians and clergy that initially received support from prominent doctors, including James Jackson Putnam and Richard C. Cabot. Coriat's affiliation was more than nominal. With the movement's two ministers, he wrote *Religion and Medicine* in 1908, and joined them that year in a summer institute to train ministers and other laymen in the principles of psychotherapy.

Coriat was genuinely interested at this time in the healing properties of religion, a fact unknown to his psychoanalytic colleagues in the late 1920s. Even after he became a psychoanalyst, Coriat ignored Freud's own hostility to religion. In an article on "The Future of Psychoanalysis" that could have been entitled "Psychoanalysis and Ethics," he quoted a patient who believed that "the experience of psychoanalysis contributes towards a living faith." He continued: "I am beginning to believe that as a type of emotional sublimation, religion, using the term in its broadest sense without any reference to any particular dogma, offers one of the most effective and satisfactory routes."[16] Coriat's strong ethical concerns, and his interest in the sublimating possibilities of religion, link him with other New England analysts, notably Putnam.

Coriat's participation in the Emmanuel Movement is perhaps the most puzzling phase of his career. The young neurologist continued to support the movement after it came under heavy attack by Boston's neurological establishment, including Putnam and Philip Coombs Knapp, one of Coriat's chiefs at Boston City Hospital. Putnam repudiated the movement because it involved nonmedical personnel in healing roles. The entire episode pointed up the difficulty of maintaining distinctive professional roles once psychoneuroses were regarded as psychogenic in origin. Whatever private doubts Coriat may have had about lay psychotherapy—and, like other American analysts, he later opposed lay analysis—he consistently held "that the fundamental principle of the entire movement is absolute medical control."[17] He insisted that ministers could be helpful in cases presenting "moral and ethical problems."[18] His ability to hold fast, despite heavy censure, indicates a toughness and determination that were helpful later when medical colleagues attacked psychoanalysis. Perhaps Coriat enjoyed being something of an iconoclast, probably a necessary trait for all first-generation analysts. In later years he seemed to take pleasure in depicting himself as a courageous and lonely fighter for the truth of psychoanalysis.

Probably the most striking aspect of the episode—that a young Jew was chief medical consultant to a movement of Christian healing—seems to have been noted only by Elwood Worcester, the movement's founder. In an autobiography published in 1932, Worcester described Coriat as "truly learned," and "well-nigh infallible" as a diagnostician. He noted their fruitful collaboration over the years, despite the fact that, as he said, "He is a Hebrew. I am a Christian. He is a Freudian...I am not a Freudian."[19]

The significance of this for Coriat can only be conjectured, but the available evidence suggests that he was no stranger to the insecurity felt by many second-generation Jews who have begun to assimilate into American society. Coriat did not repudiate his past; although there is no record of any formal religious affiliation in his adult life, he held memberships in several Jewish social and cultural organizations. But his lower-class and Jewish origins seem to have troubled him. In addition to retouching his father's occupation for a biographical encyclopedia, he added a note on his family history to a self-portrait in the third edition of *Who's Who in American Jewry*. He reported that he was descended from an "ancient Spanish family" and that an ancestor, Thomas Coryat, author of *Coryat's Crudities* published in 1611, introduced forks into England. There *was* a distinguished Coriat family; they were rabbis and scholars who lived in Morocco from the sixteenth through the nineteenth century.[20] That Isador chose to mention an ancestor who had helped to "civilize" the English is therefore significant.

An interpretation of the specimen dream in *The Meaning of Dreams*, a popularization of Freud's theories published in 1915, further supports the hypothesis that Coriat experienced anxiety among his new colleagues. The dream paralleled Freud's Irma dream, and it is possible that Coriat was also the dreamer. Noting that some of the material had been disguised, Coriat identified the dreamer as a medical friend, an internist, who was Jewish. Whether or not the dream was Coriat's, the interpretation unquestionably was. The wife of a medical colleague of the dreamer had remarked: "We don't want any more rabbis in here." In real life the dreamer had often feared that because he was Jewish he was "only tolerated" by these friends. Coriat interpreted the dream with characteristic optimism. The "disparaging" remark, made in the dreamer's presence "and without hurting his feelings," indicated that he had indeed attained the desired intimacy with the family. Although they might not want any other Jewish friends, he was to be the exception.[21] The psychology of the minority group member who is glad to be perceived as different from the others is familiar.

Nor would insecurity about one's Jewishness have been inappropriate in Boston in the early years of the century. The prejudiced founders of the Immigration Restriction League were Bostonians, and sought support for their program in their native city. Anti-Semitism had increased, as the arrival of Russian Jews swelled Boston's previously small Jewish population. Even Richard C. Cabot, a fellow Emmanuelian who was eager to overcome his prejudices, confessed how difficult it was to view his Jewish patients as individuals rather than as generic types.[22] Given the prevalence of anti-Semitic stereotypes, as well as Coriat's own insecurities, it seems likely that the young man enjoyed his status as chief medical consultant to a project supported by an Episcopal congregation, described by Worcester as "a church of the refined, of the socially respectable, in fact, of the elite of Boston."[23]

Coriat must also have benefited personally from his participation in the movement. He kept a scrapbook recording press coverage; at the height of its popularity, in mid-1908, there were almost daily entries. Given popular enthusiasm for psychotherapy at the time—some considered it "a Boston fad"—Coriat's prominence could not have hurt his developing practice. Then in his early thirties, he appeared in the press as a "well-known Boston neurologist." A few years later, a reviewer referred to him as "one of the most brilliant of the new school of morbid psychologists." Perhaps the ultimate accolade came in 1917, when a correspondent for the *Boston Evening Transcript* heralded him, despite his Philadelphia birth, as "a thorough Bostonian."[24] Surely the status and prospects of the young physician had markedly improved since his departure from Worcester in 1905.

Coriat's personal acquaintance with psychoanalysis apparently began in December 1908, when controversy over the Emmanuel Movement was at its height. Ernest Jones spoke to the psychopathologists who met periodically at Prince's home, a group that at various times included Putnam, Edward Willys Taylor, George Waterman, August Hoch, Boris

Sidis, Hugo Münsterberg, and William James—a veritable who's who of Boston psychopathologists. Many years later Coriat noted that Freud's ideas, particularly the concept of infantile sexuality and the use of free association to determine the latent meaning of dreams, had initially seemed "nonsensical." He subsequently maintained that this antagonism was "not due to any failure of intellectual grasp, but rather to inner resistances" of the sort encountered by all revolutionary scientific theories.[25]

Coriat claimed he had been extremely impressed by Freud at the Clark conference, but his conversion actually came several years later, the result of growing experience with the method and gradual acceptance of its principles. In 1910 he still conceived of hysteria in essentially Meyerian terms, as "unhealthy biological maladjustment." Within this framework, he believed that childhood experiences, "usually of a sexual nature," often caused hysteria. But he also thought that "Freud applies the term sex and its symbolic equivalents, in too broad a sense." The following year, he warned that the analyst's enthusiasm for interpreting dreams might cause distortion, and considered wish fulfillment a secondary rather than primary motive.[26]

This ambivalent attitude prompted Ernest Jones to write Putnam, shortly before the founding of the American Psychoanalytic Association in May 1911: "Coriat is evidently running with the hare and coursing with the hounds, and he is further hampered by a terrific Ich-complex. I doubt that we shall make much out of him."[27] Jones need not have feared; two years later Coriat made his profession of faith at the International Medical Congress in London. Responding to Pierre Janet's criticism of Freud, Coriat announced that he was convinced of the "complete validity of the psycho-analytic theory," including the sexual etiology of the psychoneuroses. This he considered "not so much a sexual trauma as the development of an Oedipus or Electra-complex in childhood." He further denied that symbols were read into dreams: "The symbols are already in the dream and it is the duty of the psychoanalyst to find out these symbols."[28] Thus did Coriat attempt to elucidate the points he had earlier found "nonsensical."

What did Coriat find in psychoanalysis that convinced him of its "complete validity?" Surely this was a strong statement from a man whose own painstaking research contributed to the decline of the autointoxication theory of mental illness, and who was well aware that chemical studies of the cortex had revealed nothing valuable about the etiology of dementia praecox.[29] Undoubtedly his own familiarity with the limits of contemporary biochemical research made him receptive to psychological explanations, yet it does not in itself explain his commitment to psychoanalysis.

Although biographical information about how Coriat overcame his resistances is lacking, his early papers suggest something of the intellectual appeal of the new discipline. Like others who had experimented with various therapies, he found that psychoanalysis offered the only consistent and "logical" explanation of *why* patients became ill. Too often physicians had explained their own failures by labeling the contradictory behavior of hysterics, for example, as "a form of inexplicable stubbornness," or they had fallen back on "the unsatisfactory term of functional, which is equivalent to expressing a total ignorance." Earlier Coriat, who was eager to establish a "rational basis" for psychotherapy, had helplessly confessed: "The reason for the selective action of any emotional storm, in dissociating one group of memories and sparing others, cannot even be conjectured."[30]

By contrast, psychoanalysis cast a "flood of light" on neurotic symptoms. "The value of the analytic method," he maintained, "lies in the fact that one is able to discover suppressed material, and thus establish a definite psychological connection between symptoms and repressed experiences, a real continuity in the psychic series. The entire psychical complex may be constructed through the data furnished by psychoanalysis. All the heterogeneous symptoms thus fall into a certain law and order."[31]

The deterministic explanation of psychological data provided by psychoanalysis apparently met the laboratory researcher's need for scientific certainty. Long before his conversion, Coriat maintained that there were no chance occurrences and that mental events could be interpreted just as rigorously as physical ones. Only the correct key was missing, and this psychoanalysis amply provided. Throughout his career, Coriat utilized metaphors drawn from the exact sciences; dream work was "a chemical formula," and psychoanalysis itself penetrated human thought as the x-ray penetrated tissue.[32]

Coriat also emphasized the deeper therapeutic properties of psychoanalysis. It was, he claimed, the only system that really cured. Suggestion merely removed symptoms temporarily, but psychoanalysis effected permanent cures "by eliminating the unconscious ideas or complexes which caused the psychoneurotic disturbance." Dream interpretation particularly seemed to provide the precise technique for which Coriat had been searching, and it gave medicine "the most potent instrument which it has ever possessed" in treating the psychoneuroses. Where earlier systems had led to improvisation and experimentation, he said many years later, "in a prolonged analysis, there can be predicted with almost mathematical precision, the course and development of the analytic material."[33]

Coriat's total commitment to psychoanalysis followed a pattern common to first-generation analysts. Ernest Jones called the early analysts "converts" because the "approach to psychoanalysis cannot be effected by reason alone, however much it may speak the final word; it is necessarily an emotional process involving important inner mental changes of a more than coldly rational order." Coriat may have had something like this in mind when he claimed that for trailblazers like himself "analysis became deeply assimilated into the personality and [was] not a mere intellectual superstructure." To the extent that this was true, the fierce pride that many analysts took in their early identification with the movement and their ability to withstand attack can be more readily understood.[34]

Psychoanalysis also provided Coriat with a new world view. "Deeper than any philosophy," its universal explanations of human behavior revealed that "there is 'one mind common to all individual men'...and this universal mind is the unconscious." Psychoanalysis was also "beginning to found a new ethics as well as a new psychology, a new neurology and a new school of literary criticism." Thus the scholarly Coriat permitted himself to give free rein to his many scientific and cultural interests.[35]

In the new system of ethics the analyst was the high priest. The observation of one of Coriat's patients that "the relation between physician and patient seems to me to have much in common with God's dealings with man" appealed to him. Coriat took pride in the superior skill required of the analyst, whom he considered a "paleopsychologist" who could make as much out of the fragments of a dream as the archaeologist of the fragments of a skull. He must have knowledge of "his own resistances and complexes as well as his various social, religious and political prejudices." His "mind must be clean as a surgeon's hands before an operation, his attitude towards the neurosis should be that of the physician whose task it is to help and not that of the moralist who thinks it his duty to criticize."[36] Despite this disclaimer, it seems likely that Coriat now viewed the analyst as capable of combining the roles of physician and minister—roles that had been distinct in the Emmanuel Movement.

Coriat's early work exemplified the optimism and social conformity of many first-generation American interpreters of Freud. Coriat expected much of psychoanalysis. He also ignored the tragic implications of

Freud's own work—the profoundly disturbing disjunction between primitive, unconscious desires, and the demands of civilization.[37]

Typical, perhaps, were his early views on the Oedipus complex. He believed that the complex developed only in children "exposed to an over-exuberant love from the parents, or who themselves have shown a parental affection of abnormal intensity." Prophylaxis and cure seemed simple. Coriat claimed that a case of homosexuality, prompted by the boy's love for his mother, could have been prevented: "If he had been corrected on this subject...this Oedipus trend could have been nipped in the bud." The therapy for another boy, a kleptomaniac, was "to break up the Oedipus complex so that the boy would have as much to fear of stealing from his mother as from his father." Parents, particularly mothers, could be instructed "against too strong an attachment and too much indulgence in their children."[38] The child thus became less the victim of his biological drives, and more a creature of a social environment that could be altered.

Coriat's optimism was most evident in his writing on the unconscious and sublimation. He considered the unconscious a repository of the repressed, "a sort of elemental Titan," but he denied that it embodied only man's lower and more primitive qualities. He claimed that the unconscious of a former patient, with a personality prone to shell shock, "had been so well educated by the previous psychoanalysis" that he adjusted well to life in the military. For Coriat a psychoanalysis was "an education" that "raises the unconscious to a higher cultural level." Like other Americans, he emphasized the almost unlimited possibilities of sublimation about which Freud remained skeptical: "A successful psychoanalysis should leave the patient completely sublimated, that is, it should enable him to utilize the unconscious energy for the higher purposes of life."[39]

In his popular works, Coriat remained reticent about sexuality, a stance characteristic of other Americans as well. He often explained that in psychoanalysis "the word 'sexual'...has the same broad meaning as the word 'love.' " A psychoanalytic critic was dismayed by the absence of sexual interpretation in *The Meaning of Dreams*, which contained only dreams personally analyzed by Coriat. To *The Nation*'s reviewer, on the other hand, this was a blessing, for the book could "safely be used...in a young ladies' seminary." In interpreting a "typical" dream of nakedness, Coriat observed: "This dream cannot express the fulfillment of an adult wish, since social conventionalities and the restraints imposed by culture and adult modesty would be decidedly against such a wish being fulfilled, even in a dream. The dream must, therefore...have had its origin in the past life of the individual, when such a desire existed."[40] This surely was reassuring to anyone who found such dreams distressing.

Coriat undoubtedly found it distasteful to break through Victorian cultural reticence, a difficulty that Putnam acknowledged openly. Psychoanalysis did not prompt him to challenge conventional "civilized" morality—in the interest of abjuring sexual impurity, he recommended "keeping the mind clean; that is, away from the subject"[41]—nor the goal of adjusting to the immediate environment. Perhaps more radical conclusions could have been drawn only by one who was more alienated from his society than Coriat, a man who had personally experienced the assimilating powers of American life.

Coriat later described the training of the pioneer analysts as largely a matter of reading, analysis of their own dreams, and "a more or less fragmentary personal analysis." He participated in whatever psychoanalytic activities Boston had to offer, but these were slow to develop. In 1914, the Boston Psychoanalytic Society was formed, with Putnam as president and Coriat as secretary. Putnam informed Freud of the group's meetings: "Although we are not geniuses, yet we do fair work, and, I think, keep our heads level." These informal educational activities ceased on Putnam's death in 1918; they were resumed in 1924, when Coriat invited some analysts to meet at his home for informal study. The group consisted of Jungians and Rankians, with Coriat perhaps the only one considered an orthodox Freudian. There were few analysts in Boston then, and orthodoxy was not an issue.[42]

During the 1920s Coriat attended meetings of the New York and the American Psychoanalytic Associations, and in 1924 he became president of the national body. He maintained ties with many medical groups, informed them about psychoanalysis, and attempted to reinterpret new theories, such as gestalt psychology, in the light of psychoanalysis. His interests remained broad and he was one of the few Americans interested in character types at the time.

Initially, his views were more eclectic than his reputation for orthodoxy would suggest. For some time he was attracted to the ideas of Alfred Adler, perhaps because of his own reticence about sexuality, perhaps, too, because of a lifelong interest in psychosomatic medicine. As late as 1920, Coriat referred to Adler as "one of the greatest thinkers of the Freudian school," a remark that was repudiated by the reviewer in the *International Journal of Psycho-Analysis*. Coriat applied Adler's concept of organ inferiority to amaurotic family idiocy, Kaiser Wilhelm's belligerent behavior, and stammering, the subject that he considered his greatest contribution to psychoanalysis. By the time he published his book on stammering in 1928, he was in closer touch with European developments, and the concept of organ inferiority had disappeared.[43]

By the late 1920s, a major change was under way in Boston, leading to the establishment of psychoanalysis as a profession. Coriat was active in reorganizing the Boston Psychoanalytic Society in 1930, an outgrowth of the meetings he had been holding in his home for some years. He served as president for two years. The fierce debates of this time concerned not only what training standards should be upheld, but who should determine them. Always in the background was the implicit threat to the leadership of the first generation. Older analysts like Coriat and Brill in New York apparently wished to vest this authority in the training analyst rather than in the educational committee, as required by the International Psychoanalytic Association. Under the leadership of the younger analysts, recently returned from Berlin and Vienna, the Boston Society was reorganized in 1933 to meet the standards of the American and international associations.[44]

Despite his initial reservations, and the perhaps understandable reluctance of a man who still regarded himself as a pioneer to seeing leadership pass to a younger generation, Coriat participated fully in the new organization. A younger colleague has recalled the intensity and eagerness of all Boston analysts at this time to deepen their knowledge and establish psychoanalysis on a sound professional basis. Men of "tunnel vision," old and young alike, devoted themselves to one goal—psychoanalysis. Teachers were also students then, and members attended each others' classes and met frequently to discuss their work.[45] Perhaps glad that he finally had colleagues with whom he could share his psychoanalytic interests, Coriat served as instructor, trustee, and member of the Education Committee of the Boston Psychoanalytic Institute, founded in 1935. He was also reelected president of the society in 1940–41 and again shortly before his death, an indication that he had successfully bridged the generation gap.

His greater involvement with psychoanalytic colleagues made him more insistently orthodox. In his presidential address to the Boston society in 1930, following some organizational controversies, Coriat maintained:

> Whatever may be our differences of opinion, it has been the experience of others as it has also been of mine, that through these difference [*sic*] of opinion one becomes more and more Freudian, instead of less so....Above

> all, and I feel that this is of paramount importance, we must be very careful about the admission of new members, their qualifications must be minutely scrutinized, adhering strictly to the plans which have been formulated through the acceptance of the Constitution. Any new member who is proposed must be convinced of the basic truths of psychoanalysis: we cannot accept any who have an ambivalent attitude, that is, the frequently encountered attitude of "getting together" of analysis and academic psychology....such individuals are far more dangerous to the cause of psychoanalysis than those who are out and out antagonists.

A few years later he claimed that "there have been no really constructive criticisms but only superannuated opinions," a far cry from his praise of Eugen Bleuler's "constructive criticism" in 1924.[46]

Coriat's remarks seemed to draw a curtain over his own past, his slow evolution as a psychoanalyst, and his earlier receptivity to new trends in psychoanalysis as well as the related work of psychologists, psychiatrists, and neurologists. Perhaps his need to remain in the vanguard of a movement that meant so much to him, combined with the stated or implied challenge to his psychoanalytic credentials by younger and better-trained colleagues, prompted these remarks. In any case, the insistence on orthodoxy by Coriat and his colleagues marked the transformation of American psychoanalysis from an optimistic and reformist creed to a professional specialty.

If Coriat's interests became narrower in some respects, his later clinical studies were more probing. His presidential address to the American Psychoanalytic Association in 1937 struck a deeper vein than his earlier talk on "Psychoanalysis and Literature" in 1925, and expressed his mature views on the significance of psychoanalysis.[47] Placing less emphasis on the cultural role of psychoanalysis, he noted, perhaps regretfully, that Freud's psychology of the unconscious had, "up to the present, been unable to fulfill its ideal wishes to become a world view of life." Instead, Coriat stressed its impact on psychiatry: "Psychoanalysis belongs to clinical psychiatry; it is the logical outgrowth of psychiatric thought and evolution."

The future scientific development of psychoanalysis, in Coriat's view, depended on its continued close alliance with medicine, maintenance of rigid training standards, establishment of scholarships for psychoanalytic training by institutes, and additional psychoanalytic education for academic psychologists. At the same time he wanted to expand therapeutic opportunities by developing psychoanalytic clinics for the less affluent, and accepting patients in such clinics because they needed help rather than "because they represent valuable research material." This was consistent with his human therapeutic interest in the Emmanuel Movement, which had also welcomed working-class patients. Coriat also considered the "mental hygiene of the analysts." It was too much to expect total "emotional immunity" from their patients' difficulties, for "analysts, like their patients, are human beings." The admission of the humanity of the analyst contrasted with his earlier view of the analyst as a godlike figure.

In his later years, Coriat could have looked back with some equanimity on the course of his life and that of the specialty to which he had devoted himself so completely. He had reestablished himself as a valued member of the Boston Psychoanalytic Society and Institute, and he had worked closely with younger American analysts and the distinguished Europeans who arrived in Boston in the late 1930s and early 1940s. He continued to welcome new psychoanalytic trends, notably ego psychology, and worked eagerly to improve psychoanalytic education. C.P. Oberndorf has described his lingering image of Coriat: "His peering eyes behind thick lenses...tended to increase the impression of one insistently searching for greater light and more truth."[48] Perhaps it was this quality that kept him in harness until his death in May 1943.

References

[1] A.A. Brill, "In Memoriam: Isador H. Coriat, 1875–1943," *Psychoanalytic Quarterly, 12* (1943), 402. I wish to thank Phyllis Ackman for reading an earlier draft of this paper, Sanford Gifford for providing me with material from the archives of the Boston Psychoanalytic Society and Institute, and Richard J. Wolfe and his staff for assistance in using the Isador H. Coriat papers in the Francis A. Countway Library of Medicine, Boston.

[2] George B. Wibur, "Isador H. Coriat, M.D.," *Psychoanalytic Review, 30* (1943), 479.

[3] For biographical information about Coriat and his father, see "Isador Henry Coriat," *The National Cyclopaedia of American Biography, 32* (1945), 190; *Philadelphia City Directory, 1872–1875; Boston City Directory, 1879–1895;* Albert Ehrenfried, *A Chronicle of Boston's Jewry: From the Colonial Settlement to 1900* (1963), 443–444, 751.

[4] See Benjamin Spector, *A History of Tufts College Medical School.* Prepared for its semicentennial, 1893–1943. (Boston: Tufts College Medical School Alumni Association, 1943), pp. 104–105, 116–120, 146–147.

[5] Brill, *Psychoanalytic Quarterly*, p. 400.

[6] The discussion of Meyer's years at Worcester in the next few paragraphs is based on Gerald N. Grob, *The State and the Mentally Ill: A History of Worcester State Hospital in Massachusetts, 1830–1920* (Chapel Hill, N.C.: University of North Carolina Press, 1966), pp. 263–316, and Barbara Sicherman, "Adolf Meyer: Profile of a Swiss-American Psychiatrist," *Swiss American Historical Society Newsletter, 5* (1969), 5–7.

7 Arthur E. Austin and Isador H. Coriat, *A Laboratory Manual of Physiological and Clinical Chemistry and Toxicology* (Boston: Lamson, Wolffe, 1898).

8 Isador H. Coriat to Adolf Meyer, March 21, 1905. Adolf Meyer Papers, William H. Welch Library, Johns Hopkins University, Baltimore, Maryland.

9 Brill, *Psychoanalytic Quarterly*, p. 400.

10 Isador H. Coriat to Adolf Meyer, May 10, 1905; Adolf Meyer Papers.

11 Abraham Myerson, "Morton Prince, M.D." in Spector, *A History of Tufts College Medical School*, pp. 206–210.

12 Isador H. Coriat, *Abnormal Psychology*, second ed. rev. (New York: Moffat, Yard, 1914), p. xii.

13 Morton Prince and Isador Coriat, "Cases Illustrating the Educational Treatment of the Psycho-Neuroses," *Journal of Abnormal Psychology, 2* (1907), 166–177; Isador H. Coriat, "The Lowell Case of Amnesia," *ibid., 2* (1907), 93. (This journal will hereafter be cited as *JAbP.*) The dedication appears in *Abnormal Psychology*, first ed. (New York: Moffat, Yard, 1910).

14 Coriat, *Abnormal Psychology*, second ed. rev. (1914), p. 3.

15 Coriat's ideas on psychotherapy appear in Elwood Worcester, Samuel McComb, and Isador H. Coriat, *Religion and Medicine, The Moral Control of Nervous Disorders* (New York: Moffat, Yard, 1908), pp. 260–265, and Isador H. Coriat, "Psychotherapy," in Parley Paul Womer, ed., *The Relation of Healing to Law* (Chicago: Magnum Bonum, 1909), pp. 193–212.

16 Isador H. Coriat, "The Future of Psychoanalysis," *Psychoanalytic Review, 4* (1917), 385, 383. Interview with Dr. M. Ralph Kaufman, November 13, 1970.

17 The scrapbooks kept by Coriat contain numerous clippings about the movement. They are in Isador H. Coriat Papers, in the Francis A. Countway Library of Medicine. For Coriat's remarks, see the entry entitled "Dr. Putnam Replies to Dr. Worcester," from *Boston Herald* (November 22, 1908), Scrapbook no. 3, p. 36.

18 Coriat in Womer, *Relation of Healing to Law*, p. 202.

19 Elwood Worcester, *Life's Adventure. The Story of a Varied Career* (New York: Scribner's, 1932), p. 306.

20 *Who's Who in American Jewry, 1938–1939*. III, 193; *The Universal Jewish Encyclopedia*, III, 369. I wish to thank Jacob R. Marcus of the American Jewish Archives for calling my attention to the entry in *The Universal Jewish Encyclopedia*.

21 Isador H. Coriat, *The Meaning of Dreams*, "Mind and Health Series" (Boston: Little, Brown, 1915), pp. 13–42.

22 Barbara Miller Solomon, *Ancestors and Immigrants: A Changing New England Tradition* (New York: Wiley, 1965), especially pp. 145, 167, 175, 37–41; (originally published in 1956).

23 Worcester, *Life's Adventure*, p. 296.

24 Review of *Abnormal Psychology*, in *British Journal of Inebriety 3* (1911), Scrapbook no. 3, p. 80; Isaac Goldberg, "The Hysteria of Lady Macbeth," *Boston Evening Transcript* (June

13, 1917), p. 5, Scrapbook no. 1, p. 36.

25 Isador H. Coriat, "Some Personal Reminiscences of Psychoanalysis in Boston: an Autobiographical Note," *Psychoanalytic Review, 32* (1945), 2–3. Coriat had been familiar with Jung's association tests since 1906.

26 Isador H. Coriat, "Hysteria in the Light of the Analytic Method," *Saint Paul Medical Journal, 12* (1910), 414–415, 420, 421; Isador H. Coriat, "A Contribution to the Psychopathology of Hysteria," *JAbP, 6* (1911), 33–65.

27 Ernest Jones to James Jackson Putnam, April 15, 1911. Nathan G. Hale, Jr., ed., *James Jackson Putnam and Psychoanalysis* (Cambridge, Mass.: Harvard University Press, 1971), p. 266.

28 Quoted in Coriat, "Some Personal Reminiscences," p. 4.

29 See especially Isador H. Coriat, "Recent Trends in the Psychopathology of Dementia Praecox," *American Journal of Insanity, 70* (1914), 669–682.

30 Coriat, *The Meaning of Dreams*, p. 167; Coriat, "The Lowell Case of Amnesia," *JAbP*, II (1907), p. 110.

31 Coriat, "Hysteria in the Light of the Analytic Method," p. 415; Coriat, "Contribution to the Psychopathology of Hysteria," *JAbP, 6* (1911), 65.

32 Coriat, *The Meaning of Dreams*, p. 67; Isador H. Coriat, "The Eightieth Birthday of Sigmund Freud." Unpublished remarks made at a meeting of Jewish Book Week at Boston, May 17, 1936, p. 8, The Coriat Papers.

33 Coriat, *The Meaning of Dreams*, pp. 164, xi; Coriat, "Current Trends in Psychoanalysis," *Psychoanalytic Review, 25* (1938), 446.

34 Ernest Jones, *Free Associations. Memories of a Psycho-Analyst* (New York: Basic Books, 1959), p. 212; Coriat, "Some Personal Reminiscences," p. 8. See also Paula Fass, "A.A. Brill—Pioneer and Prophet." Unpublished master's essay, Columbia University, 1968.

35 Isador H. Coriat, *Repressed Emotions* (New York: Brentano, 1920), pp. 182–183, 181–182.

36 Coriat, "The Future of Psychoanalysis," p. 384; Coriat, *Repressed Emotions*, pp. 37–38, 41–42.

37 My knowledge of the history of American psychoanalysis in this section and throughout the paper has been deeply influenced by Nathan G. Hale, Jr., *Freud and the Americans: The Beginnings of Psychoanalysis in the United States, 1876–1917* (New York: Oxford University Press, 1971), see especially pp. 332–396.

38 Isador H. Coriat, "The Oedipus-Complex in the Psychoneuroses," *JAbP, 7* (1912), 176; Isador H. Coriat, "Psycho-analysis and the Sexual Hygiene of Children," reprinted from *The Child, 2* (1912), 4; Coriat, "Future of Psychoanalysis," p. 387; Isador H. Coriat, "The Psychoanalytic Approach to Sex Hygiene," in Milton J. Rosenau, *Preventive Medicine and Hygiene* (fifth ed.; New York and London: Appleton, 1927), p. 82.

39 Coriat, *Repressed Emotions*, pp. 5, 142, 154, 151–152.

40 Isador H. Coriat, *What is Psychoanalysis?* (New York: Moffat, Yard, 1917), p. 53; Bar-

bara Low, review of *The Meaning of Dreams* in *International Journal of Psycho-Analysis, 3* (1922), 394–395; review of *The Meaning of Dreams* in *The Nation* (September 16, 1915), in Coriat, Scrapbook no. 1, p. 16; Coriat, *The Meaning of Dreams*, p. 132.

41 Coriat in Rosenau, *Preventive Medicine*, p. 84.

42 Coriat, "Some Personal Reminiscences," p. 5; Putnam quoted in Hale, *James Jackson Putnam and Psychoanalysis*, p. 38. Accounts of the psychoanalytic activities in Boston discussed in the next few paragraphs may be found in Coriat, "Some Personal Reminiscences," and in Ives Hendrick, *The Birth of an Institute*, twenty-fifth anniversary of the Boston Psychoanalytic Institute, November 30, 1958 (Freeport, Maine: Bond Wheelwright, 1961), *passim*.

43 Coriat, *Repressed Emotions*, p. 43; D.B., review of *Repressed Emotions*, in *International Journal of Psycho-Analysis, 3* (1922), 235; Isador H. Coriat, "Stammering as a Psychoneurosis," *JAbP, 9* (1914), 417–429; Isador H. Coriat, *Stammering: A Psychoanalytic Interpretation* (New York and Washington: Nervous and Mental Disease Publishing, 1928).

44 See Hendrick, *Birth of an Institute*, especially pp. 14–23, 31–33, 38–39, 41, 46–48, 75, 78–79. For discussions of education, see Bertram D. Lewin and Helen Ross, *Psychoanalytic Education in the United States* (New York: Norton, 1960), and Ives Hendrick, "Presidential Address: Professional Standards of the American Psychoanalytic Association," *Journal of the American Psychoanalytic Association, 3* (1955), 561–590.

45 Interview with M. Ralph Kaufman, November 13, 1970.

46 Isador H. Coriat, "Presidential Address before the Boston Psychoanalytic Society, November 12, 1930." Typescript in Library of the Boston Psychoanalytic Society and Institute, p. 2; Coriat, "Some Personal Reminiscences," p. 1; Coriat, "Progress in Psychiatry: Interpretive Psychiatry," *Boston Medical and Surgical Journal, 191* (1924), 499–501.

47 Coriat, "Current Trends," *passim*.

48 C.P. Oberndorf, "Obituary: Isador Henry Coriat," *International Journal of Psycho-Analysis, 24* (1943), 94.

Solomon Carter Fuller

ROBERT H. SHARPLEY

The obituary in the *Journal of the American Medical Association, 151*:1122, read in part: "On January 16, 1953, Solomon Carter Fuller, M.D., died at the Framingham Union Hospital, following a long illness from diabetes mellitus and gastrointestinal malignancy. Dr. Fuller, who was 81 years old, was Professor Emeritus of Neurology at Boston University."

This obituary gave notice of the end of a man's life. Paradoxically, it signaled the birth of a new approach to life as professional colleagues and scientists, who had not known Solomon Fuller, later learned and then sought to perpetuate the principles that had guided his life. These principles included a commitment to search for, understand, and assess all available pertinent knowledge when involved in the process of problem solving or considering an unfamiliar subject. Fuller's insistence on maintaining an open, inquiring mind and pursuing data in the most scholarly and broadest way possible came to mark the mode of life and the reputation of this man. It should be clear that these habits were not newly acquired professional habits, but seemingly traits that were developed from his earliest years.

Historical records show that the Fullers were a slave family who lived in Virginia, more particularly in the area of Norfolk.[1] John Lewis Fuller, the grandfather of Solomon, was a cobbler. His proficiency at his trade as well as his ability to manage the business of his owner resulted in his sharing the profits and eventually buying himself out of slavery. His continued diligence allowed him to earn a sufficient income to buy his future wife's freedom as well and to establish their home. John Fuller's progressive discontent with the existing political and social freedom, or lack thereof, and the growing restrictive measures he experienced during the years following the Nat Turner insurrection caused him first, in 1847, to send a son to Liberia and later, in 1849, to emigrate there with the rest of his family. He continued working as a shoemaker; however, he later became a carpenter in response to the greater need for skills to build the colony. John Fuller again demonstrated his organizing skill as well as his concern for and desire to aid others in founding the Charitable Mechanics Society of Monrovia, an organization similar to the Masons. It was a protective society that helped provide care for retired artisans, the feeble, and the sick.

Dr. Fuller defined his grandfather's other major contribution as that to his family. It is interesting to note that he regarded this input as a distinct contribution and one that deserved praise. It was probably the elder Fuller's attitude and example which developed the family ethos of emphasizing service.

John Lewis Fuller's son, Thomas (Solomon's uncle), who preceded the family to Liberia, would possibly be called a militant in today's terminology. The family's concern that Tom's "hotheadedness" might result in loss of his own safety caused them to send him to Africa in 1847. In Liberia, Tom channeled his energy into useful occupations. He became a probate judge in his early career and later mayor of Monrovia, through which he significantly helped to develop the city.

Dr. Solomon Carter's father, Solomon, was a successful planter and later high sheriff of Monstrado County, Liberia. He also served on the Boundary Commission of Liberia and worked for settlement of land claims between his country and Sierra Leone. His offices not only gave him significant power and control, but also encouraged habits of detail and precision. Although he was given a generous salary, equivalent to the salaries of hospital superintendents in Massachusetts, he frequently was paid in land. By this means the family acquired large holdings, some of which were leased to the Firestone Company after the discovery of rubber. The Fullers were one of the leading families in Liberia and lived in a manner commensurate with their status. Dr. Solomon Fuller was raised in a family with servants and had a personal servant as constant companion and bodyguard until he came to the United States.

Reviewing the course of his life four years prior to his death, Dr. Fuller said, "There are many things which influence a man's life...and I guess that my grandfather was quite significant in mine."

Information about Fuller's mother is being researched. It is known that she came from an educated family and was apparently well educated herself. She had a vibrant interest in acquiring knowledge, and especially in seeking education for her children. Fuller visited her once after coming to America; this was in 1904. They maintained a correspondence over the years until her death in 1921.

The Fullers lived on Ashman Street in Monrovia, Liberia, when Solomon Fuller started school at age five. Three years later, in 1880, they moved twelve miles up river to Calwell. Schooling was continued through lessons taught by Solomon's mother, who not only had mastered the basic learning skills, but also was competent in Latin. A year or so later, when Solomon was approximately nine or ten, he and his brother were enrolled in a small private school which was directed by a West Indian Episcopal missionary minister, Mr. Gibson. This was a positive experience but also the source of later disillusionment. While attending the school, Solomon went to church services regularly. He was enthralled by reports about the United States, the opportunities for education and growth, and the various freedoms that purportedly existed there. When he later arrived in this country and witnessed as well as experienced discrimination and racism even in the church practices, he severed his connection with the church except for conversations he had with various clergymen whom he knew socially or professionally. Indeed, he was unhappy with his sons' involvement in the church and church activities. He urged them to carefully analyze and consider the words and then the actual facts.

When Solomon was in his tenth year he was sent to Monrovia so he could get a better education at the College Preparatory School of Monrovia. He distinguished himself academically and at sixteen was enrolled in the subfreshman class of the school. A good example of his interests lies in the following anecdote. He reported that when he was to be punished, the instructor or headmaster would send him to his room to complete a specified number of pages of Latin, unaware that this gave young Fuller the opportunity to engage in something he enjoyed. He stated that he was reading Caesar's *Gallic Wars* in Latin at age ten. His study of Latin was an interest he pursued throughout his lifetime.

Near March of his subfreshman year, Solomon's father died; the details of his death are unknown. Three months later, in June 1889, Solomon was sent to the United States to gain further education at Livingstone College, Salisbury, North Carolina, from which he graduated in 1893 with a bachelor of arts degree. His memories and stories about the college as recalled by family and friends were very positive except for the racial problems. His academic performance was one of continued excellence; he was named class speaker, and salutatorian, and graduated with honors. Although he had no particular athletic skills, his interest was shown in his management of the football team. He received minimal or no financial support from his mother while in college and met his obligations by working in the printing office of the Livingstone College Press as a typesetter. This was a busy job, for the press was responsible for the publication of the A.M.E. Zion Church newspaper.

Medicine was a discipline which first of all required scholarship in Latin; Dr. Fuller was a Latin and Greek scholar. He was directed into medicine because it had been the profession of his maternal grandfather and thus a discipline to which he became attracted early in childhood. In 1894 he enrolled in the Long Island College Hospital Medical College, where he remained until March of that year when he transferred to Boston University Medical School. Here again, his seeking admission caused him some traumatic memories. He reported that he was offered entrance into the school with financial aid if he would agree to return to Africa as a medical missionary following graduation. He refused; yet his forthright statement that he would not accept or promise to follow such an agreement gained him entrance into the school, but without financial aid.

While a medical student he drew the attention of Dr. Edward P. Colby, a professor of neurology, who was impressed by Solomon Fuller's understanding and seeming facility for work in this specialty. Following Fuller's graduation in 1897, Dr. Colby arranged for him to meet Dr. George Adams. This was a fortunate event, for Fuller did not have a job and was trying to determine where he would go and what he would do to advance a medical career.

Dr. Adams was the superintendent of Westborough State Hospital. He offered Dr. Fuller two choices: he could come to the hospital and work as an intern for a three to six month period without pay, or he could come to the hospital, work as an intern, and also be an official helper in the developing pathology laboratory. The laboratory was then run by Dr. Edward L. Mellis. Dr. Fuller would receive board, lodging, laundry, and twenty dollars per month.

The decision was not as easy as it would appear. The first offer held unwritten and unspoken understanding that successful completion of a short internship would lead to the opportunity of progressing to a permanent staff position if, in Dr. Fuller's words, "one were an ordinary person."[2] It can easily be seen that this first offer appealed to Fuller, who realized that in intellectual competence he was more than a little capable. It also appealed to his spirit of meeting a challenge and gaining a position on the basis of his merit. This opportunity and his ideals were of necessity thwarted because of the realization that he was not "ordinary" and thus could not hope for full advancement on the basis of competence.

His decision to accept the second offer was influenced by many factors. His early training in classics and his knowledge of significant historical figures in medicine had fostered the spirit of using observation and reason as a means of gaining answers and advancing scientific knowledge. There was the challenge of working in a new and developing field where he could exercise his old habits of reading, reflecting, searching, and associating in a scholarly way. A third factor was that by the mid-nineteenth century medicine was incorporating physics, chemistry, and psychology in an effort to explain disordered behavior in terms of disrupted nervous structure and function. Virchow had published his paper, *Omninus Cellula e Cellula*, which suggested that all pathology could be understood in terms of cellular disease. Medical science in the last half of the nineteenth century, as Selesnick and Alexander said, "was devoted to intensive study of pathological anatomy and biochemical investigations were carried on by men of great acumen."[3] Wernicke equated "the analysis of emotional disorders with descriptions of the neurological conditions."[4]

Perhaps the most immediate conscious determinant was Solomon Fuller's attendance at the fiftieth annual meeting of the American Medico-Psychological Association, where the noted neurologist S. Weir Mitchell was the keynote speaker. Indeed, Fuller later attributed his interest in pursuing a career in neuropathology and psychiatry to this address. Mitchell took the hospitals to task for not actually doing anything in the study of mental disease or the advancement of knowledge pertaining to it. He characterized the hospitals as custodial institutions without laboratories or facilities for scientific approaches.

Mitchell raised many questions and made many recommendations that today would be regarded as commonplace. Included in his list of faults and needs were: the need for residents; the need for teaching young nurses facts about mental illness, with the suggestion that young doctors be utilized as the teachers; the inclusion of training schools in mental hospitals; the incorporation of psychology and neurology in preparing doctors for the field of psychiatry; the removal of restraints in mental hospitals; the need for a more aesthetic environment; initiation of a process that would encourage and demand the development of original research by medical staff; and greater awareness of the influence of heredity, marriage, physical locations and environment, social pressures, and race on mental illness.

Perhaps his strongest attack, or at least the one that attracted and fixed Fuller's attention, was the following:

> The question we ask at starting is if you, who are so powerful within these alien camps, are really doing all that might be done without serious

> increase of expenditure. Frankly speaking, we do not believe that you are so working these hospitals as to keep treatment or scientific precedent on the first line of medical advance...Where, we ask, are your annual reports of scientific study, of the psychology and pathology of your patients? They should be published apart...Believe me, the best hospitals of any kind are those where the most precise scientific work is done. There the treatment becomes accurate, the results best.[5]

It is reported that some were enthusiastic over Dr. Mitchell's remarks and reacted by establishing or setting in motion procedures that would lead to the development of scientific laboratories. Westborough State Hospital, which had been established in 1886, did not have a pathology laboratory at the time of the speech in May 1894. By 1897 there was a change. In the Thirteenth Annual Report of the Trustees of Westborough Insane Hospital, which described operations of the hospital for the calendar year 1897, there appeared the following paragraphs:

Pathology

> Dr. E.L. Mellis was appointed as pathologist to the hospital in March, and at once began to make microscopic examination of the effects of mental disease upon the cortex of the brain, and continued this special work until September 28, when he resigned to accept a position at the Johns Hopkins Hospital in Baltimore.
>
> Work in another department of pathology has been furthered by the appointment of an interne, whose whole time is given to the examination of pathological conditions in the living, taking up the work in this direction heretofore done by the assistant physicians; to which has been added, since April first, the examination of the blood of each patient admitted. While not expecting immediate results from the blood examinations, it is hoped that when a large number of cases have been collected they may be tabulated, and perhaps lead to valuable conclusions. Some interesting phenomena have already been observed, which, if verified later, will be given to the public.[6]

As these paragraphs indicate, Fuller worked with Mellis for less than a year before he was left with the responsibility of continuing the work and developing what became the neuropathology department. He accepted the challenge with a realistic humility and an awareness of and interest in its potential.

The first feeling, that of humility, was reflected in his statement that "there was no one more conscious of his inadequacy for the job than myself."[7] Nevertheless, Dr. Fuller determined to prepare himself for the work and attacked it with an uncompromising diligence. He also realized the newness of the field, and apparently was intrigued by this fact and by his being one of the pioneers. "It was a time when it was popular to explore things in this area [neuropathology] and I was one to begin."[8] His overriding feeling was that through the laboratory some answers would be found to help supply knowledge about mental illness.

Dr. Adams was interested in developing the neuropathology laboratory of the hospital and in the next few years supported the growth of the physical facilities. His remarks in the annual reports to the trustees and to the state indicate his concern that appropriate attention be given to the role of neuropathology and the work of Dr. Fuller in developing this specialty. In the report for 1898 he wrote, "Dr. S.C. Fuller has been appointed pathologist to the hospital, and I call your attention to this report and the statistical table showing in condensed form the results of his work,"[9]—a not particularly notable statement, except that the report included his formal six-page pathologist's report, the longest section in the entire annual report, as well as a three-page paragraph elsewhere in the report also describing his other work and discoveries.[10]

To illustrate: the report contained statistics giving the precise number of laboratory procedures of various types and some of their results; it also gave an indication of his attempts to find significant data that might correlate with clinical syndromes. For example, he collected and analyzed laboratory results on patients with diagnoses of mania, paranoia, melancholia, and pernicious anemia (diseases common in the Westborough census) to see if there were any significant indications of differences that should be explored. He looked for any possible influence of diabetes on mental illness. Finally he noted and began to study carefully the urine of morphine and opium addicts to see if there were any signs of the addiction that might be pathognomonic. He did find some crystals in the urine of morphine addicts, wrote up his results, and initiated a research project with Dr. John P. Sutherland, professor of anatomy at Boston University, to further explore his findings.

Dr. Fuller's budding interest in brain anatomy and pathology was evidenced in remarks and laboratory notes of what he observed in various patients as he studied and compared the circle of Willis. Within a few years he enlarged upon this subject considerably. Of note was the following quotation:

> In the way of histological investigation of the brain not much has

> been done, most of the time having been given to cases not yet fatal. More of this is hoped to be done later, as we recognize that such investigation will help much to give a better idea of the pathology of mental disease.[11]

Two years later, he expanded upon this idea, indicated the inclusion of the laboratory tests as part of hospital procedure, and revealed his hope:

> During the year just completed the greater portion of the time has been devoted to work of a purely clinical nature. The improved facilities for work of this character has made the laboratory more than ever an adjunct to the ward work of the clinical physicians. If for no other reason than this, I think the laboratory justifies its raison d'être. Work in the line of research is certainly to be desired. It is in this way a better knowledge of the causes that operate against mental equilibrium is largely to be acquired—an acquisition which eventually must have a salutary effect on the body politic, and result either in a diminution proportionately of insanity or lead to effective measures of prophylaxis in many cases. I regret no work in the line of pure research has been done this year.[12]

Although Solomon Fuller's work was drawing positive critical acclaim, providing mental stimulation and excitement, he was plagued by the knowledge of inadequate financial compensation for his work, an inadequacy resulting from racial prejudice. He was pathologist for the hospital and worked under that title, assuming the full responsibilities of the job. His salary was twenty-five dollars per month. After requesting an increase a year later, he was offered only five dollars per month more. This offer was made more bitter by the knowledge that another physician, who had joined the staff a year later than he and held a lesser rank, was started at a salary twenty dollars higher than his proposed salary after the raise. His initial reaction was to quit the job and he indeed offered Dr. Adams his resignation. The latter refused to accept it and asked Fuller not to leave the hospital. Adams suggested that if Fuller remained in the neurological and pathological laboratories he would be in an area of medicine where he might encounter least resistance and have the best chance for advancement. Fuller realized the truth of this statement and did not resign. Neither did he accept the salary increase; he asked that his salary remain at the same level, but that he be given two working days off in lieu of the pay raise. The trustees accepted this offer. The next year, 1899, he was offered a salary of $800 per annum, including six weeks' leave, provided he would agree to remain with the hospital for at least a year. Fuller remained at Westborough State Hospital until 1919 as the chief pathologist, receiving more appropriate increments in salary through the years.

The year 1900 found Dr. Fuller remarking that a museum should be planned to "illustrate the not infrequent association of physical disease with mental disturbance." This was also the year he went to the Carnegie Laboratories in New York to take advanced courses in pathology and study with Dr. Edward K. Dunham in histopathology. He later recalled this as a rich experience which provided a more than adequate source of study material. He spent some of his time studying at Bellevue.

At the end of this study he returned to Westborough Hospital, remaining until 1904, when he took a leave of absence to enroll and study at the University of Munich. It was on this trip to Europe that he routed himself through Africa to visit his mother, whom he had not seen since his departure for America in 1889. It was the last time he saw her.

In the hospital's annual report for 1901, following Dr. Fuller's return from the Carnegie Laboratories, Dr. Adams wrote:

> Better accommodations are required for the pathologist. His work has been done under serious disadvantages, but in spite of this fact, many important results have already been obtained.[13]

In that same report Fuller mentioned that he was publishing a paper in the *New England Medical Gazette*. The following year, 1902, he introduced the hospital and trustees to one of his inventions in the following remarks:

> It has always been our object to keep full records of all specimens which have come to the laboratory. This year, with the aid of a simple apparatus constructed from odds and ends, the microscopical records have been enhanced by the introduction of the photomicrograph.[14]

In this characteristically modest way Solomon Fuller described a simple apparatus which was essentially a method he had invented for making photomicrographs of slides. He also reported that he had completed two more papers for publication.

By 1903 he was anxious to "introduce" studies in physiological chemistry as a means of learning the etiology of certain psychiatric disorders. The visit to Germany, which began in 1904, was one of his most pleasant memories and was marred only by his having the flu upon arrival. Even then, the treatment he received, the open hospitality and concern that he experienced quickly counteracted his disappointment over his ill health.

He was initially interviewed by Emil Kraepelin, was later taken on a tour of his laboratory and clinic, and while in Munich enjoyed conversation at Kraepelin's home. Fuller was impressed by Kraepelin's command of English. Although he described him as a "distant, entirely impersonal man," Fuller must have made a positive impression on Kraepelin to receive a card to attend his lectures. While he was enrolled at the institute and studying under Kraepelin, he took courses in general pathology from Professor Otto von Bollinger, and on the spinal cord from Dr. Schmaus. Dr. Schmaus noted Fuller's interest in brain pathology, and by working with him became sufficiently impressed to refer him to Alois Alzheimer.

When Fuller visited Alzheimer in Frankfurt, he had worked for some time in Kraepelin's institute; thus he was not initially anxious over the interview. He reported, however, that when he walked into the reception room, already full of young applicants wanting to study and work with Alzheimer, his anxiety grew as he realized he was the last person to be seen and he repeatedly heard Alzheimer tell applicants, "Nicht reif genug" (not ripe enough). His experiences at the Carnegie, his ability to cut and mount brain sections, his capability as verified at the institute in Munich, and finally his interview resulted in his acceptance as one of five students. He found Alzheimer "a delightful, sweet, warm, unassuming, most unassuming man...the poorest lecturer I ever heard at the clinic but excellent when conferring at the microscope." He found his study with him "the most productive period insofar as learning about techniques and the structure of the cortex that I ever had."[15] He worked with him for most of an academic year. As a result of his work there he later published his work on Alzheimer's disease in English. Fuller commented years later that although Betts at Buffalo had published a paper, he had "missed the most characteristic features" of the disease.

While studying with Alzheimer, Fuller visited Weigert at his laboratory, where he met and became friends with Ludwig Edinger who later encouraged him to publish. Before leaving Germany Fuller visited with Paul Ehrlich. As a result of that visit he agreed to bring some mice, which Ehrlich had infected with tumor cells, back to the United States where they would be studied by Dr. William T. Councilman at Harvard Medical School. In Fuller's papers there are letters from Ehrlich which indicate his appreciation and also anxiety about the transport.

The trip to Europe and the groups of people Fuller chose to acquaint himself with certainly give some indication of where his interests lay and what he felt was worth exploring. It should not be overlooked that in studying under Kraepelin he selected a person who was in some circles known as the head of Imperial German Psychiatry because of the marked respect accorded him and his insistence on order, authority, and organization. We should also not fail to observe that both men believed in the importance of detailed observation, careful description, and an organic approach to understanding mental illness.

While Fuller was studying in Europe, action was being taken on plans he had helped to draw for a new pathology laboratory. The annual report of the hospital for 1905 included these paragraphs:

> Dr. S.C. Fuller, our pathologist, was absent from the hospital from November 1904, to August 1905, going to Munich, Germany, and having an opportunity, while there, of studying under Kraepelin. He returns to the hospital with well-earned knowledge and increased interest in his work...
>
> We note with special satisfaction that the new pathological building is nearly completed, and we feel that it will be of great service to the hospital. The pathological work for some years has been of a high order, and has deserved better accommodations than any previously furnished; and the new building, with the work rooms it contains, will make possible still better work, both of a routine nature and also original investigation into new and unknown fields of medicine.[16]

And cryptically in 1906 George Adams noted: "Building complete and Solomon C. Fuller moving in."[17]

That same year Fuller reported on studies he had conducted in 1902 and 1903 on histological changes after the administration of belladonna. The next few years witnessed the writing of papers dealing either with neuropathology or with clinical neurology. In 1912 he edited a book of fifteen chapters, several of which were written by him. The purpose of this book was to honor George Adams. From 1901 to 1929 Fuller published regularly.

When he left Westborough Insane Hospital in 1919 he did so to devote more time to teaching at Boston University. He had been teaching there for several years: in 1899 he was instructor in pathology; in 1909, instructor in neurology; in 1914, lecturer in neurology; in 1919, associate professor of neuropathology; in 1921, associate professor of neurology; and in 1933 he retired as professor emeritus of neurology. His experience in the academic world held the same limitations as the clinical. This was an issue that perpetually depressed, angered, and frustrated him. He was embittered that both full academic status and financial compensation were limited by the color of his skin.

Besides the influence history had in shaping Solomon Fuller's professional career and contributions, of further interest is the influence he had on medicine, most particularly on psychiatry, and to the nonprofessional factors in his life.

He took an organic approach to studying and trying to identify the physical and chemical factors that influenced or had some role in mental illness. Much of this work was represented in the papers he published. Another dimension of his life, that of the clinical neurologist and neuropathologist, was exemplified by his appointments: for twenty-three years as consultant at Westborough State Hospital after he resigned as pathologist; for eleven years as visiting neurologist at Massachusetts Memorial Hospital; for ten years as consultant neurologist at Massachusetts General Hospital; as consultant at Framingham Marlboro Hospital and the Allentown, Pennsylvania, State Hospital; and as a court psychiatrist in later years. Concurrently with his duties as pathologist at Westborough State Hospital he served as director of the Clinical Society Commission of Massachusetts.

He maintained a lively interest in the advent and growth of the psychoanalytic movement. He read papers pertaining to this field, discussed its development with contemporaries, and eagerly attended Freud's lectures at Clark University. In fact, one of the now famous and familiar photographs of Freud, G. Stanley Hall, and others standing in front of Clark during the time of the lectures includes Fuller. According to one of his colleagues, Fuller had definite questions he wanted to explore with Freud while he was here, but it is unclear whether he did so.[18] Through the years he continued to read and follow developments in psychoanalysis, but never felt he wanted to subscribe to it personally. Not surprisingly, he viewed it as a tool which should be refined for understanding behavior and emotional disturbances, but not as a theory that should necessarily become doctrine.

His other legacy to the field of psychiatry resulted from his training and teaching roles. Prominent men he took under his personal tutelage were Winfred Overholser, George Branche, Simon Johnson, Drew King, and Karl Menninger. The first went on to become the superintendent of St. Elizabeth's Hospital in Washington, D.C. Branche, Johnson, and King were instrumental in providing the means by which black physicians became psychiatrists.

When the government was establishing the Veterans Administration Hospital at Tuskegee, Alabama, in 1923, Dr. Fuller was asked by General Frank T. Hines to accept a staff position and develop a neuropsychiatric unit at the hospital, but he declined. He was approached twice more, and his response again was that he could not accept the offer but that he would see what he could do to help achieve the goal. He then gathered together Drs. Branche, Johnson, and King in a kind of training group. He became responsible for their grasp and knowledge of neurology and psychiatry, and he arranged for some additional psychiatric training under Dr. Sutherland. In later years, these men would often recall not only the instruction they received from Fuller and Sutherland, but also the group experience with Fuller and the positive influence he exerted. This influence later helped them to establish and develop the new department, to understand and be better able to meet confrontations from Dr. Fuller himself, and to act effectively as a group at Tuskegee. Most significant, because of Fuller's work and knowledge about syphilis, these men had the tools that permitted them to accurately diagnose black World War I veterans who had been diagnosed previously as having behavioral disorders or being bad conduct cases.

Thus, Solomon Fuller is particularly remembered and appreciated by many black psychiatrists for providing a means for others to enter the field, his emphasis on approaching and trying to understand situations with an open mind, his concern to be thorough and to obtain as many facts as possible, to gather and use the knowledge of many fields which might contribute to the understanding of a problem, and not to overvalue or become so indoctrinated in any one process to the extent that it would lead to the exclusion of facts or ideas from other schools of thought. Doubtless, to achieve this goal, careful collection and organization of data and thoughts are essential. Because of Fuller's belief in as well as practice of these principles, he has served as an inspirational model.

Dr. Fuller's nonpsychiatric influence was evident in the circle of people who actively sought his friendship, advice, and counsel. They were a group who represented all professions, ethnic groups, and economic levels, and in whom he could find some kernel to relate to, irrespective of background. In fairness it must be admitted that, although he could get on well with all persons, he doted on a stimulating intellectual environment. Some of his close friends, who were either frequent guests or sometimes house guests, were Alaine Locke, Harold Fey (whom he helped in his early experiments to establish sonar devices that were later developed into radar by the Raytheon Company), W.E.B. DuBois, Phillips Brooks, Harold Burleigh, James Faulkner, William Augustus Hinton, Charles Drew, and Charles Pinderhughes. I do not mean to suggest that his friends were only famous persons, for he also was sought out by and entertained undergraduates, and directors and members of college choruses on tour from Johnson C. Smith College, Fisk University, and elsewhere.

The segment of Solomon Fuller's life which I have not touched upon is the private one. In 1909 he married Meta Vaux Warrick, a talented sculptress whose artistic ability drew critical praise in her native Philadelphia. Because of her talent she was urged to go to Paris following her graduation in 1899 from the Philadelphia School of Industrial Arts. While in Paris she studied under St. Gaudins, Collarosia, Rolland, and finally Rodin. Rodin was sufficiently impressed to help her arrange a one-woman show in Paris which drew notices in New York papers and later commissions. She remained in Paris for three years before returning to the United States. In 1907 she was commissioned to do a large piece for the Jamestown Exposition which commemorated the landing of the settlers in 1607.

Following her marriage in 1909 she retired from the art world to raise her family, but was called out of retirement to do pieces for the anniversary of the Emancipation Proclamation, the Atlanta YMCA, and the Making of America Exposition in 1921. Over the years she continued to sculpt at the studio that she built at Larned's Pond, a short distance from the Fullers' home in Framingham, Massachusetts.

The Fullers had three sons, all of whom live in the Boston area. One is an executive with the United Community Services, another a broker, and the third a businessman. They remember their home as a beehive of intellectual activity, culture, and entertainment. Entertainment in the home was very formal; it reflected both parents' culturally rich early years, and involved some degree of ceremony. Less formal activity occurred at their mother's studio, which was large enough for small theater groups to meet and perform.

Friends and students describe Solomon Fuller as a remarkable man, unusually professional in bearing and approach, a man who was a neuropsychiatrist. He presented himself as having mastered psychoanalysis, but as being interested in French. In 1942 he lost his sight but continued to study through "talking books."

There are areas I have not touched upon, some because they do not have particular relevance in the present context, others because factual data are still being gathered, and still others because substantiating material is seemingly not yet available. For example, Fuller had a long and close relationship with G. Stanley Hall. His sons have related that Hall later became a patient, and as a consequence, Dr. Fuller never would discuss him.

As I think of his devotion to completeness I am reminded of his hobbies. One was photography—a process of looking at life. Another, as he grew older, was bookbinding. So in the course of his life he set print, wrote content, and finally bound the books.

References

[1] *Journal of the American Medical Association, 151* (1953), 1122.

[2] Tape recording of Dr. Fuller.

[3] Sheldon T. Selesnick and Franz G. Alexander. *The History of Psychiatry* (New York: Harper and Row, 1966), p. 154.

[4] *Ibid.*, p. 158.

[5] *Proceedings of the American Medico-Psychological Association, 1* (1894), 108, 116.

[6] Thirteenth Annual Report of the Trustees of Westborough Insane Hospital for the year ending September 30, 1898, p. 16.

[7] Tape recording of Dr. Fuller.

[8] *Ibid.*

[9] Fourteenth Annual Report of the Trustees of Westborough Insane Hospital for the year ending September 30, 1898, p. 16.

[10] *Ibid.*, pp. 20–25, 13.

[11] *Ibid.*, p. 25.

[12] Sixteenth Annual Report of the Trustees of Westborough Insane Hospital for the year ending September 30, 1900, p. 16.

[13] Seventeenth Annual Report of the Trustees of Westborough Insane Hospital for the year ending September 30, 1901, p. 9.

[14] Eighteenth Annual Report of the Trustees of Westborough Insane Hospital for the year ending September 30, 1902, p. 18.

[15] Tape recording of Dr. Fuller.

[16] Twenty-first Annual Report of the Trustees of Westborough Insane Hospital for the year ending September 30, 1905, pp. 16, 17.

[17] Notebook of George S. Adams, Westborough Insane Hospital Library.

[18] Charles A. Pinderhughes, personal communication.

Boston Psychiatry in the 1920s—Looking Forward

JOHN C. BURNHAM

The history of psychiatry in Boston involves not only specific persons but also the changing nature of the community and the changing place of Boston in American life. The men and women who practiced medicine could escape from neither and reflected both. In the opening years of the twentieth century, Boston was clearly the most exciting location in American psychiatry. By the 1920s only a legacy was left—but it was a significant and lasting one. Boston lost its stature as the citadel of psychiatry, and yet the city exported both ideas and personnel to newer centers of activity.

Once at the very center of the national establishment, by the 1920s Bostonians were vying for a share in the funding, power, and recognition that created the modern American industrial, scientific, medical, and intellectual complex. Any number of symptoms betrayed the changing status. Early in the new century, for instance, *The North American Review* was no longer effectively maintaining its former prestige against a host of magazines based in Manhattan. By the time of the opening of the foundation era in the twenties, Boston's scientists, too, were often crowded out in the struggle for backing that meant so much then to medical endeavors. In psychiatry and neurology specifically, many Bostonians began to feel that they were following, not leading.[1] Except for the remarkable progress and prosperity of other American cities, the reasons for the decline in Boston of psychiatry specifically are still elusive. Particular institutions and general style both throw some light on the shifts that were taking place and on their national significance.

The psychiatric community of Boston was relatively well defined. Massachusetts and Boston were each heavily represented in the American Psychiatric Association (and its predecessor, the American Medico-Psychological Association)—in 1923, 137 out of its 1,093 members, one-eighth, were residents of the state, and an additional twelve were from the often affiliated area of Rhode Island. As in other parts of the country, the specialty of neurology largely overlapped that of psychiatry, particularly in outpatient practice. At the beginning of the century, nervous and mental diseases were very often lumped together, most typically for teaching purposes and in professional groups—specifically, in Boston, the Boston Society of Psychiatry and Neurology.

Two types of institutions gave a more refined identity to psychiatric practice—the medical schools and the hospitals. The hospitals were of two varities, proprietary and public. In the Boston area the proprietary-hospital psychiatrists were very prominent, especially earlier in the century.[2] Moreover, by the 1920s a strikingly large proportion of Boston-area psychiatrists were in private practice of some sort.

This dominance of private practitioners could not but have adverse effects upon institutional psychiatry, and the various hospitals in the area showed a record of fluctuating fortunes, with some years productive and inspiring and others when funds and talent and initiative ran short. Much of the best evidence we have of what happened to Boston psychiatry is to be found in histories of the three major medical schools, Harvard, Tufts, and Boston universities. Except for Morton Prince's early instruction in "psycho-therapeutics" at Tufts and Alberta Boomhower-Guibord's pioneer course in psychopathology and psychoanalysis at Boston University, during the earlier decades of the twentieth century neither Tufts nor Boston University offered any appreciable deviation from the national pattern of minimal instruction in nervous and mental diseases. Harvard Medical School, however, was tied particularly closely to the Boston elite, and, in addition, was affiliated with a university that by about 1910 clearly had become the premier institution of higher education in the United States. Harvard psychiatry therefore demands the most particular attention.

Until about 1920, Boston and Harvard produced a series of leaders in American psychiatry; perhaps this was why contemporaries seemed to sense that after World War I the psychiatric profession in the city languished, and that training at Harvard left both the medical school and the city behind the times, at least compared with the great days of the 1900s and 1910s. City and medical school are hard to separate, and it is perhaps not profitable to do so; nor should psychiatry be separated from the general history of the medical school, where all of the specialties were finding it difficult in the 1920s to maintain premier or even good status.[3] Psychiatry, however, need not have declined as precipitously as it did, even though the great days could not be maintained forever.

Psychotherapy, the first great advance over therapeutic nihilism in neurology and psychiatry, had made its way into America primarily by way of Boston. Not only did Morton Prince introduce his own variety, but Boston physicians in person welcomed both Janet in 1904 and 1906 and Freud in 1909. Harvard had reached out to McLean Hospital for prestigious clinical lecturers on mental diseases, most notably Edward Cowles, and the city felt the presence at Worcester State Hospital of Adolf Meyer from 1894 to 1902, with his adaptations of Kraepelin and his emphasis upon individualized cases. Within the city and on the Harvard faculty, James Jackson Putnam gave leadership to neurology and, later, to psychoanalysis. In addition to these stars, a number of other figures provided formidable substance to the study, practice, and teaching of psychiatry and neurology.[4]

One person who deserves particular mention is Elmer Ernest Southard.[5] As the young director of the innovative Boston Psychopathic Hospital and soon chief professor at Harvard of courses dealing with neurology and psychiatry—as well as a stunningly brilliant man—Southard exerted a dominating influence for some years. His secret was largely his personality. In his research, he was an extreme adherent of organicism, and his investigations were never fruitful, except for small, specific contributions. He concentrated many resources just after World War I, for example, on neurosyphilis, expecting a large upsurge in the disease such as followed the Franco-Prussian War, but he missed the payoff he anticipated.[6] As a teacher, he was conservative and conventional in his lectures.[7] Yet he inspired a generation of first-rate physicians to enter the field of psychiatry, apparently through his open-mindedness. For instance, although he attacked Freudianism repeatedly, he very early had a psychoanalyst on his staff and welcomed a great diversity of other viewpoints—with most of which he disagreed.

Southard and Cowles died in 1920, and Putnam before them in 1918. Another extremely influential Bostonian, the expert on mental deficiency, Walter Fernald, died in 1924. Boston psychiatry never recovered from these deaths. During a series of administrative changes that emphasized the schism between neurology and psychiatry, the new head of the Boston Psychopathic Hospital, C. Macfie Campbell, became professor of psychiatry at Harvard. Campbell, a Scot who had been second in command to Adolf Meyer at Baltimore, had the best credentials and was known to be friendly to psychoanalysis. He turned out, however, to be an uninspiring and sarcastic teacher. (The only graduates from Harvard Medical School for some years after World War I who became very well-known among psychiatrists were William Herman, Tracy Putnam, and

Bronson Crothers—a very slim list compared with the galaxy of leaders graduated in earlier days and with the numbers of Harvard undergraduates who went on to medical school and fame elsewhere.) As head of the Psychopathic, Campbell was extremely conservative and resisted the kinds of change that were taking place elsewhere.[8]

Surprisingly, others in Boston similarly moved away from psychotherapy and toward a type of rigid organicism that also suggested a general conservatism. Bostonians, for instance, were conspicuous in the movement to boycott Smith Ely Jelliffe's *Journal of Nervous and Mental Disease*, which had some psychoanalytic content, by founding the *Archives of Neurology and Psychiatry*. The local psychiatrists even explicitly voted down an effort to soften the blow against Jelliffe.[9] Others changed stances, as Campbell apparently did. A better example than he is Abraham Myerson, whose biography has long been needed. Myerson left Harvard to take a position in neurology and neuropathology at Tufts, becoming a professor in 1925. In consonance with his title, he apparently dropped his earlier strong interest in environmentalism and became organically oriented. This shift obscured his originality of mind, and he lost some of his national visibility; only recently has his pioneer work in psychopharmaceutics in the 1930s come to be fully recognized.[10]

By and large, then, there were only isolated areas of some excitement and innovation in the city's psychiatric community after 1920, and often little encouragement for the enthusiasts and innovators. Eventually the arrival of a number of Europeans in the 1930s led to a rekindling of innovation and enthusiasm in both psychotherapeutics and organic psychiatry in Boston, evidence of the continuing potential of the community to be both entrepôt for foreign ideas and a research center.[11] But after World War I, outside of the most conventional neurology, first-raters tended to be replaced by second-raters, freshness of outlook tended to wither, and many young people left to go to New York or other localities with stimulating atmospheres.[12] Indeed, one of the persistent laments of mental health leaders in Massachusetts was that their trained personnel were constantly being lured away to positions outside the state.[13]

There persisted in Boston, however, a spirit that transcended the persons and institutions involved in the practice of psychiatry, and many of those who left the city took that spirit with them. The tradition showed up best in the mental hygiene movement and was described even before the war by Southard:

> Particularly in America, it would seem, should the range of psychia-

> try advance from a medical to a medicosocial range; for particularly in America has the spirit of sociology been caught concretely in the shape of social service and its prophylactic branches, sex-hygiene, eugenics, mental hygiene, and the like.
>
> Since Boston is a hotbed of medicosocial interests (witness, to pick two examples, the Massachusetts General Hospital center with Dr. Richard Cabot and Miss Ida Cannon, and the Boston Dispensary center with its Director, Michael Davis), work cannot fail to be stimulated in these directions in the psychopathic hospital and particularly in its out-patient and after-care services.[14]

What Boston had, then, was social institutions and a social milieu that fostered cooperation of psychiatrists with other professionals, not only expert medical consultants but more typically psychologists and social workers, in a community effort to foster the mental health of individuals. This community support, for example, had been crucial in the decision of the founder of child guidance, William Healy, to come to Boston. Moreover, the cooperation between social agencies that could support psychiatric services was built into the social fabric of the city. As a contemporary observer said, "A gathering of the clans at tea time, lunch, or dinner"—Lees, Cabots, Jacksons, Lowells, Putnams, Higginsons—"could resolve itself into a council of social agencies." Nowhere else was the coordination of psychiatrist and community so well developed and institutionalized. Southard and social worker Mary C. Jarrett described their contribution at the time: "We claim no novelty or originality for the social work of the Psychopathic Hospital, but rather we would claim to have created the part that the social worker is to play in the mental hygiene movement and to have given it a name—psychiatric social work."[15]

Although Bostonians, except for William James, were not deeply involved in the founding of the mental hygiene movement (the movement at one point, in the early years, was dominated by the so-called Yale group), they quickly became its leaders. Frankwood W. Williams, for example, moved from being medical director of the Massachusetts Mental Hygiene Association to direct the national organization in the 1920s. In that same period the mental hygiene movement seemed to absorb most of the interest of Campbell at the Psychopathic and at Harvard, and it was of extreme importance in the careers of some of the more prominent newcomers, such as James V. May, who became superintendent of Boston State Hospital in 1917. In a time when psychotherapy was not flourishing as before the war, neither were prevention and a search for causation inappropriate preoccupations for a psychiatry in which there was available precious little therapy.[16]

What Boston had to offer to mental hygiene was the team concept. Most typically formulated by Healy at the Judge Baker Foundation for children, the system was based on individual case reports and discussion by a psychiatrist, a psychologist, and a social worker. Healy patterned his case conferences after those of Richard Cabot at the Harvard Medical School, which were afterward reported in the *Boston Medical and Surgical Journal.* (Healy of course had to do without the pathologist's report that crowned Cabot's case conferences.) Southard's noon staff meetings at the Psychopathic Hospital, in which laboratory technicians and nurses participated with psychologists and social workers as well as with medical personnel, may have been another inspiration. But, in either case, Boston was the source of the idea of a psychiatric team.[17]

The team concept provided American psychiatry with great resilience. Whoever new came along—endocrine specialists, dieticians, shock therapists, psychoanalysts of several varieties—could simply be added to the team without displacing the neurologist or psychiatrist or someone else.

The mental hygiene movement affected all of American psychiatry. It was Thomas W. Salmon and his colleagues in mental hygiene, many from Boston, who in World War I got neuropsychiatry, as it was then called, instituted as a major element in U.S. military medicine and who continued after the war and the shell shock sensation to suggest effectively to the American public the importance of neuropsychiatry (a specialty that turned out in practice to be mostly psychiatry.) In the postwar era mental hygiene was fundamentally characterized by the team concept, exported from Boston. As Bronson Crothers at Harvard put the case in 1932:

> It seems clear to me that one of the most urgent problems facing the pediatrician today is that of intelligent team play. The child guidance movement, chaotic as it is, ought to be studied by pediatricians. Unless doctors in general cooperate they will find that parents and teachers are looking to them in case of physical disorders and to another group for advice on "emotional" disturbances.[18]

Particularly conspicuous also in the methodology of the mental health movement in the 1920s was an emphasis upon the child, reflected, for example, in the founding of the American Orthopsychiatric Association. Again, Boston took a leading position, particularly with Healy, although many others, such as Crothers, reflected this interest, in large part because it was consonant with the social interests of Boston medicine in general. The post-World War I rise of the intelligence test fitted in with an existing preoccupation of some of the local prominent families and established physicians with mental deficiency, and the key figure, Walter Fernald, was not only the leader in the field, but quite powerful in the Boston psychiatric community. The emphasis upon children was reinforced everywhere, of course, by the effective influence of psychoanalysis and then of dynamic psychiatry in focusing upon genetic factors in personality formation and mental disease.[19]

The mental hygiene approach and the team concept did have disadvantages and hazards. Much energy, for example, that in later years appeared grossly disproportionate, went into the study of the psychological well-being of a very small sector of society, college students. In this not-very-fruitful endeavor Bostonians were once more major movers. More particularly, the team concept tended to break down the barriers between the physician and the paraprofessional personnel, in fact encouraging lay competition with psychiatrists. As Paul E. Bowers of Los Angeles recalled at the end of the decade:

> While attending clinical lectures at the Boston State Psychopathic Hospital in 1922, I frequently heard the professors of psychiatry and members of the staff caution the social workers at this institution not to make diagnoses of mental cases when they were compiling or reading their sociological reports. On many occasions I have heard social workers making diagnoses of psychiatric cases in other institutions and at various clinics...In other words, the practice of labeling mental cases by unqualified persons is quite a common one.[20]

On the whole, however, Boston physicians were less upset about incursions into the medical domain than their colleagues elsewhere, and it was this respect for other professionals that left them flexibility and, in particular, exposed them sooner to influences not strictly medical.

The bulk of Boston's psychiatric practitioners did not themselves change remarkably from the generally (and relatively) conservative-organic stance that characterized the specialty in the 1920s. Interest in brain surgery (spectacularly represented locally by Harvey Cushing), such phenomena as the aftereffects of encephalitis, and particularly neuroendocrinology and other physiological studies provided ample prima facie justification for their professional theories. But either the subject matter was uninspiring or the personnel, as I have suggested, lacked the quality of those of an earlier period, for the contributions of Boston to psychiatric theory and therapy in the 1920s were not outstanding, no more notable than those of other provincial metropolises.[21]

The presence of nonmedical personnel interested in psychiatric problems—the other members of the team—provided a substantial base for newcomers with new ideas, a base that the psychiatrists by themselves would not have provided, however tolerant they were compared with, for instance, the psychiatric community in Philadelphia. By the late 1920s the meetings of the Boston Society of Psychiatry and Neurology were consistently crowded with guests when papers appeared on the program dealing with psychoanalysis. Foreign visitors such as Adler and Rank packed the hall, and only the discussions of war service and the Leopold-Loeb case rivaled in popularity the increasingly frequent discussions of psychoanalysis by local physicians.[22]

By 1930 or so Boston was becoming once again an exciting place in the world of psychiatry. Except for occasional contributions, usually in collaboration with nonpsychiatric physicians, organically oriented psychiatrists, however open to new methods, were not contributing to the ferment. Rather, the interest was in psychoanalysis and social and psychological areas. To some extent external factors contributed to this differential development. First, Boston was particularly cordial and receptive to the growing numbers of Europeans who came to the United States, and, second, psychoanalytic, social, and psychological endeavors did not usually require the huge sums of money that modern medical laboratories involve. Bostonians were able increasingly to command funds in the social sciences, but suspicions about the effectiveness of the psychiatric community persisted.

The institutional deficiencies and the assets of tradition therefore together marked the way in which Boston psychiatry developed for many years.[23] At first, community involvement and lack of orthodoxy were unable to make up for the loss of inspirational leadership just after World War I, but a decade or two later, the spirit of a team approach had become familiar throughout the country and laid the basis for Boston's reentry into the foundation and research establishment and, in the process, created a psychiatric community notable for its liveliness.

References

[1] See in general Joseph C. Aub and Ruth K. Hapgood, *Pioneer in Modern Medicine: David Linn Edsall of Harvard* (Cambridge, Mass.: Harvard Medical Alumni Association, 1970). E.E. Southard specifically had in mind in 1915 three models for the Boston Psychopathic Hospital: Germany, the Rockefeller Institute Hospital and the Johns Hopkins

Hospital; see his account of the administration of the Psychopathic, in Box 8, E.E. Southard Papers, Francis A. Countway Library of Medicine, Boston. The place of Boston in foundation support can be seen, for example, in the printed reports of the Carnegie Institution of Washington and in the files of the National Research Council, National Academy of Science Archives, Washington.

2 The records of the Boston Society of Psychiatry and Neurology, Countway Library of Medicine, reveal considerable competition among the groups. See also L. Vernon Briggs, *A Victory for Progress in Mental Medicine, Defeat of Reactionaries, The History of an Intrigue* (Boston: Wright and Potter, 1924).

3 Aub and Hapgood, *Pioneer in Modern Medicine.*

4 See, for example, "The Department of Neurology and Psychiatry," *The Bulletin, Harvard Medical Alumni Association, ns 6* (July 1908), 64–68. A general account of these events is contained in John C. Burnham, *Psychoanalysis and American Medicine, 1894–1918; Medicine, Science, and Culture* (New York: International Universities Press, 1967).

5 F.P. Gay, *The Open Mind: Elmer Ernest Southard, 1876–1920* (Chicago: Normandie House, 1938).

6 *Annual Report of Massachusetts Commission on Mental Diseases*, 1917, p. 45; 1919, pp. 13–14.

7 See materials preserved in the Southard Papers.

8 Based on the writer's personal collection of interview material as well as official publications of the Harvard Medical School.

9 Smith Ely Jelliffe, "Glimpses of a Freudian Odyssey," *Psychoanalytic Quarterly, 2* (1933), 318–329, and records of the Boston Society of Psychiatry and Neurology.

10 *Catalogue of Tufts College*, 1911–1929. Abraham Myerson, "Effect of Benzedrine Sulfate on Mood and Fatigue in Normal and in Neurotic Persons," *Archives of Neurology and Psychiatry, 36* (1936), 816–822. Compare Myerson's pre-World War I publications with, for example, "Sanity in Mental Hygiene," *Mental Hygiene, 17* (1933), 218–225.

11 Other papers in this volume deal with the rise of psychoanalysis especially.

12 Specific ratings of psychiatric research talent in Boston are to be found in the National Research Council files.

13 For example, *Annual Report of the Massachusetts Commission on Mental Diseases*, 1928, p. 38.

14 E.E. Southard, "Contributions from the Psychopathic Hospital, Boston, Mass. Introductory Note," manuscript, Box 8, Southard Papers, p. 3.

15 William Healy and Augusta Bronner, oral history interviews with John C. Burnham, 1960–1961. The quotation and interpolation are from Roy Lubove, *The Professional Altruist: The Emergence of Social Work as a Career, 1880–1930* (Cambridge, Mass.: Harvard University Press, 1965), p. 50. E.E. Southard and Mary C. Jarrett, *The Kingdom of Evils: Psychiatric Social Work Presented in One Hundred Case Histories, Together with a Classification of Social Divisions of Evil* (New York: The Macmillan Company, 1922), p. 521. An undated and anonymous memorandum apparently written in 1930, in the office of the Massachusetts Commissioner of Mental Health, Boston, summarizes the state of mind: "In 1916 the present Department of Mental Diseases entered upon a program of preventive work and re-organization. This also marked the Department's general entrance

into the welfare of the community. From 1916 to the present time great progress has been made in psychiatry, particularly in Massachusetts."

16 Albert Deutsch, "The History of Mental Hygiene," in J.K. Hall, ed., *One Hundred Years of American Psychiatry* (New York: Columbia University Press, 1944), pp. 325–365; Barbara M. Sicherman, "The Quest for Mental Health in America, 1880–1917," unpublished doctoral dissertation, Columbia University, 1967; and *Mental Hygiene* for these years. The hostile or, at best, ambivalent Bostonian, Bronson Crothers, "The Mental Hygiene Campaign as Seen by an Outside Observer," *Boston Medical and Surgical Journal, 187* (1922), 861–867, shows well how hard it was to resist the pressures generated by mental hygiene advocates.

17 Healy and Bronner, oral history; Gay, *The Open Mind*, p. 123.

18 Bronson Crothers, "Certain Pediatric Doubts About Modern Psychiatry," *New York Academy of Medicine Bulletin, 8* (1932), 515. This aspect of the mental hygiene movement is covered from another viewpoint in John C. Burnham, "The Struggle Between American Psychiatrists and Paramedical Personnel, 1917–1940," *Journal of the History of Medicine and Allied Sciences, 29* (1974), 93–106.

19 *Mental Hygiene* and *American Journal of Orthopsychiatry* for these years.

20 Paul E. Bowers, "William Edward Hickman, A Psychiatric Study," *Medical Journal and Record, 130* (1929), 79; Burnham, "The Struggle."

21 Boston psychiatry can be evaluated, for instance, in the annual articles on "Progress in Psychiatry" in the *New England Journal of Medicine*, in which local pride obviously skewed the sampling; or in the sources of authorship of articles even in the congenial *Archives of Neurology and Psychiatry*; or in the quick way in which the 1920s were covered by Henry R. Viets, "Fifty Years of the Boston Society of Psychiatry and Neurology," *New England Journal of Medicine, 203* (1930), 914–917, and Walter E. Barton, "Boston's Contributions to Psychiatry," *Hospital and Community Psychiatry, 19* (1968), 108–110.

22 Records of the Boston Society of Psychiatry and Neurology.

23 See, for example, the editorial, "A New Era in Psychiatry," *New England Journal of Medicine, 208* (1933), 98–99.

DISCUSSION

Sanford Gifford, presiding

ARCANGELO D'AMORE: I have found Professor Hale's two books and his presentation informative, rich, and interesting. I do differ from him on one point. He said that not until 1913 did White speak publicly, and gingerly, about psychoanalysis, whereas Putnam was discussing it earlier. Actually White had two problems. One was that he was superintendent of the Government Hospital for the Insane and was constantly being subjected to congressional investigations, and so he had to be careful about what he said publicly. The other problem was that he did not know German well and had to rely on translations. As nearly as we can determine, this was why he did not go to Clark University in 1909.

However in 1909 there was a tremendous amount of correspondence between Brill and White and Jelliffe to get Freud translated and published before his arrival at Clark. It is obvious from their correspondence that they wanted to make this as big and successful a publishing event as possible and they were quite worried as to whether they would get the publication out on time. And there were questions pertaining to the translation. For instance, Brill asks White how to translate *Abreagierung*—should he translate it as "off reaction," should he just call it "abreaction," and so on. I think that White was interested in informing the public about psychoanalysis, but was burdened with those governmental inquiries and with his halting German. In regard to Putnam, it should be noted that he was in approximately the last decade of his life when psychoanalysis was gaining momentum, from 1909 until his death in 1918, whereas Jelliffe and Brill and White and others were younger. William James died in 1910, and G. Stanley Hall in 1924, so that psychoanalysis in the Boston area almost disappeared for a time because these men were older than their colleagues in New York and Washington.

JEAN CURRAN: I have a vivid memory as a callow medical student over half a century ago, of Morton Prince. And I've entitled it, An Evening with Morton Prince. Some fifty-five years ago, during the transition from the administration of Dean Edward H. Bradford to that of David L. Edsall, the Harvard medical students, in small groups, enjoyed the hospitality of the Bradfords at delightful informal evening receptions; thereby we had unique opportunities to meet various distinguished Harvard figures, including, on one memorable occasion, Dr. Morton Prince. I recall quite clearly what he said in reply to Dr. Bradford's suggestion that he tell us about his investigation of the claims of mediums using hypnosis. Prince began by explaining his hypothesis that the messages claimed to have been received from the dear departed in the spirit world were in fact recollections of long-forgotten memories buried in the unconscious. He illustrated by explaining that newspaper articles, for example, that had been read ten, twenty, or even thirty years before, could be brought back through the reader's associations by hypnotism. To illustrate, he gave us an account of a young woman from St. Louis, genuinely convinced of her powers as a medium, who, as a patient, had been willing to submit herself to Dr. Prince's tests of the validity of her revelations from the world beyond the grave.

According to her story, a few years previously her father had died, leaving her and her mother in very straitened circumstances. In search of saleable assets, they discovered in the attic an old forgotten painting badly in need of cleaning. Hoping it might prove valuable after restoration, the girl decided to seek spiritualistic guidance via an Ouija board. It obligingly spelled out an answer: "See Paul Harne." When she asked where, the reply was, "At the Lexington Hotel." When she asked there for Paul Harne, a gray-haired clerk reacted with surprise and some shock, saying, "Yes, he used to live here, but he's been dead for years." She went back to her Ouija board and asked the name of the fluid used by Harne to clean old paintings. The reply was an incomplete word, s-a-l- and then a blur. When she asked for clarification, she was told she was not yet sufficiently attuned to the spirit world to receive the complete answer. Undismayed, she went to St. Louis's long-established art store and asked for the liquid used by the painter Paul Harne to clean old canvases. She was handed a bottle containing a yellow fluid. Filled with doubt, she asked sharply, "Are you sure this is what Mr. Harne used?" An older clerk overheard and broke in to say, "Why no, that isn't the right one," and handed her a bottle with dark brown liquid. The name on the label was salamander oil. With this convincing evidence of her mediumistic powers, one evening over her Ouija board she asked, "May I see you, Mr. Harne?" The answer was, "Look into that dark corner across the room," and there she had a distinct vision of a tall, slender figure having distinguished features, with pointed moustache, a red bow tie, and a gray suit.

The next morning she went to the leading photographic studio in the city and asked if there was a picture of Paul Harne. The proprietor replied, "Yes, I can find you one in that pile on the shelf there." She said, "Wait, let me do it myself." She went through the pile and found Mr. Harne's photograph without guidance. Now convinced of her genuine mediumistic capability she decided to make a career of it, but because of emotional difficulties she was referred by her doctor to Prince for a consultation.

The first finding under hypnotism was getting her to recall reading the morning paper of years before in which Mr. Harne's obituary appeared, with the usual details—his artistic career, residence at the Lexington Hotel, and a picture, but not the one of her vision. During further sessions, Dr. Prince was able to get his subject to remember an occasion some years earlier when she was taken by her escort for a Sunday dinner at the Lexington Hotel. As they were walking through the crowded lobby, a porter standing nearby called out, "Good day, Mr. Harne!" She turned to see a tall, distinguished-looking man, identical with her vision. As to the salamander oil revelation, Prince could find no explanation other than that it was merely a fortuitous encounter with a knowledgeable clerk.

The fact that I remember these details so clearly is evidence enough of the vivid impression made upon me by the charismatic Morton Prince. I assure you that in this instance my recall has not been aided by a session with hypnotism. I might add that that same evening Dr. Bradford and Dr. Prince joined in a description of a successfully painless major orthopedic operation performed by Bradford, with Prince as a hypnotic anesthetist. This may give us some food for thought today in view of the current excitement over acupuncture as an anesthetic.

GEORGE GARDNER: I wish to add two items, one relative to Morton Prince and the other relative to Dr. Coriat. I was a member of Morton Prince's last class at Harvard in 1926. I remember very well how Prince could induce an asthmatic attack in a young lady by bringing in some paper roses, which of course had nothing to do with the asthmatic factor itself. He was always presenting us with these odd things, and he took great delight in them.

Now, as to Dr. Coriat, I think it should be a matter of record that in 1929 he was refused membership in the Boston Society of Psychiatry and Neurology, I think, for the second time. Whether this was due entirely to the fact that he was an analyst who was perhaps anathema or whether it had to do with his association with the Emmanuel Movement, I do not know.

JULIUS SILBERGER: I want to turn again to Professor Marx's paper because it relates to something Professor Sicherman said. The development of a research program often seems to require the invention of a research tool that offers access to a hitherto unavailable body of phenomena. In Newton's instance, presumably this would have been the calculus; in Freud's, the free-association technique. Of course the method is often devised to validate a hypothesis, as apparently it was in Newton's case, and so there is some interpretation of the hypothesis and development of the technique. What made me think of it was Professor Sicherman's comment about Coriat having left the laboratory bench for the practice of clinical psychiatry, because it seems to me that this is not so odd as it might at first seem. In clinical psychiatry one works very much as in the laboratory with a method of making new discoveries; we have a number of examples in clinical psychiatry of people who did both. Coriat presumably was one, Stanley Cobb was a second, and Freud did the same, having started off in neuroanatomy and then moved into another area of interest.

OTTO MARX: There are various schools in the history of science. I like to believe that tools are more important. Lakatos is a theoretician who developed his ideas relative to theories. I think it is not fair to call the calculus a tool in that sense. I have given much thought to the question of what was different in regard to Freud, and I think one of the crucial things was first, the shift from what you tell the patient to what the patient himself tells, and it turns out that you can observe so much more if you do that much less. But much more important than that, I think, is a shift away from the patient. Everybody had been concerned with patients, and the hypnotists were concerned in the greatest detail, but what was new here was a concern with the relation. For the first time there was a move away from the traditional idea that you have to have a good relation with people, toward understanding that no matter what relation you have, you can use it therapeutically, so that it is just as useful whether the patient dislikes you or you dislike the patient. Then suddenly we are getting away from a more moralistic point to a much more scientific one, where you examine whatever goes on. And of course this is where Freud then moves into the interpersonal, when the analytic aspect is what matters.

SANFORD GIFFORD: I want to add one descriptive detail about Dr. Coriat for which I am indebted to Dr. Dalrymple. She was a member of the study group that met in the late twenties before the founding of the institute. She described these meetings at which Dr. Coriat sat in a high-backed Spanish chair and his pupils sat on the floor around him. Whether the Spanish chair is a reference to his Sephardic background, I leave to the audience.

M. RALPH KAUFMAN: C. Macfie Campbell was one of the most brilliant teachers that I have ever encountered. He had a basic philosophy in relation to psychiatry and to life. He was not one who accepted things because somebody said they were so. He was responsible for the best eclectic training that I know of anywhere. Campbell took the best in psychiatry as it was then known and as he projected it.

In relation specifically to analysis, many people may not know that Campbell wrote two excellent psychoanalytic papers early in the 1900s. He was responsible for a large group of his students becoming psychoanalysts and dynamic psychiatrists. He also placed a tremendous amount of emphasis on teaching and on the opportunity for his fellows to practice psychotherapy.

NATHAN HALE: I would like to defend Professor Burnham, whose work I admire immensely. Let me suggest that he was working from the written record. I have read all of C. Macfie Campbell's papers in order, and I think they become thinner in the 1920s. I have also just gone through most of the inpatient records at Massachusetts General Hospital for the period. There is a marked decline in the use of psychotherapy there in this period under James B. Ayer. It is clear and remarkable. Perhaps the decline was less precipitous because the eminence was less real, that is to say, in Boston psychiatry there was no golden age up to 1918 and then a precipitous decline; it was pretty solid all the way along.

Finally, in this period there was the rise of other important centers: in New York, at Hopkins and, notably, in Washington at St. Elizabeth's. I would add that the vitality in American psychoanalysis in this period was not within the orthodox analytic group but with people outside it, like Sullivan, who were working with White at St. Elizabeth's.

DAVID SHAKOW: As a resident psychologist, or intern, at Boston Psychopathic Hospital during that middle period, the twenties, I might add a few words to what has been said. I was very much excited by what I got at the "Psycho" while I was there, but I must say that most of it was from Freddie Wells and not so much from Macfie Campbell, with whom I took a seminar. I was living in the hospital at the time and used to attend some of the lectures that Campbell gave to the freshmen students of the Harvard Medical School. Once as I was going out following a group of students, one said, "How wonderfully he puts things; the way in which he uses language is just overwhelming," and another one replied, "Yes, that really is true, but what did he say?" I am afraid that for the younger people, at least, the quality of his speech and of his particular performance caused a negative reaction compared with that of older and more experienced psychologists. But I did not get the impact from Campbell that I had expected.

MILTON GREENBLATT: I thought that Campbell was an absolutely brilliant teacher, with a tremendous mastery of the literature. When we discussed cases on rounds, we had to choose our words carefully or we would get sliced up. He taught us to be critical and careful, especially in descriptive analysis. However, in the early forties the Boston Psychopathic Hospital was not a good place to be admitted to as a patient, and in this I think Campbell was remiss. He permitted poor patient care to go on. While he might have been indignant at what he saw, he did little to correct it. Seclusion, wet sheet packs, and all that were carried on to an absurd degree. Concern for the details of the patient's life was terribly neglected, and the man who taught us that this was so was the man who succeeded Campbell, Harry Solomon.

THOMAS CADWALLADER: The influence that the psychological views of Charles S. Peirce had upon both William James and G. Stanley Hall should be extended to Adolf Meyer and E.E. Southard.

Adolf Meyer himself pointed to Peirce's influence. He also specified how, during his Chicago years (1892–1895), he was introduced to the writings of Peirce by the German-American philosopher Paul Carus (1852–1919), who was then editor of *The Monist* and *The Open Court.* Peirce published in Carus's two journals from 1891–1908; e.g., in 1892 he published an important paper, "The law of mind," in *The Monist.* While Peirce's influence on Meyer has been pointed to by some commentators, e.g., Leighton and Lidz, the question of how important it is would seem to merit serious study.

Although Southard presumably had been introduced to Peirce's thought by William James, it was through Josiah Royce's seminar in comparative methodology that Southard really learned to appreciate Peirce's genius. Southard attended Royce's seminar for many years and in fact carried it on during Royce's absence from the seminar in 1912 following his stroke.

Peirce's influence on Southard may be seen, for example, in Southard's 1916 paper "On the application of grammatical categories to the analysis of delusions." It seems probable that Peirce's thought inspired the paper, "Pragmatic Psychiatry," which Southard delivered to the New York Neurological Society only five days before his death in 1920. After Royce's death in 1916, the editing of Peirce's papers fell to Southard. Just three days before he died, Southard wrote about the challenge of this project to Frederick P. Gay, who was later to become his biographer: "I feel that my own intellectual life is going to be made over by the work."

Although Charles Peirce's role in the intellectual heritage of the United States in general and of New England in particular has been at least partially recognized, his influence upon psychology has only recently come to light,[1] and although there has been some recognition of his influence on psychiatry through that on Meyer and Southard, and recently on Rabkin and Percy, Peirce's influence on, and his implications for, psychiatry still seem largely unexplored.

Reference

[1] Thomas C. Cadwallader, "Charles S. Peirce (1839–1914): The first American experimental psychologist," *Journal of the History of the Behavioral Sciences, 10* (1974), 291–298; Cadwallader, "Peirce as an experimental psychologist," *Transactions of the Charles S. Peirce Society, 11* (1975), 167–186; Cadwallader and J.V. Cadwallader, "America's first modern psychologist: William James or Charles S. Peirce?" *Proceedings of the 80th Annual Convention, American Psychological Association*, 1972, pp. 773–774.

Illustrations

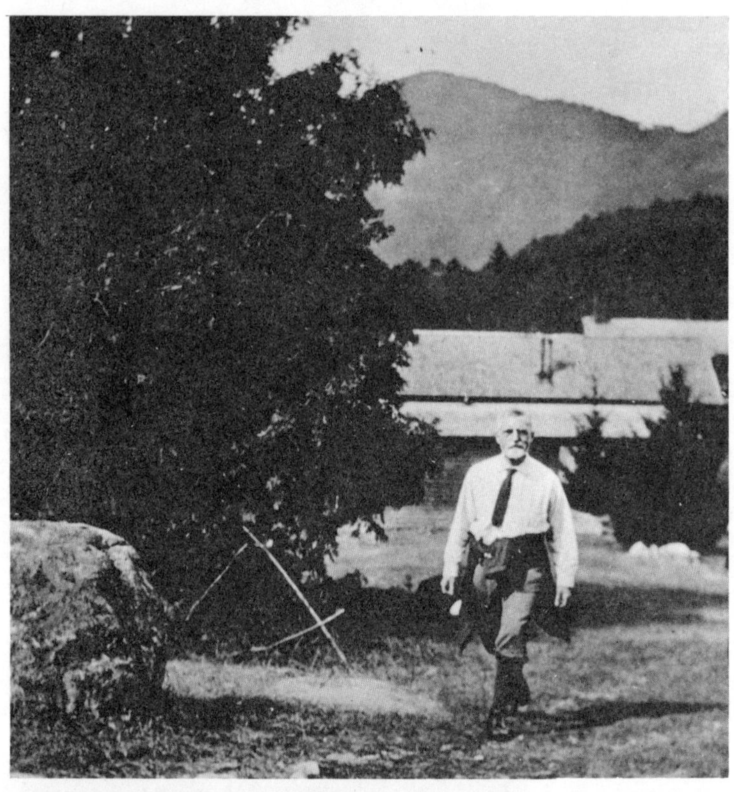

15. James Jackson Putnam at his Adirondack camp. *Putnam Collection, Countway Library.*

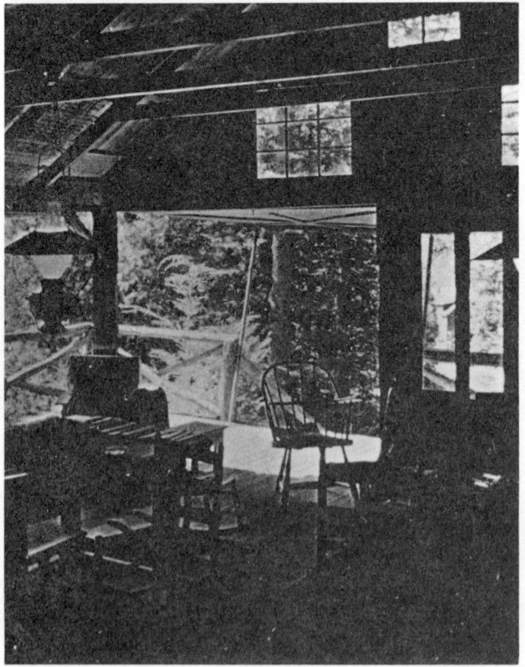

16. "The Stoop" at the Putnam camp, where Freud stayed in 1909.

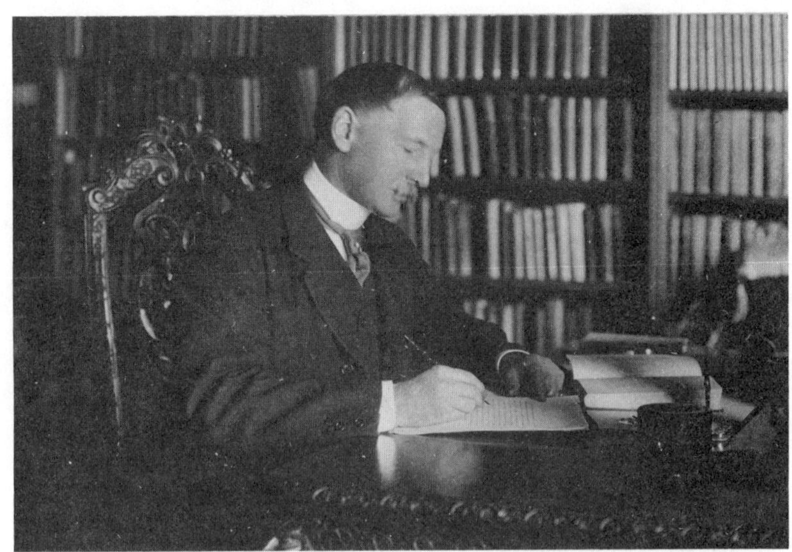

17. Morton Prince. *Boston Medical Library Collection, Countway Library.*

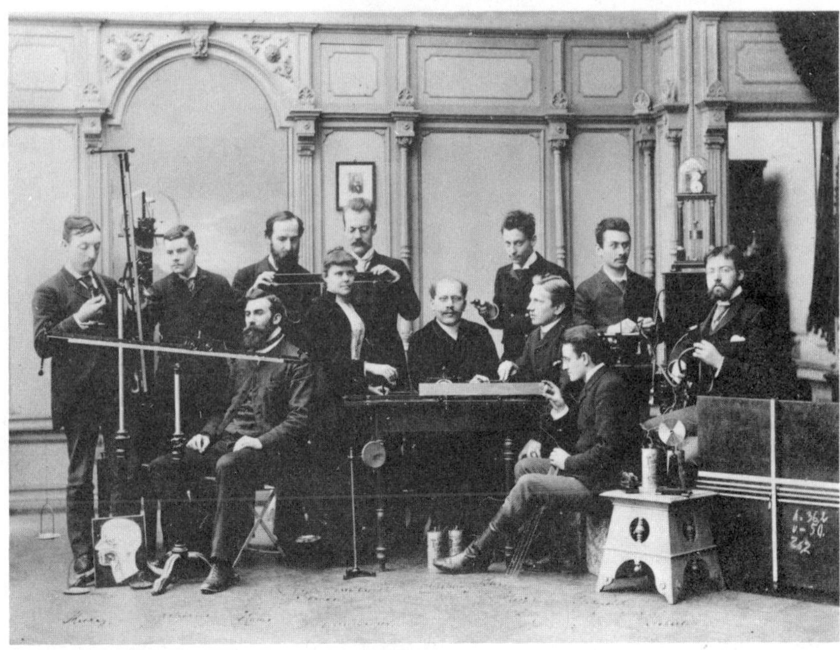

18. Hugo Münsterberg's Freiberg Laboratory in the 1890s. The laboratory was in two rooms of Münsterberg's house. Dr. Münsterberg is seated at the table. *Harvard University Archives.*

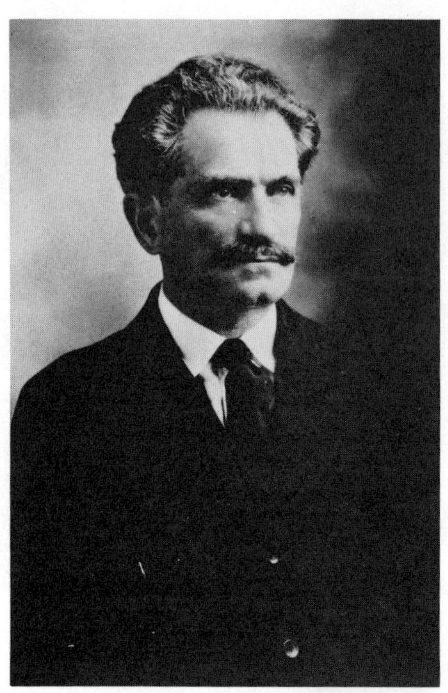

19. Boris Sidis. *Courtesy of Dr. Jacob Goldwyn.*

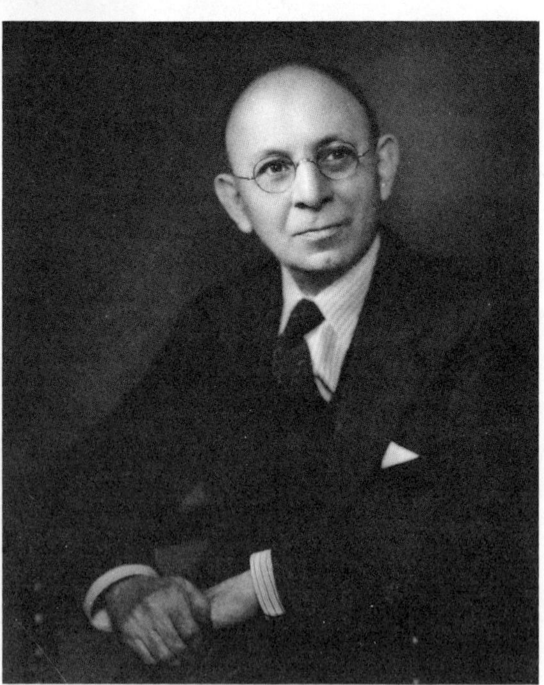

20. Isador Coriat. *Boston Medical Library Collection, Countway Library.*

21. Solomon Carter Fuller. *Solomon Carter Fuller Institute, Cambridge, Massachusetts.*

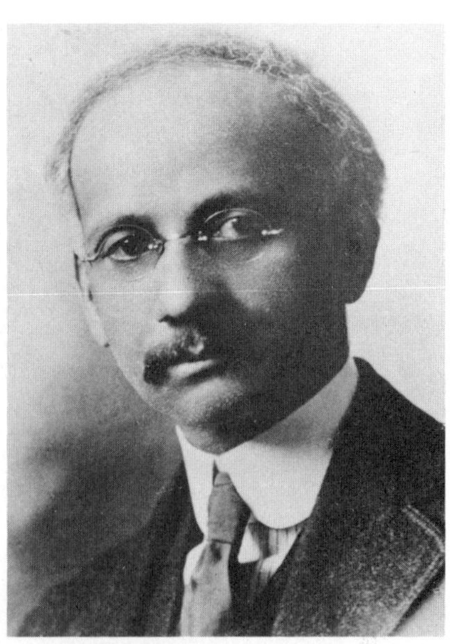

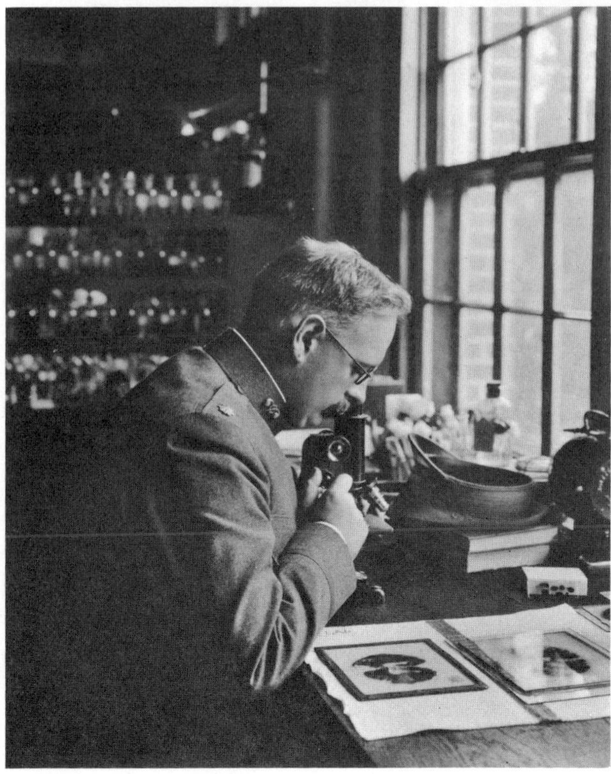

22. Elmer E. Southard. *Countway Library.*

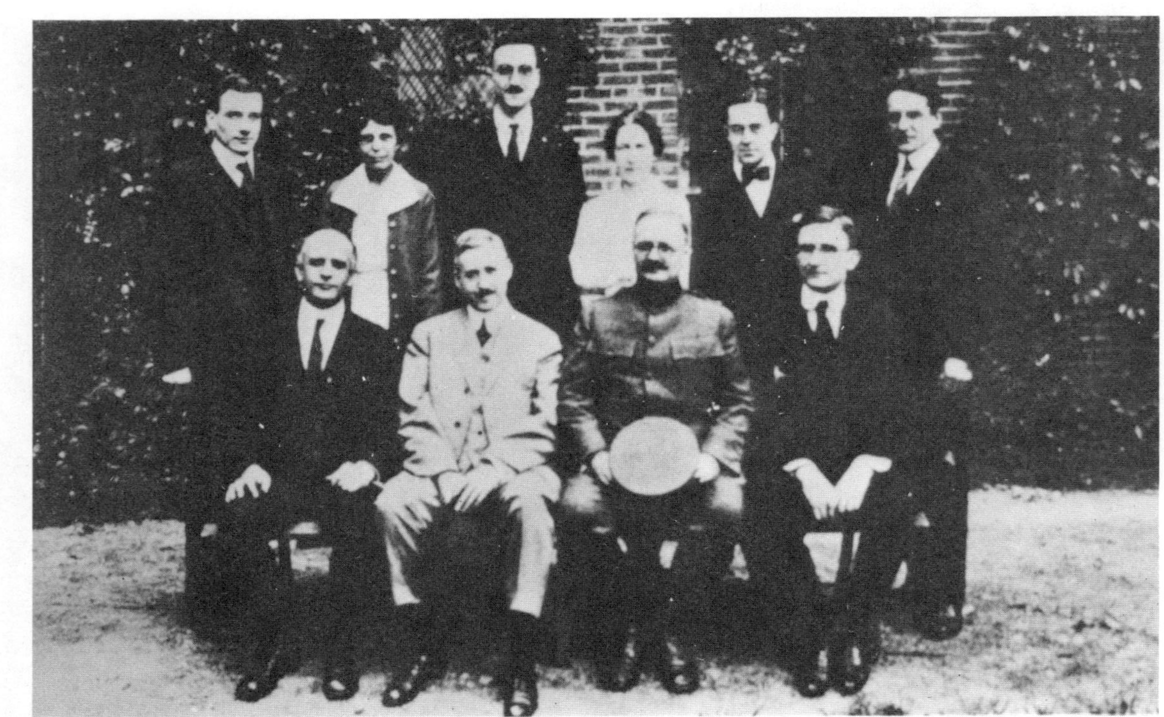

23. The group that was connected with the Boston Psychopathic Hospital, 1918. *Left to right, seated:* Abraham Myerson, James V. May, Elmer E. Southard, Lawson G. Lowrey; *standing:* Richard H. Price, Annette M. McIntire, Karl A. Menninger, Esther S.B. Woodword, Edwin R. Smith, Clifford G. Rounsefell. *Greenblatt Collection, Countway Library.*

24. Frederick Lyman Wells, for many years chief of the Psychology Laboratory, Boston Psychopathic Hospital, made numerous and significant contributions to his field. *Greenblatt Collection, Countway Library.*

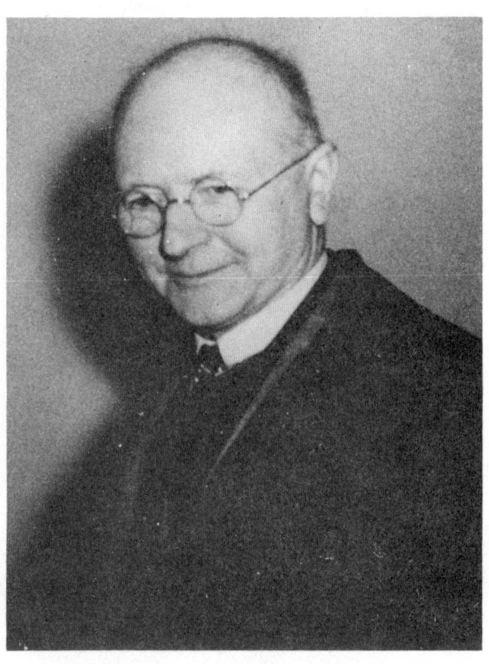

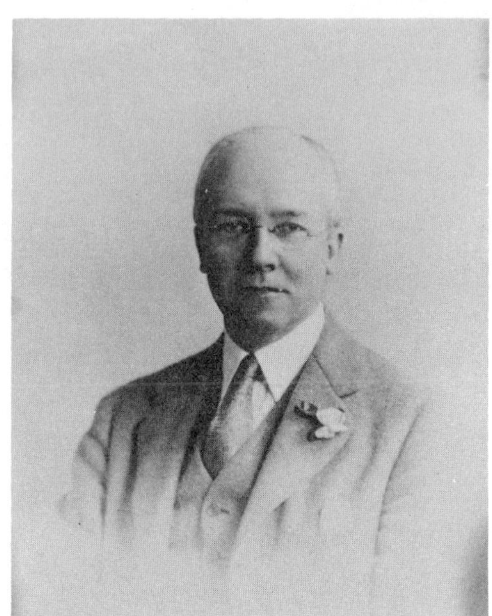

25. L.E. Emerson, psychologist at the Massachusetts General Hospital. *Courtesy of Eugene Emerson, Cambridge, Massachusetts.*

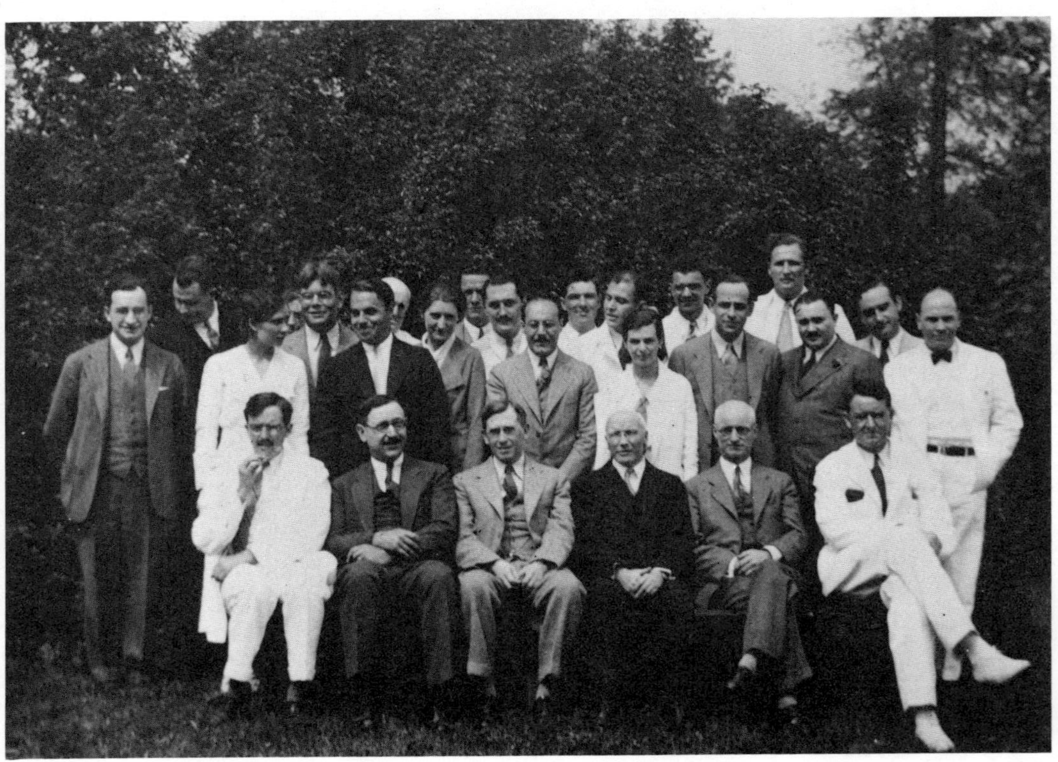

26. *a.* Staff picture at the Boston Psychopathic Hospital at the time of C. Macfie Campbell. *Left to right, seated:* Edgerton Howard, Harry Solomon, Karl Bowman, C. Macfie Campbell, Oscar Raeder, Robert Fleming; *standing:* Israel Kopp, Merrill Moore, Sara Thompson, unidentified man *(partly hidden),* Irma Bache, William Roth, unidentified man, Joseph Michaels, two unidentified men, Marjorie Meehan, unidentified man, Samuel Epstein, Samuel Kraines, Gaylord Coon, Jacob Finesinger, Waldo Winekoop. *Ives Hendrick Archives, Boston Psychoanalytic Society and Institute.*

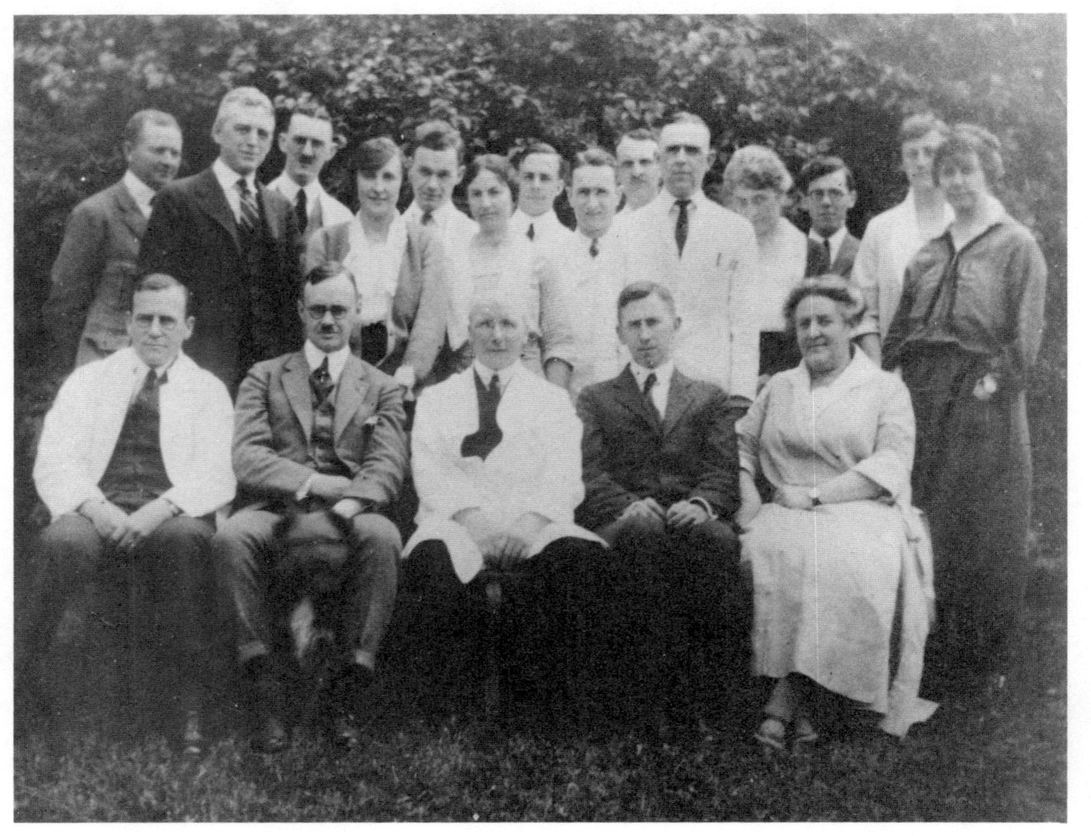

b. Left to right, seated: Alfred Ehrenclou, W. Franklin Wood, C. Macfie Campbell, Karl Bowman, Marianna Taylor; *standing:* Frederick Wells, Martin Peck, Sidney Smith, Olive Cooper, Arthur Young, Ella Wakeman, Lewis Hill, Richard Wilson, George Daniels, Thomas Houlton, Myrtle Canavan, Don MacFarlane, Cora Morris, unidentified woman. *Courtesy of Mrs. Martin Peck, Archives of the Boston Psychoanalytic Society and Institute.*

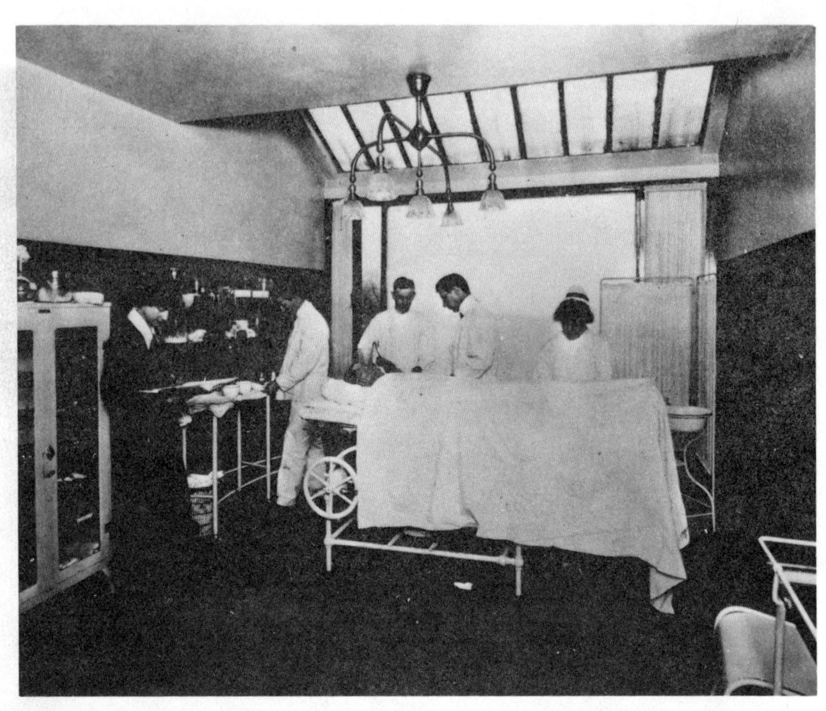

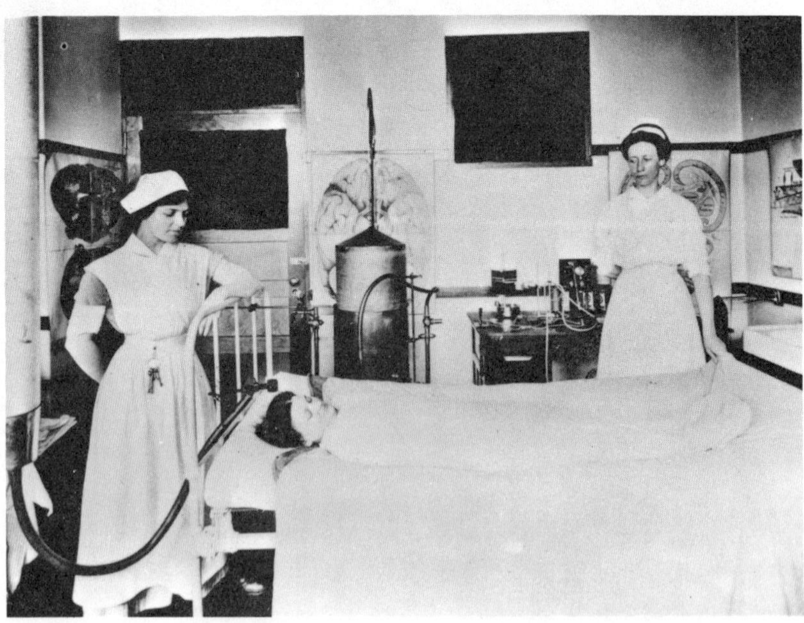

27. Somatic therapies at the Boston Psychopathic Hospital.
a. Harry C. Solomon, second from right, at the neuro-syphilis clinic. Maida H. Solomon is at left.
b. Studies of basal metabolism rate in mentally ill.
c. Hydrotherapy tubs.
d. Insulin unit.
Greenblatt Collection, Countway Library.

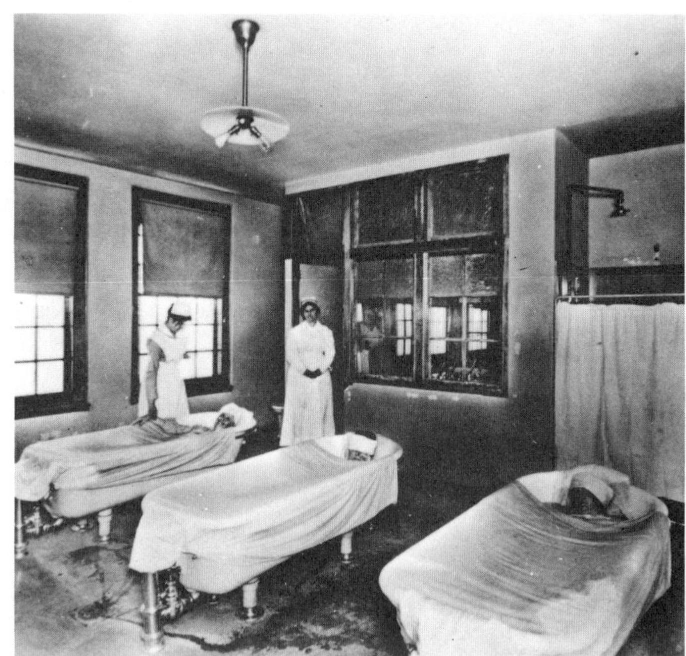

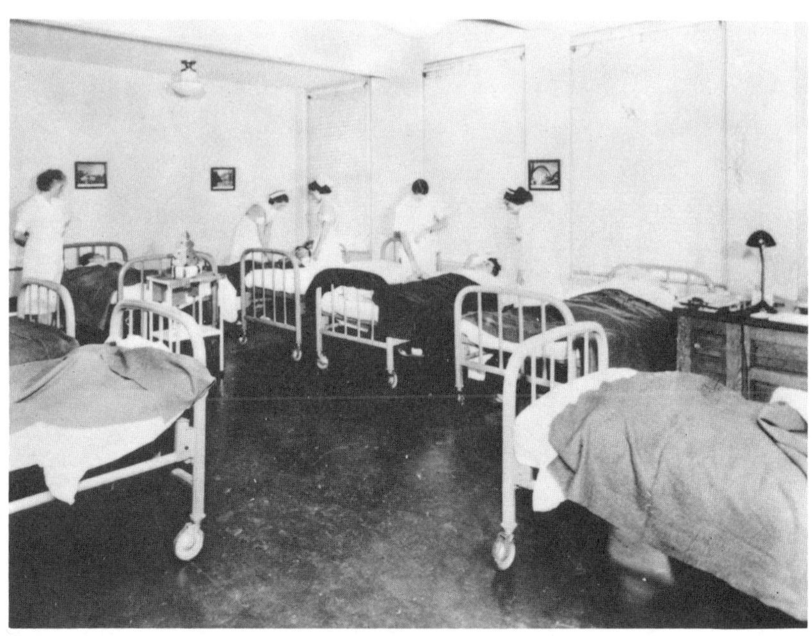

The 1920s and 1930s

George Arthur Waterman, 1872–1960, and Office Psychiatry

G.E. GIFFORD, JR.

George Arthur Waterman was born in Viola, Illinois on December 14, 1872, "in a little shack on the open prairie."[1] The same year, the patrician Dr. James Jackson Putnam (1846–1918) returned from postgraduate medical studies in Europe and was appointed "Electrician to the Massachusetts General Hospital." This appointment followed the directive, "There shall be appointed annually by the trustees, an Electrician, whose duties shall be to take charge and proper care of all the magnetic and electrical apparatus of the Hospital, and administer magnetism and electricity to patients, whenever called upon by the Physicians and Surgeons."[2] It was also in 1872 that a sixteen year old boy named Sigmund Freud was leading his class at Sperl Gymnasium in Vienna. The lives of these three diverse men would have one common goal—the treatment of the psychoneurotic patient.

George A. Waterman was to become "probably Boston's leading psychotherapist."[3] He was the joint protégé of both James Jackson Putnam and Morton Prince. Although Waterman made no major contributions to psychiatric thought, his career reveals the education and training of a neurologist, the resistant reaction to analytic psychology, and the methods of psychotherapy from the early 1900s to 1940. Perhaps more sympathetic to Freudian theory in his earlier years, Waterman later became eclectic in his approach.[4] This account will deal with that continuing medical psychotherapeutic tradition.

In 1877 the Waterman family moved from Illinois to East Cliftondale, Massachusetts, described by Waterman as "a beautiful village until horse cars from Lynn came there but life was peaceful under apple trees —Sundays jackknife on the lawn. Beautiful, lovely childhood."[1] Waterman's father was secretary and treasurer of the then small concern of Waite and Bond, manufacturers of the Blackstone cigar. Waterman attended Saugus High School, dropped out to work for a year, and then attended Chelsea High School, living with Mrs. Harriman, his mother's sister. He was graduated from Harvard College in 1895, and from Harvard Medical School, *cum laude*, in 1899.

James Jackson Putnam had progressed from "Electrician" at Massachusetts General Hospital to being designated "Physician to the Out patients with Diseases of the Nervous System" in 1873. A department of neurology was created in 1874 and Putnam was appointed lecturer. As professor of neurology (1893–1912) at the hospital, it was he who established one of the first neurologic clinics in America,[5] and in 1875 he was one of the founders of the American Neurological Association, along with William Alexander Hammond (1828–1900), Edward Constant Sequin (1843–1898), Meredith Clymer (1817–1902), James Steward Jewell (1837–1887), Roberts Bartholow (1831–1904), and T.M.B. Cross.

Neurology finally became required study in 1895, the year Waterman entered Harvard Medical School and the year Morton Prince was appointed clinical instructor in neurology (1895–1898). Prince, who had been graduated from Harvard Medical School in 1879, had practiced general medicine, but his interest gradually shifted when in the 1880s he took his mother to Paris to be seen by Charcot for a "neurotic ailment"; later, his wife also suffered from the same difficulty. Prince became interested in the work of Charcot's student, Pierre Janet, who published a series of papers on hysteria. As a medical student, Waterman had both James Jackson Putnam and Morton Prince as instructors.

After graduation, Waterman spent eighteen months as an intern on West Medical at Massachusetts General under Reginald Fitz and William Richardson. He vividly described Putnam's habitat:

> When I was a House Officer, in 1900, the old X-ray room was just starting in the little room under the arch, at the left of the main entrance of the old original building [this was not the earliest location of X-ray]. It was in this room that Dr. Putnam first started the Department of Neurology, when he came back from Europe in 1872. Dr. Shattuck (Visiting Physician to the MGH, 1849–1885), used to picture Dr. Putnam as sitting in this little room under the arch with an electric battery. They used to send him all cases that nobody understood. On account of the appearance of the arch and the inflow of patients not understood, and not desirable for this reason, Dr. Shattuck said they used to call it the "cloaca maxima."[6]

The *cloaca maxima* was the great sewer in Rome; here we have an early example of classically phrased medical hostility and resistance. Perhaps it was owing to space limitations in "the little room under the arch" that Putnam established a small personal laboratory in his own home that may be "looked on as the antecedent of the present endowed neuropathologic department of the Harvard Medical School."[5]

In 1901, Waterman was appointed "assistant physician to the outpatient department at MGH,"[7] and it was noted that "the teaching force has been further increased by the appointment of Dr. S.A. Lord (1900–1901), Dr. George A. Waterman (1901), and Dr. E.W. Taylor (1904) as Assistants [Neurology]."[8]

The case-method system of teaching had been introduced by W.B. Cannon[9] in 1900 at Harvard Medical School. In order to carry out more completely and systematically the case method in neurological teaching, J.J. Putnam and G.A. Waterman published *Studies in Neurological Diagnosis*,[10] a book of actual cases that was to be used by third-year medical students as a modified textbook.

At this time, both Putnam[11] and Prince[12] were developing their interest in the psychological aspects of medicine. Prince was involved in the seven-year treatment of a young woman whose case would become psychiatric history with the publication of *The Dissociation of a Personality*, and the patient, Miss Christine or Sally Beauchamp (Beecham) would become a celebrity (the case was a sort of early *Three Faces of Eve*). It was also at this time that Waterman became associated with both Putnam and Prince in their respective private practices.

For Waterman the neurological resources at Massachusetts General were indeed meager. In 1903, two beds were assigned to neurology, whereas in the same year Putnam reported "that Long Island Hospital (Boston) has a 'thriving neurological ward'"[13] where Waterman and Putnam conducted a joint study of cerebellar tumors and their treatment.[14]

In 1904 Janet came to Boston as part of a speaking tour on psychopathology, which included stops at St. Louis and Chicago. This trip was arranged through Dr. Edward Cowles, superintendent and director of McLean Hospital (1879–1904), and Adolf Meyer.[15] In 1906 Janet was invited by Harvard Medical School to give a series of lectures on hysteria.[16]

In 1905 Putnam and Waterman suggested that physicians undertake a careful investigation of the psychological state of the epileptic such as had already been undertaken for the hysteric. Perhaps, they suggested, a painstaking investigation would show a connection between psychological processes and the symptomatic acts that occurred during an epileptic attack.[17]

In 1906 Prince founded and became the editor of the *Journal of Abnormal Psychology*; the associate editors were Hugo Münsterberg, James

Jackson Putnam, August Hoch (Bloomingdale Asylum, New York), Boris Sidis, Charles L. Dana (Cornell University Medical School), and Adolf Meyer (Psychiatric Institute, New York Hospitals.)

In the second volume (1907), Waterman wrote a book review on *Hysteria in Children*[18] and in volume three (1908), he and Putnam wrote a prefatory note to an article by "B.C.A.," "My Life as a Dissociated Personality." "We are convinced," they said, "that the patient is a truthful witness, a conscientious observer, an intelligent and right-minded person...We believe that what she describes as memories were memories and not vaporings or fabrications...Furthermore, a number of her statements were susceptible of verification and were verified by us."[19]

Volume four (1909) of the *Journal of Abnormal Psychology* included another contribution by Waterman, "The Treatment of Fatigue States."[20] This was included in a symposium on psychotherapy, read before the American Therapeutic Society at the annual meeting in New Haven, May 6, 1909. The papers in this symposium were published as a book, *Psychotherapeutics* (1910). Waterman's article mentions some physiological references: Hodge, 1892; Halliburton, "The Chemical Side of Nervous Activity." On the psychological end: James, "Energies of Man"; Prince, Janet, Tissie, and Féré. But obviously, the most influential was Dubois and *The Psychic Treatment of Nervous Disorders* (1905). There was also a mention of Mitchell's rest treatment modified by Déjerine. Typically, Waterman espoused both methods—the eclectic approach.

The unhumble Ernest Jones in his *Life of Freud* tells us how it was in Boston in 1908:

> New England was by no means unprepared to listen to Freud's new doctrines. In the autumn of 1908, while staying with Morton Prince in Boston, I had held two or three colloquiums at which sixteen people were present: among others, Putnam, the Professor of Neurology at Harvard University; E.W. Taylor, later his successor; Werner Münsterberg, the Professor of Psychology there; Boris Sidis; and G.W. Waterman [Jones got the middle initial wrong]. The only one with whom I had any real success was Putnam.

Jones also tells of "his" role in the formation of the American Psychopathological Association:

> The time not yet being ripe for a purely psychoanalytical society, I proposed to Putnam that a wider association be formed where psychoanalytical ideas could be discussed. I then approached Morton Prince, promis-

> ing him that he should be the first president, and circulars were sent out to suitable people. Since psychiatrists were at that time even less interested in psychology than were neurologists, we decided to hold our meetings immediately after the annual meeting of the American Neurological Association. So on May 12, 1910, at the Willard Hotel in Washington, the American Psycho-pathological Association came into being. There were forty present at the meeting. The following officers were elected: President, Morton Prince; Secretary, G.A. Waterman (his private assistant in Boston).[22]

It was at this meeting that Jones took a dislike to Waterman because of his obvious resistance to Freudian theory. Neither Prince nor Waterman appears in the famous photograph of Freud surrounded by his American coterie at the Clark lectures.

After its first meeting in 1910, the American Psychopathological Association took the *Journal of Abnormal Psychology* as its official organ with the following slate of papers presented to the organization: "The Sex Symbolism in Dreams," James Jackson Putnam; "The Action of Suggestion in Therapeutics," Ernest Jones; "The Anxiety Neurosis," A.A. Brill; "Dreams as a Cause of Symptoms," George A. Waterman; "Mechanism of Dreams," Morton Prince. They were duly published in volume five.[23] At the second annual meeting of the American Psychopathological Association in Baltimore, May 10, 1911, there was a symposium on the pathogenesis of morbid anxiety, and again Waterman revealed his reservations about the sexual etiology of anxiety. He reported two cases that were reactive anxiety states.[24]

In September 1910, Jones suggested that Putnam send a "little circular" to a few chosen people "inviting their adherence" to psychoanalytic theory. Jones suggested "Stanley Hall, Hoch, Macfie Campbell, Holt, Hart, White, Coriat. We must take in Meyer *if he desires it*, but need hardly ask him. Karplus and Ricksher I am rather against."[25] In a letter to Putnam, October 11, 1910, Jones expressed his more explicit feelings toward Waterman:

> I should be against either Taylor or Waterman being asked to sign [the circular], for we want not so much a petition, as in the case of the A.Pp.A. [American Psycho-pathological Association] as a more authoritative document. I am even very dubious about the wisdom of accepting them at all, at least for the present. Taylor is a broad-minded and highly capable man, and has a sympathetic attitude, though he does not seem very interested in psychological questions. Is he taking up psychoanalysis any more than before? Waterman, on the other hand, is rather disappointing. Last May 1910 he showed to me very great resistances against psychoanalysis (I

> think personal, for he has strong complexes), and a complete ignorance of the subject. When one finds a young neurologist so wrapped up in practice that he won't even take the trouble of learning German—and how can one begin neurology without that first indispensable step?—it is not very hopeful. However, it is our duty to be as charitable as possible, and personally I should like nothing better than to hear of some evidence that he was taking a real interest in psychopathology, especially psychoanalysis.[26]

Putnam replied to Jones on October 14: "I think better of Waterman than you do. He certainly has complexes but he is interested and does fair work."[27] Perhaps a beginning wedge was deepening in the relation between Waterman and Putnam.

At any rate, Putnam did think better of Waterman than did Jones. When Putnam was made chief of neurology at Massachusetts General in 1911, Henry C. Baldwin and Edward W. Taylor were appointed neurologists. Walter W. Paul, Joseph H. Pratt, and George A. Waterman were appointed "assistant neurologists." When Putnam retired from active service and was appointed to the Board of Consultation in 1912, E.W. Taylor was made chief of neurology and again Waterman was elevated to associate neurologist at Massachusetts General and instructor in neurology at Harvard Medical School.[28]

The first General Executive Committee Report for 1912 on Neurology reported, "Excellent work is being done in the study of psychoneuroses by the analytic methods; and there is no doubt that results of importance will proceed from the clinic in this increasing important region of research...An assistant [L.E. Emerson] has recently been appointed with special reference to the cases of mental disease which may appear at the clinic."[29] It would not be until 1926 that there would be a full "Neurological and Neurosurgical Ward"—"Bulfinch West."

It was also in 1912 that Waterman married Mrs. R.E. Forrest (Claire Brenner) and they lived at 535 Beacon Street, on the water side. It was an open secret that the lady was none other than the famous patient of Morton Prince, Sally Beauchamp. Waterman had married a lady whose psychodynamics were in book form! The Countway Library has Waterman's copy of Prince's *Dissociation of a Personality*, inscribed "G.A. Waterman, 2 Marlboro St." All this adds credence to Henry James's classic verdict, "hardly passionate Marlborough Street," as quoted by Robert Lowell in *Life Studies*.

> Prince described Sally as "extremely reticent and said she dislikes any discussion of herself or her circumstances. She is even reticent in reference

> to her physical ailments, so much so that it is never easy to discover any temporary indisposition from which she may be suffering. She dislikes the publicity which her physical trouble tends to draw upon her, and has sought jealously to guard her secret. Indeed, all three personalities have endeavored by every artifice to conceal the knowledge of their trouble from friends, and have done so with a success that is astonishing. It has been at the expense of being considered a strange, incomprehensible person, "unlike other people."[30]

Those who remember her recall her as a large woman, who was abrupt and "ran a tight ship" with the Waterman patient retinue. Omnipresent, she sat "like a Chinese Ancestor portrait." She avoided children, as was explained by an associate: "She had reached maturity without having any of the children's diseases and in adult life she feared being exposed to them." This "symbiotic" doctor-patient, husband-wife relation must have strongly influenced Waterman's own doctor-patient relations.

In 1911 the Boston Psychoanalytic Society was founded and in 1915, Waterman was appointed "Neurologist" at Massachusetts General. But in 1916 he severed all academic connections and went into private practice. According to G.C. Caner, this was due to the fact that "his private practice became so large and demanding." Waterman never affiliated with a psychiatric hospital, possibly because he did not have psychotic patients. No hospital in the area in the 1920s had an outpatient psychiatric department. From 1904 to 1919, the McLean Hospital was under joint administration with Massachusetts General Hospital. An outpatient department was opened in 1917 for a short time, until the first World War; it was not reopened until 1951 and not established permanently until 1963. It was clear that Waterman was treating outpatient psychiatric patients and that "official" medicine had essentially ignored this need. He was, however, on the medical advisory board of the Austen Riggs Foundation from 1921 to 1946, whose original members were: Stanley Cobb, Walter B. James, James A. Miller, Bruce W. Paddock, Moses A. Starr, E.W. Taylor, W. Sidney Thayer, and Frederick Tilney.[31]

Waterman gathered around him a brood of wealthy, dependent psychoneurotics who followed him from Palm Beach to Pooduck, his summer home in Brooklin, Maine. Brooklin is situated on a peninsula, fingering into Penobscot Bay to the west and Blue Hill and Jericho bays to the east. Here the boundaries between social ties and the doctor-patient relation were blurred. The scene was reminiscent of the Newport and Bar Harbor days of S. Weir Mitchell[32]—the moral treatment days when patients were taken into the family life of the superintendent of the early asylums.[33] The "en famille" approach made the symptoms less alien and more respectable, encouraged social interaction, and covered it all with the aegis of taste, culture, and refinement. Lobster was served on silver plates on the beach at Pooduck Farm. There was much philosophizing and the leader was Waterman, a magnetic, tall man, a handsome man with cornflower-blue eyes, who acted like an "ancient Roman." The architecture in Maine was studiedly rural—and to those of us in this age for whom reality is severe, the Henry James epoch sounds like fantasy. A friend of Waterman's recalled the scene:

> The Pooduck Farm Road ran through a grove of pointed firs, white pine and birch, by a well-kept garden of many kinds of vegetables and a cutting garden of flowers on to a white clapboard farm house surrounded by flowers. In front there was a rose garden and a guest house (I believe it was used largely for visiting patients) behind which there was meadow pasture and a flock of sheep. Like most all Maine farmhouses, the barn was near or attached to the house. White fan-tailed pigeons fluttered in and out of the dove-cote. White Chinese silky chickens roamed in and out of the barn drinking at a marble basin bird bath Dr. Waterman had brought from a miner's cabin near a marble quarry in Vermont. The clipped lawn swept to the shore at Pooduck Point and a flock of White Holland turkeys was feeding and strutting across it...The table was set beautifully with elegant simplicity, and the menu included a rack of lamb and a festive molded steamed blueberry pudding with sweetened light cream—nothing left undone, nothing overdone. A menu card was at Dr. Waterman's place so he could anticipate the food he most liked...A friend told us a lovely story about the visiting patients. She was walking from the summer colony of Haven to the Watermans' home and in the red raspberry patch came upon an elegant lady in a Paris costume wearing a famous strand of black pearls, reputedly valued at $100,000 in local gossip, around her neck and clutching a wooden pint berry box. She looked up with a smile and said, "Dr. Waterman says I cannot have dinner until I fill this."[34]

Waterman's nephew, Stanton, also recalled life in Maine:

> I considered him the epitome of the Renaissance Man...philosopher, poet, humorist, epicurean, naturalist, brilliant conversationalist and profound humanitarian. In his gun room at Pooduck Farm in Maine, or sitting by a tidal pool in his south beach, or by his beach cabana in front of the Breakers Hotel in Palm Beach, his conversation would always include the objects around him or the natural phenomena of the moment to illustrate his philosophy and flower his counsel. In his later years he took few select

> patients, with whom he mostly talked about life and behavior. I mentioned the south beach in Maine. He had a tidal pool there in which he reclined, bronzed and often naked like Socrates. He illustrated his talks about life with examples of life in the tidal pool and the microcosm of the low tide beach. We used to have Shakespeare readings in his boat house, and he loved to draw young people into his world of the classics. His vast fund of original Greek and Latin classics, on which he frequently drew from memory, seemed inexhaustible.[35]

As his nephew mentioned, the Watermans wintered in Palm Beach, Florida. Their house was designed by the architect Marion Sims Wyeth, in the American version of Italian Renaissance. It was near the waterfront at 2000 El Bravo Way, where Waterman had a collection of fifty different kinds of palm trees. It was here that he became a founder of the Society of Four Arts.[36] He was chairman of the Library Committee of the Society for a number of years and was instrumental in the enlargement of the library structure as well as generous in his donation of books.[37] He also became a shell collector of note,[38] and continued to see patients who had followed him from Pooduck Farm to Palm Beach.

A pungent insight into Waterman's impact on patients is to be found in a letter of Robert Frost's (March 12, 1940):

> I have been very sick largely we now think from some very drastic medicine that doctors tried on me for cystitis. I went crazy with it one night alone and broke chairs and ——— til a friend [Merrill Moore] happened to save me. I have had a strange two years—not all as bad as it might have been and perhaps should have been. I was in one bed or another pretty much all of December and January and in one pain or another...You can see from this paper where I have quietly been. I got out Sunday.
>
> R.F.[39]

The letter was written on stationery bearing the printed letterhead, "2000 El Bravo Way, Palm Beach, Florida." Frost was even more explicit in a later letter to a close friend: "I'd be a bad man as well as a bad author if I wouldn't squeeze a report for you out of my pen on how I came out after I left you. Dr. Waterman at Palm Beach thought he didn't think me too bad yet didn't think me quite good enough to face the lectures in North Carolina and Virginia."[40] The best example of the ambivalent rapport between Waterman and Frost is in a letter from the poet to Louis Untermeyer:

[Boston, Mass.]
March 31, 1940 Eve of departure for
Western Pennsylvania, Iowa, Utah, Indiana, etc.

Dear Louis:

In all that concerns me trust your poetic imagination more than anything you hear from my over-anxious friends. I was willing the doctors down in Florida (Dr. Waterman to be precise) and the doctors up here (Dr. Moore to be precise) should have me as sick as they pleased if it would get the prescription out of them that I wanted, namely, that I should "go back north where I was born bred look to die." I told Dr. Waterman's wife in his presence and hearing that he had better look out for me: I wasn't above using him merely to get out of work or get around a woman. She answered I would have to be a pretty smart man to get anything out of her husband that he didn't see me getting and intend me to get. I ventured to say I was a pretty smart man when I have been up awhile and was well awake. Well the result of our fencing was that my aches and pains were authenticated and I got my order to go North for my health instead of further South. Looking each other wickedly in the eyes we both laughed. No money passed between us. In exchange for his treating me I treated him for not knowing infallibly enough how to tell a good quatrain from a bad quatrain; a discrimination I demonstrated that lies at the very root of all poetry appreciation. A bad quatrain consists of an epigram of about the extent of two lines which the poet thinks of first but saves for the last and two lines preliminary labored into some semblance of validity or at least plausibility to round out the form. A good quatrain keeps you from knowing which member of the rhyme-twins the poet thought of first. I had the doctor's acknowledgement of value received.

Ever and steadily yours,
Robert[41]

It is clear from these letters that Merrill Moore sent Frost to Waterman. At that time, Moore, a member of the Fugitive Poets, who had done a residency in neurology at Boston City Hospital and held the post of assistant physician at the Boston Psychopathic Hospital from 1932 to 1935, went into private practice and affiliated with Harvard Medical School, Boston City Hospital, and Massachusetts General Hospital.[42] Moore was a friend of Waterman's and at one time considered taking over his practice. In 1937 he had repeated interviews with Waterman and jotted down notes on his cases and on his psychotherapeutic ploys. The techniques were those of suggestion and hypnosis. Waterman made no attempt at insight, but rather placed a strong emphasis on the patient leading a productive life and accepting the world as it is. One of his favorite quotations from Epictetus captures this belief: "When will the westwind blow? When it pleases Aeolus, my good man. For the Gods have not made you the manager of the winds, but Aeolus." Of Waterman, Moore has written:

> In trying to understand Dr. Waterman and his techniques of working with mentally sick people I am impressed by these three factors in his technique which are not important as techniques in general but which are important actually in the way he works and the results he gets:
>
> (1) His unusually strong, active and vivid memory which is characterized by a very high or powerful pictorial or visual sense.
>
> (2) His immense knowledge of classical thought, literary background and scientific facts.
>
> (3) His skill and power as a teacher and his subtle use of didactic method in gaining insight or more importantly directing the flow of the patient's libido away from anxiety towards a balanced and satisfactory ideal or life aim.[43]

As he aged, Waterman's mind began to wander and he took to keeping a notebook and to collecting pictures of people to correlate facial characteristics with psychic states. He had become a physiognomist. Perhaps it was a function of his own mental state that he ended his days on an organic note.[44]

Toward the end, his practice, which had included such patients as General George Patton, Maude Howe Elliott, daughter of Julia Ward Howe, Miss Louise Guyol of New Orleans, and Mrs. Larz Anderson, was taken over by G. Colket Caner, associate in neurology, Massachusetts General Hospital, and psychiatrist in the department of hygiene, Harvard University, who dedicated a book, *It's How You Take It,*[45] to "George A. Waterman, M.D., Friend and Teacher." Waterman died in 1960 at the age of eighty-eight at 282 Beacon Street, Boston.

George Arthur Waterman was a disciple of James Jackson Putnam and Morton Prince. After he gave up his academic affiliation with Harvard in 1916, he became a diligent practicing physician who used suggestion, encouraged relations of dependence, and was a forceful father figure to his patients. In the 1920s he was the "leading psychotherapist" in Boston; it suited Boston. He did not subscribe to Freudian tenets. Waterman developed a wealthy clientele who moved with him from Blue Hill, Maine, to Palm Beach, to Beacon Street. He was a powerfully charismatic figure who drew no lines between friends and patients. He obviously did not use transference to resolve his patients' problems. Colket Caner has written:

> His private practice became so large and demanding that he gave up his hospital work after only a few years. He was an eclectic in his methods, focusing mainly on educating his patients to attitudes that made for maturity, emotional stability and good human relationships. He made skillful use of suggestion, frequently relieving severe symptoms by suggestion after only one or two interviews; but he was not content with the relief of symptoms, always striving to effect changes in attitudes and philosophy. He made use of inspiring poems, and his own personality and philosophy had an inspiring effect. The trust and admiration which his patients felt toward him contributed greatly to his psychotherapeutic success. Most of his patients were devoted to him, as well as almost all who knew him.[46]

Waterman was a neurologist who treated psychoneurotic patients. His affiliations with the Boston Society of Psychiatry and Neurology, the American Neurological Association, and the Association for Research in Nervous and Mental Disorders reveal his sustained and dominant neurological orientation.

Beginning in the 1920s, psychiatry and neurology became more and more separated, each discipline harboring some hostility toward the other. This is evident in the evaluation of Waterman, the old-style practitioner, by more recent neurologists and psychiatrists. The late Henry Viets, neurologist, said of Waterman: "He could talk longer and say less than any man I ever knew." Stanley Cobb, the psychiatrist, wrote to me in October 1966:

> I am glad you are writing on Dr. Waterman. I did not know him well, but admired him for his devotion to his patients. He seemed to be a satellite of Dr. Putnam's who quietly went about kind and good things for neurotic patients. In fact I think he "spoiled" many of them by too much personal kindness that was not in the professional line of duty. He struck me as a saint, but I don't get along well with saints!

References

[1] Merrill Moore Papers, Library of Congress. Waterman discussed his cases and psychotherapeutic ploys with Merrill Moore who kept notes of the conversations through the year 1937. (The first note to Moore from Waterman is dated May 4, 1937.) There are also four typed manuscripts of notes on Dr. G.A. Waterman by Moore, September 2, 3, 4, and 6, 1938, in Maine. The folder also contains a notebook filled with shorthand, presumably the original of which the typed documents are transcripts. Permission to use this material was given by Anne Leslie Moore, Moore's widow. The information footnoted is a Merrill Moore interview with G.A. Waterman, September 6,

1938. Biographical material about Waterman is given in: (a) obituary by G. Colket Caner, *New England Journal of Medicine, 263* (1960), 1032, 1090; (b) obituary in *Harvard Medical Alumni Bulletin, 35* (1960), 68; (c) Harvard College, Class of 1895, *Twenty-fifth Anniversary Report*, Number VI, 1895–1920 (printed for the Class; Cambridge, Mass.: University Press, 1920), pp. 511–512; Report VII, 1925, p. 315; *55th Anniversary Report*, 1945, pp. 669–670; (d) Thomas Francis Harrington, M.D., *The Harvard Medical School, 1782–1905* (Boston: Lewis, 1905), vol. III, p. 1630; (e) Frederic A. Washburn, M.D., *The Massachusetts General Hospital, Its Development, 1900–1935* (Boston: Houghton Mifflin, 1939), p. 314.

2 Washburn, *Massachusetts General Hospital*, pp. 603, 619.

3 John A.P. Millet, "Psychoanalysis in the United States," reprinted from Franz Alexander, Samuel Eisenstein, and Martin Grotjahn, *Psychoanalytic Pioneers* (New York: Basic Books, 1966), p. 551.

4 *Ibid.* John C. Burnham, *Psychoanalysis and American Medicine 1894–1918: Medicine, Science, and Culture.*, Psychological Issues, vol. V, no. 4, monograph 20 (1967), p. 25.

5 Cecilia Mettler and Fred A. Mettler, *History of Medicine* (Philadelphia: Blakiston, 1947), p. 592.

6 Washburn, *Massachusetts General Hospital*, p. 175.

7 Archives of the Massachusetts General Hospital.

8 Harrington, *Harvard Medical School, 1782–1905*, pp. 138, 141, 198; Washburn, *Massachusetts General Hospital*, p. 318.

9 Walter Bradford Cannon, *Boston Medical and Surgical Journal*, January 11, May 31, 1900.

10 James Jackson Putnam, M.D., and George A. Waterman, *Studies in Neurological Diagnosis* (Boston: George H. Ellis, 1902, 2nd, 1909).

11 Nathan G. Hale, Jr., *James Jackson Putnam and Psychoanalysis* (Cambridge, Mass.: Harvard University Press, 1971), Introduction, pp. 1–63; Nathan G. Hale, Jr., *Freud and the Americans: The Beginnings of Psychoanalysis in the United States, 1876–1917* (New York: Oxford University Press, 1971).

12 Merrill Moore, M.D., "Morton Prince, M.D. (1854–1929), a Biographic Sketch and Bibliography," *Journal of Nervous and Mental Diseases, 87* (1938), 701; H.A. Murray, "Morton Prince, Sketch of His Life and Work," *Journal of Abnormal Social Psychology, 52* (1956), 291–295; Otto Marx, "Morton Prince and the Dissociation of a Personality," *Journal of the History of Behavioral Sciences, 6* (1970), 120–130.

13 Washburn, *Massachusetts General Hospital*, p. 317.

14 George Arthur Waterman and James Jackson Putnam, "A Contribution to the Study of Cerebellar Tumors, and Their Treatment," read at the meeting of the American Neurological Association, September 15–17, 1904. Boston, 1904, pp. 49–75.

15 Henri F. Ellenberger, *The Discovery of the Unconscious* (New York: Basic Books, 1970), p. 344.

16 The lectures of Pierre Janet were published in a volume, *The Major Symptoms of Hysteria* (London: Macmillan, 1907).

17 J.J. Putnam and George A. Waterman, "Certain Aspects of the Differential Diagnosis Between Epilepsy and Hysteria," *Boston Journal* (May 4, 1905) 509–516. See Hale, *Freud and the Americans*, p. 89.

18 *Journal of Abnormal Psychology, 2* (1907), 134–137; Review of *Hysteria in Children* by D'Orsay Hecht, M.D., *Journal of the American Medical Association*, February 23, 1907.

19 *Journal of Abnormal Psychology, 3* (1908), 314.

20 *Journal of Abnormal Psychology, 4* (1909), 128–139.

21 *Psychotherapeutics, A Symposium* (Boston and Toronto: Richard G. Badger, Gorham Press, 1910). Contributors were: Morton Prince, Professor of Diseases of the Nervous System, Tufts College Medical School; Frederick H. Gerrish, M.D., Professor of Surgery, Bowdoin College; James J. Putnam, M.D., Professor of Neurology, Harvard Medical School; E.W. Taylor, M.D., Instructor in Neurology, Harvard Medical School; Boris Sidis, M.D.; George A. Waterman, M.D., Assistant in Neurology, Harvard Medical School; John G. Donley, M.D., Physician of Nervous Diseases, St. Joseph's Hospital, Providence; Ernest Jones, M.D., Demonstrator of Psychiatry, University of Toronto; Tom A. Williams, M.D.

22 Ernest Jones, *Life of Freud*, vol. II, *Years of Maturity, 1901–1919* (New York: Basic Books), pp. 56, 57.

23 *Journal of Abnormal Psychology, 5* (1910), 196–210.

24 *Journal of Abnormal Psychology, 6* (1911), 170–171.

25 Hale, *James Jackson Putnam and Psychoanalysis*, letter from James to Putnam, September 9, 1910, p. 227.

26 *Ibid.*, Jones to J.J. Putnam, October 11, 1910, p. 233.

27 *Ibid.*, Putnam to Jones, October 14, 1910, p. 236.

28 Archives, Massachusetts General Hospital.

29 Washburn, *Massachusetts General Hospital*, p. 319.

30 Mark Antony De Wolfe Howe, *A Venture in Remembrance* (Boston: Little Brown, 1941), p. 225; Robert Lowell, *Life Studies*. (New York: Farrar, Straus and Cudahy, 1959), "Memories of West Street and Lepke," p. 85.

31 Lawrence S. Kubie, *The Riggs Story* (New York: Hoeber, 1960), p. 139.

32 Ernest Earnest, *S. Weir Mitchell, Novelist and Physician* (Philadelphia: University of Pennsylvania Press, 1950).

33 Norman Dain, *Concepts of Insanity in the United States, 1789–1865* (New Brunswick, N.J.: Rutgers University Press, 1964); Ruth B. Caplan, *Psychiatry and the Community in Nineteenth Century America* (New York: Basic Books, 1969).

34 Letter from Elizabeth B. Patton, October 24, 1966, to George E. Gifford, Jr.

35 Letter from Stanton A. Waterman, July 2, 1966, to George E. Gifford, Jr.

36 See obituary, *Harvard Medical Alumni Bulletin, 35* (1961), 68.

37 Letter from James R. Knott, West Palm Beach, August 4, 1966, to George E. Gifford, Jr.

[38] G.E. Gifford, Jr., "A Scallop-Shell of Quiet," *Harvard Medical Alumni Bulletin, 48* (1974), 28–31.

[39] Laurence Thompson, *Selected Letters of Robert Frost* (New York: Holt, Rinehart, and Winston, 1964), letter to Sidney Cox, March 12, 1940, p. 487.

[40] *Ibid.*, letter no. 378 to Harvey Allen, March 31, 1940, Boston, p. 488.

[41] *Letters of Robert Frost to Louis Untermeyer* (New York: Holt, Rinehart and Winston, 1963), pp. 321–322.

[42] About Merrill Moore, see Joseph Garland, "Doctor's Afield: Merrill Moore," *New England Journal of Medicine, 251* (1954), 230–231.

[43] Merrill Moore, interview with G.A. Waterman, September 2, 1938, p. 6. Merrill Moore Papers, Library of Congress.

[44] Waterman's physiognomical collection is deposited at the Francis A. Countway Library of Medicine, Boston.

[45] G. Colket Caner, *It's How You Take It* (Bungay, Suffolk: Richard Clay, 1956).

[46] ———, obituary, see reference 1.

Abraham Myerson

PAUL G. MYERSON

As you might well imagine, I have found it difficult to write in a detached way about my father, Abraham Myerson. I shall try to remain objective in this exposition, but quite apart from the obvious problems a son has in discussing his father, Abraham Myerson was a passionate man and his presence evoked intense reactions in every one who knew him well. Those who loved him, and there were many, loved him with intensity, and those, fewer in number, whose feelings he had hurt rarely forgave him. He was a fascinating man, not only because of his great wit, intelligence, and erudition, but especially because of the many contradictory aspects of his personality. He was truly generous-hearted, contributing freely of his time, interest, and purse to many causes and people; however, where his beliefs were at stake, he could react with breathtaking pugnacity and show little concern about the sensitivities of his opponents. He was generally ebullient, lively, highspirited. At times when he took a hard look at what was becoming of the twentieth century, those of us close to him were aware of his fatalistic state of mind, which sometimes bordered on depression. No one was more cynical about the foibles of mankind, yet more convinced that he should dedicate himself to do the best he could to alleviate the lot of others. He had heroic prejudices, while being extremely receptive to new ideas.

And so it went. In fact there was one supreme paradox that characterized him: the many facets of his personality suggest an unfathomable complexity, yet he was basically a simple man—simple in the sense that he was open, direct, and completely unambiguous. He would sometimes state that to exert any position of power one needed to have the strength of the lion, the wisdom of the owl, the wiles of the serpent, and the gentleness of the dove. He was strong and wise, and at times gentle, though not cunning in any way. He was as honest as any man could be with himself and with every one else.

I deeply wish I could do justice to the essence of this unique man.

Yet I am afraid there are too many parts of him in too many diverse and contradictory parts of myself to accomplish this task. How can I depict an idealized introject when I must make allowances for the way my father has influenced my identifications, my counteridentifications, my superego, and my ego ideal? Perhaps one may be able to get some sense of what he was like, how he affected the people he loved and who loved him, yet who were confronted by his powerful character, through the way I, his son, write about him.

My father was born in the ghetto village of Yanova, Lithuania, in 1881 and was brought to this country in 1886. He was fortunate in that his parents were hardworking, intelligent, and loving people. His father had originally been educated to be a rabbi but rebelled against his religion and became an agnostic and a socialist. The first chapter of my father's last book, *Speaking of Man*, is entitled, "My Father and I Discuss Matters," an unqualified tribute to his father's beneficial influence. His mother was a spunky and shrewd woman, enormously and justifiably proud of her children. My father looked back on his childhood with great relish. It was presented to me as a series of amazing adventures and heroic events: the gang war with the Broadway street gang, the battle with the bully, of course won by him, the time he and his brother almost joined the circus as professional acrobats, and so on. These tales sounded somewhat strange to my admiring and admittedly somewhat envious ears, which had been protected through his growing affluence from the jarring decibels of Boston's slums. I was far from miserable, although I had my share of childhood Weltschmerz and wondered how his boyhood could have been such unalloyed pleasure. I believe now, however, that his supreme natural endowments, both physical and mental, and the special role he played in his family constellation enhanced his self-esteem and fostered a remarkable zest for living.

That notwithstanding, my father faced many hardships. His father was a scholar but not a successful businessman and there was no money for a college education. After graduating from high school, he worked for the biblical seven years in his brother's shop, cutting pipe to save enough money to go to medical school. (He did not go to college.) He enrolled in Columbia Medical School, but his money ran out at the end of the first year and he was forced to work for a year as a substitute streetcar conductor under unbelievably oppressive circumstances. He came face to face with the ruthless ways workers were treated at the turn of the century and he told me that many years later when the streetcar employees went out on strike he experienced a triumphant glee at the discomfiture of the bosses—a rare type of reaction for him. Being young and ambitious, he went back to medical school, first returning to Columbia and then transferring to Tufts where he graduated in 1908. There he came into contact with Morton Prince. His great interest in brain anatomy called him to Prince's attention, and he joined and later was president of a club Prince organized for discussions on psychology. He had a lifelong admiration and respect for Prince and it was with considerable satisfaction that he eventually held the chair in neurology at Tufts that had been his.

After graduation he worked for two and one-half years as an assistant in the Department for Diseases of the Nervous System at the Boston City Hospital. He then spent six months in neuropathology in Southard's laboratory before going to St. Louis where he was resident neurologist at the Alexian Brothers' Hospital under the benevolent auspices of William Washington Graves, whom he chose to be my godfather.

Graves was a magnificent Dickensian character, who frequently came to Boston for treatment of radiation burns which he sustained during his pioneering work in radiological studies of the scapula. He clearly adored his distinguished student and frequently interrupted his conversations with my father by suddenly putting his hands on his shoulder and expostulating, "my dear, dear Abe." There were also asides to me in the form of K Y P I Y P which stood for, I was subsequently told, keep your pecker in your pants, an admonition I at first found shocking and then, as I became more sophisticated, delightfully quaint. Graves was apparently a superb neurologist and a first-rate physician, but he had a lifelong belief that the size and shape of the scapula reflected intelligence, character, and the potential for mental illness.

What influence Graves had upon my father's continued interest in the inheritance of mental disease I cannot say. I am inclined to believe this developed more from the circumstances he found himself in when he became clinical director and pathologist at the Taunton State Hospital, a position he held from 1913 to 1917. My father was an enormously curious, energetic, and pragmatic individual, determined to discover whatever he could about the phenomena he was presented with. What he was presented with at the Taunton State Hospital were thousands of psychotic individuals, hundreds of brains, and a myriad of patient records going back many decades. The microscope, alas, did not reveal the mysterious flaw in cerebral structure that was responsible for what in those days was called dementia praecox. He had too much clinical responsibility for far too many patients to make systematic observations upon their behavioral characteristics and indeed the winds from Zurich had not reached a rural state hospital in the second decade of the twentieth century. But the records which he pored over assiduously did show that of all the patients who had been in the hospital since it was founded in 1854, roughly ten percent had one or more relatives who had also been hospitalized there.

These observations were published in 1917, the first of a series of such studies that occupied him all his professional life. His enormous clinical practice—where he examined over a thousand new patients a year for many years and observed on many occasions members of the same family with severe mental illness—convinced him of the importance of the inheritance factor in mental illness. He was concerned about the long-term social dangers of an increasing genetic pool of defects leading to mental impairment, and at times was sympathetic to a program of limited eugenical sterilization. Yet he also recognized the frequent connection between individuals of great talent in families that were tainted with emotional illness. He argued against the measures proposed by the more ardent eugenicists.

In line with his interest in genetics, my father was convinced that some day a biological basis for mental illness would be found, and despite the fact that he had had no fundamental training in physiological research, undertook to hasten that day. In 1927 he became director of research at the Boston State Hospital and soon thereafter developed a technique for obtaining blood from the internal jugular vein and the internal carotid artery. "It seemed theoretically correct," he wrote "that if one could study the blood directly before it reached the brain, and then could study it directly as it came from the brain...something might be learned of what takes place within the brain." While the mysterious flaw in cerebral metabolism responsible for schizophrenia, as it was by then called, once again, alas, did not yield to his earnest and most careful scrutiny, his approach has been of great value in many and varied physiological studies of the brain. In 1933 the Commonwealth of Massachusetts completed the laboratory at the Boston State Hospital, which is now called the Myerson Building, and a grant from the Rockefeller Foundation in 1935 supplied the funds for many of his projects. That same year he was appointed clinical professor of psychiatry at Harvard. In the period that followed, he and his associates made many significant studies of the effects of the sympathetic and parasympathetic drugs upon such bodily functions as the heart rate, blood pressure, and the gastric juice.

Yet even though his interest in ascertaining the biological basis of mental illness never weakened any more than his conviction that it would one day be found, his major concerns were with the wide and exciting world around him—the consulting room, the ward, the jails, the courts, the lecture hall, with all the fascinating and confused human beings he met every day. He was the supreme participant-observer. For example, in accordance with Briggs' law, he examined thousands of prisoners over a period of eight years for the Commonwealth of Massachusetts to ascertain their sanity. He was meticulous in his assigned task, but was primarily concerned with trying to determine the genesis of criminality. It is of considerable interest that despite his predilection for an inherited basis of mental disease and his exposure to the Lombrosian traditions where the criminal was considered to be mentally sick, he came to believe that society—rather than the genes—was in large measure responsible for the disorganized and unintegrated behavior of the imprisoned men he met.

He was continually preoccupied with the nature of the clinical phenomena that he observed daily. Much of his writing in later years was directed towards ferreting out the interrelationships of the various syndromes he encountered. This is suggested by the titles of some of his papers, "Neuroses and Neuropsychoses: The Relationship of Symptom Groups," "Scrutiny, Social Anxiety, and Inner Turmoil in Relationship to Schizophrenia." He frequently emphasized the importance of recognizing and studying the minor forms of the major clinical syndromes. He was convinced that it was often possible to prevent severe mental conditions from developing by alleviating some of the physiological components apparent in the early stages of these disorders, in particular through reversing the disturbance of the sleeping and waking mechanism. I was in practice with him after World War II for two years and we had many discussions about the transitions of one symptom complex to another, for example the relationship of obsessional states to depressive and paranoid conditions. His clinical records of his last years in practice are replete with extremely meticulous observations, and still can be read with great interest.

One of his most important publications advocated the use of total push for the schizophrenic patient. He had come to believe that many of the schizophrenic phenomena which could be observed in the back wards of state hospitals were iatrogenic or at least enhanced by the apathy of the staff toward schizophrenic patients. In the late thirties he initiated a program at the Boston State Hospital in which schizophrenic patients were actively treated by having them exercise, interact with each other and with the staff, as well as by the use of energizing drugs that were available at the time. He found that a number of patients responded favorably to what he called a total push approach and several improved to the point where they could be discharged.

My father had a passionate eagerness to understand the world around him and he was continually shifting his focus. In 1934 he published *Social Psychology*, in which he emphasized the influence social forces have over attitudes, desires, pleasures, and even bodily functioning. His final work published posthumously, *Speaking of Man*, is a collection of essays that elaborates this theme. The book has many passages rich with insights and presented in Abe Myerson's inimitable style. Perhaps I had best allow my father to speak for himself. In a chapter entitled "Social Ambivalence" he states: "I have used 'biological' and 'social' and the related nouns as if they were opposites or, at least, markedly different. Broadly speaking, biology includes sociology, since it is a prime biologic characteristic of man to be social. It is biologic for men to use tools, and therefore all mechanical development and the artificialities of the machine age are as much a part of the biology of man as his glands; it is biologic for 'Homosapiens' to think, and therefore all the seemingly fantastic restrictions and inhibitions he has placed on his more primitive urges are as biologic as the forebrain, which does his thinking. There are men who preach with passion against the uses of medicines as nonnatural, yet they shave, wear clothes, brush their teeth, and use eyeglasses, to itemize a few of a thousand departures from nature, whatever that may be. I use the term 'biological' to mean the expression of primitive bodily activities and needs and the term 'social' to denote those processes and demands which are represented by man's institutions and often show the dominance of tradition, custom, and taboo. There are psychologists who question whether man really has social instincts, yet the psychologists are men who live in groups and who could not survive or remain sane without sociality. There is no real dichotomy of biologic and social.

"With no solution for this apparent disharmony, I still deny the validity of a scheme which balks and declares obscene man's fiercest cravings, those which build up the continuity of life. There is something wretchedly wrong in the whole ideal of chastity; it is something of an incubus on human life. St. Paul's contemptuous saying that it is better to marry than to burn has been amplified into a whole code of life which relegates sex, its pleasures, and its results to the position of necessary evils.

"I am not wise enough to know how we shall establish a valid social psychology and social psychology of morality. Not, I am sure, on the authoritative thunderings of men who did not know about the ovum, the sperm, or the hormones; or of men who thought that plagues, floods, failure of crops, mental disease, and death came because God was displeased by some failure to observe rites. We would not run railroads by the notions of people who knew only about ox-carts." Vintage Abraham Myerson!

But above all else, more than his laboratory search for the biological basis of mental illness or his writing delving into the effect of social institutions upon human nature, or the inspiration he knew he communicated to his students, my father valued himself as a practicing psychiatrist—and he had every right to. Even today, a quarter of a century after his death, I and members of my family meet individuals whom he treated and who speak of him with enormous affection and gratitude. He was the master of the short-term contact or crisis intervention, as it is now called. While he used drugs and shock treatment extensively, he was a general psychiatrist to whom people turned when they had severe disorders—he had an unusual capacity for truly establishing rapport. He would sit across from his patient, smoke his pipe, and with a few well-chosen remarks communicate his understanding, his wisdom, and his humanity. He was, I believe, in intimate contact with the preconscious and could clarify for his patient what they both were experiencing. He was extremely pragmatic as well as enormously experienced and would often make usually judicious, and by and large cautious, suggestions about how his patients might remedy their situations.

This is not the place nor am I the person to speak of the limitations of his approach. We obviously had a fundamental disagreement about the importance of psychoanalysis, although this in no sense disturbed our relationship. Temperamentally, he was the activist, the doer, best suited to tracking the many roads to knowledge, to meet and help thousands of patients, rather than sit quietly and explore the hidden depths of the few. He was a man who gave unstintingly of himself—and most of his patients came away at least a little wiser and a little more aware of themselves. Those of us who knew him well were vastly inspired by what he gave to us.

Bibliography

BOOKS

The Nervous Housewife (Boston: Little, Brown & Co., 1920), 273 pp.

The Inheritance of Mental Diseases (Baltimore: Williams & Wilkins Co., 1925), 336 pp.

When Life Loses Its Zest (Boston: Little, Brown & Co., 1925), 218 pp.

The Psychology of Mental Disorders (New York: The Macmillan Co., 1927), 135 pp.

The Foundations of Personality (Boston: Little, Brown & Co., 1931), 406 pp.

The German Jew—His Share in Modern Culture (with Isaac Goldberg) (New York: Alfred A. Knopf, 1933), 161 pp.

Social Psychology (New York: Prentice-Hall Co., 1934), 640 pp.

Eugenical Sterilization—A Reorientation of the Problem. By the Committee of the American Neurological Association for the Investigation of Sterilization, Abraham Myerson, Chairman. (New York: The Macmillan Co., 1936) 211 pp.

SELECTED SCIENTIFIC ARTICLES

"Psychiatric Family Studies," *American Journal of Insanity, 73* (1917), 355–486.

"Anhedonia," *American Journal of Psychiatry, 2* (1922), 87–103.

"Technic for Obtaining Blood from the Internal Jugular Vein and Internal Carotid Artery" (with R.D. Halloran and H.L. Hirsch), *Archives of Neurology and Psychiatry, 17* (1927), 807–808.

"Researches in Feeblemindedness with Special Relationship to Inheritance," *Bulletin of the Massachusetts Department of Mental Diseases, 14* (1930), 108–229.

"Studies of Biochemistry of Brain Blood by Internal Jugular Puncture," *American Journal of Psychiatry, 10* (1930), 389–406.

"Physiological Approach to the Psychoneuroses," *Bulletin of the Massachusetts Department of Mental Diseases, 15* (1931), 1–9.

"Insulin Hypoglycemia; Mechanism of the Neurologic Symptoms" (with W. Dameshek), *Archives of Neurology and Psychiatry, 33* (1935), 1–18.

"Neuroses and Neuropsychoses. The Relationship of Symptom Groups," *American Journal of Psychiatry, 93* (1936), 263–301.

"Human Autonomic Pharmacology. XII. Theories and Results of Autonomic Drug Administration," *Journal of the American Medical Association, 110* (1938), 101–103.

"The Legal Phases of Psychiatry," *American Journal of Jurisprudence, 1* (1938), 73–78.

"Theory and Principles of the 'Total Push' Method in the Treatment of Chronic Schizophrenia," *American Journal of Psychiatry, 95* (1939), 1197–1204.

"The Attitude of Neurologists, Psychiatrists, and Psychologists towards Psychoanalysis," *American Journal of Psychiatry, 96* (1939), 623–641.

"The Social Psychology of Alcoholism," *Disorders of the Nervous System, 1* (1940), 1–8.

"The Rationale of Amphetamine (Benzedrine) Sulphate Therapy," *American Journal of Medical Science, 199* (1940), 729–737.

"Experience with Electric Shock Therapy in Mental Disease" (with Louis Feldman and Isadore Green), *New England Journal of Medicine, 224* (1941), 1081–1085.

"The Incidence of Manic-depressive Psychosis in Certain Socially Important Families, Preliminary Report" (with Rosalie D. Boyle), *American Journal of Psychiatry, 98* (1941), 11–21.

"The Sale of Alcoholic Beverages. A Proposal for Changes in the Present Methods to Conform with the Federal Food, Drug and Cosmetic Act and to Promote Public Health" (with Leo Alexander and Merrill Moore), *Mental Hygiene, 26* (1942), 235–242.

"The Bisexuality of Man" (with Rudolph Neustadt), *Journal of Mount Sinai Hospital, 9* (1942), 668–678.

"The Sleeping and Waking Mechanisms. A Theory of the Depressions and Their Treatment," *Journal of Nervous and Mental Diseases, 105* (1947), 598–606.

"Scrutiny, Social Anxiety, and Inner Turmoil in Relationship to Schizophrenia," *American Journal of Psychiatry, 105* (1948), 401–409.

William Healy: 1869–1963*

GEORGE E. GARDNER

On a cold and blustery day in November 1878 a thin, spindly English boy of nine years came down the gangplank of the White Star-Leyland steamship *Colonian* onto the docks in New York City. He was accompanied by his father, his mother, an older brother, and an older sister. It was only a matter of a few moments before the boy's mother found her brother, Henry, who had come to welcome them to America. Eighty-five years later (at age ninety-four) this immigrant boy, William Healy, died, after making a notable contribution to our culture and creating a revolution in respect to programs relating to the proper study, care, and treatment of children and youth.

It is usually assumed that, whereas immigrants to America from Russia, Poland, and Italy were extremely poor and landed with but a few dollars in their pockets, the immigrants from England arrived with enough money to support themselves for a reasonable length of time. This assumption was definitely false in the case of William Healy's family. They were almost, if not actually, penniless. The fare for their passage had been forwarded to them by the boy's maternal uncle in order that they might escape a desperate financial plight in England and try to make a living in America.

William Healy was born January 20, 1869, the youngest of four children, near Beaconsfield, Buckinghamshire, in central England. His father (as the Healys had done for generations) tilled the soil on a small portion of a manorial estate called Penn Lands, and added to his income by making bricks and roof tiles from clay found in one area of the farm land. The father had returned to this land from an apprenticeship in London upon the death of his father and older brother.

Their marginal economic status was lost when the father's brothers challenged his primogeniture rights. William Healy, Senior, because of his strict and sincere fundamentalist religious beliefs and affiliation, refused to contest the contemplated court actions of his mother and brothers. He relinquished his rights to the family plot of land, removed himself and his family to Bournemouth on the sea in the south of England, and with borrowed money started his own brick and tile-making business. On the night of the first burning, a hurricane swept up the Channel and destroyed his kiln and all his sheds. As Dr. Healy said, "Then we were *really* poor. I can remember we had meat to eat only once a week." After numerous attempts at gainful and steady employment in and near Bournemouth, the father could not support his family. At this point, the maternal uncle, Henry Hearne, who had emigrated to America some years before, came to the rescue and, with his help, the family was able to go to America.

Knowing Dr. Healy's later contribution to the understanding of the problems, the anxieties, and the difficulties of the poor and particularly of poor children, one wonders what effect these intrafamilial and financial problems had upon his young spirit. As far as can be ascertained from his own memories of his early childhood, these experiences seemed to have had no serious effect. His was a happy childhood. He was well loved by his mother and he loved her devotedly in turn. A close relation existed between himself and his sister, but he never mentioned his relations with his brothers, both of whom were older than he.

The Healy family spent but a few months with Uncle Henry in Buffalo and then moved to Chicago, where a maternal aunt and her American-born husband lived. It is clear that there were no jobs in Buffalo for which the elder William Healy could qualify. And, indeed, there were few, or none, in Chicago either. Eventually the father became a supervisor of a street-sweeping gang—an employee of the city. The older brother also found employment. The family lived on the top floor of a tenement house with no central heating.

Nothing is known of the educational background of the father and mother, but the latter read frequently and extensively to young William and his sister. In England, he attended the rigid, old-fashioned, conventional school of that era and on arriving in America, he was at the appropriate third- or fourth-grade level in school achievement expectancies. In Chicago he attended school for only four more years (until age thirteen). The next institution of learning he attended was Harvard College, which he entered in the fall of 1893 as a "special student." Dr. Healy was not only a high school dropout; he was a grammar school dropout as well.

Some time *before* his fourteenth birthday (1883), William Healy was offered a job (through a church friend of the family) as an office boy in the Fifth National Bank on LaSalle Street, at five dollars a week. After assuring his mother that he would continue his education at night, he was allowed to accept this job, mainly because the family desperately needed the money. He remained in the employ of this bank until the fall of 1893, when he left to enter Harvard College.

I am sure that the question immediately arises in the reader's mind, as it did in mine, "How was it possible that this immigrant boy, who never finished grammar school and who went to work at thirteen, prepared himself so that he was accepted at Harvard College, proceeded to the Harvard Medical School, and graduated with an M.D. from Chicago?" In my limited excursions into the field of adult biography I have concluded that two prerequisites exist to account for such a phenomenon. The first necessity is that the individual must be exceedingly bright and inquisitive; the second is that, given these attributes, the individual must have the all-important good fortune to become a protégé of an adult who, in the first place, becomes an object of motivating identification for the youth and, in the second place, himself identifies with the promised abilities of the youth and has the determination and the power to forward that youth's aspirations through practical help.

William Healy, the bank office boy, had the necessary individual attributes. From earliest childhood he was motivated to learn the secrets of nature, beginning when, to his amazement, he found through a pamphlet that all of the wild flowers of his English boyhood environment could be classified on the basis of the differences in stamens and pistils. That such order through classification was possible in botany was exhilarating and forever motivated him to learn more about life at all other levels, particularly at the human one. Here was a boy who, even at ten years, was innately curious about the world and its varied organic components. Such were the individual attributes, genetically or experientially determined.

What of the second necessity—the identification figure and his motivation and help? Before this person emerges, consider for a moment the milieu into which this thirteen-year-old was thrown at the bank. From his own account of it, the Fifth National Bank of Chicago from 1883 to 1893 must have been populated with extraordinary employees, men who had wide cultural interests and who recognized the brightness and the receptivity of the office boy and messenger, William Healy. For example, there was one bookkeeper, a Scot, who involved Healy immediately in the works of Robert Burns in their noon-hour lunches; a second bookkeeper was a devotee of Shakespeare and read the plays of the bard with Healy when work was slack. There was a third office employee who taught him the basic theories of economics, a fourth who sang part time in operas, and a fifth, Reginald de Koven, who later became a world-famous musician and composer, and who, while doling out greenbacks as a cashier, would surreptiously write musical scores on his broad white English cuffs and discuss and hum them with his bank colleagues. (In case you have forgotten, de Koven was the composer of that deathless ballad, "Oh, Promise Me.")

Hence on the basis of all he heard from these bank colleagues, and on the added basis of all the books that they suggested that he read (and he *did* read them), William Healy became, in truth, a self-educated man. In fact, without a day's formal education beyond the seventh grade, when he entered Harvard College, Healy was far, far ahead of his classmates in his knowledge of English literature. That he knew nothing of Greek, Latin, and mathematics and had but a smattering of science was a handicap—but his bank colleagues and the city library had served him well.

The crucial identification figure that it is my custom to search for in an attempt at biographical understanding emerges through the person of the Reverend William M. Salter. For years Healy had been a disbeliever as far as organized religion was concerned—an overreaction (as he noted) to his father's strict orthodoxy and a position on the part of the son that distressed the father greatly. Two years after he entered the bank he discovered the Ethical Culture Society, and within it he found emotional comfort and exciting intellectual discussions. The leader of this society in Chicago was the Rev. William M. Salter who, previously identified with the (then considered) leftist Unitarian Church, moved even more to the theological left and the liberalism of the Ethical Culture Society. Salter was, basically, a philosopher rather than a theologian, and Healy studied and discussed problems at length under the tutelage of this man and his group. He also was impressed by the fact that here was a man who took to the streets and the public platforms, and to the halls of the legislature and its committees, to fight for the causes of people victimized by social and economic injustices. Healy was an enthusiastic follower of Salter's and Salter, in turn, noted the extraordinary brilliance of the self-educated William Healy.

This could have been the end of it and Healy could have become (and was promised he would be) a successful and highly placed Chicago banker and presumably a wealthy and highly regarded citizen. But here enters one of those extraordinary coincidences that seals the fate of men destined to greatness—a coincidence that at the moment of its effectiveness seems irrelevant. The Rev. Mr. Salter was a Harvard alumnus and was married to the sister of William James, the already renowned professor of philosophy and psychology at Harvard. The perceptive Salter recognized a genius when he saw one, and he enlisted the good services of a prominent Harvard graduate, an official of the bank where Healy worked, and the attendant help of Professor William James himself through letters to him, to effect the acceptance of William Healy at Harvard.

Healy himself never commented upon these personal interests and influences, but a biographer has a right to a between-the-lines interpretation of probable events even though the subject permits himself to attribute little or no importance to them. However Healy later dwelled upon his close relations to William James: his many evening invitations to his Cambridge home, his visits to James's summer house in Chocurua, New Hampshire, and through Professor and Mrs. James's inner group of students and Cambridge academics, his acquaintance with later outstanding figures in the fields of psychology, psychiatry, and other branches of medicine. James—through his brother-in-law William Salter's influence—looked upon William Healy as a Harvard student who was to be an object of his especial care and guidance. More important, however, William James was the figure with whom William Healy identified and this identification (as physician, psychologist, and philosopher) fixed his abiding interests. In his nineties Dr. Healy still declared his never ending interest in philosophy—and this after he had become a historically important contributor to the fields of medicine and child psychology.

William Healy's determination to become educated and to go to college *some* time is attested to by the fact that, in addition to contributing to the support of his home, by the age of twenty-three he had saved $3,000 to pay for his intended college education. He attended Harvard for three years, and spent three more years at Harvard Medical School, until his $3,000 ran out. He transferred to Rush Medical College for his senior year, living at home. As far as one can ascertain, Healy had a thoroughly pleasant and stimulating six years at Harvard. The students with whom he became personal friends (largely under William James's influence) constitute a veritable Who's Who of later outstanding personages in psychology and medicine, and particularly in neurology and psychiatry. For example, he shared a closeness with Earl Bond, later professor of psychiatry at the University of Pennsylvania, with the physiologist Walter Cannon, with E.E. Southard, later of the Boston Psychopathic Hospital, and with many others of like interests and future renown.

Interestingly enough, Healy, though always listed as a member of the Harvard class of 1897, did not graduate with his class because of a deficiency in Latin, a study to which neither his colleagues at the Fifth National Bank of Chicago nor the Rev. Salter had ever directed his attention. At the suggestion of Professor Josiah Royce, philosopher, Healy studied Latin for two summers, took an examination at the end of each summer, but failed both of them. However, in 1899 the faculty voted to give him a bachelor degree and finally he became a legitimatized Harvard alumnus.

Dr. Healy was never able to give me a convincing answer to why he went to medical school, why he wished to be a physician, and particularly why, eventually, he chose the allied specialties of psychiatry, neurology, and the behavioral development (or psychology) of childhood and adolescence for his life's work. As a matter of fact, he said that his first preference in study was philosophy and for years (like many other psychiatrists) he returned periodically to prolonged bouts of reading the philosophers, notably Plato, Aristotle, Kant, Berkeley, Hume, and, curiously enough, Nietzsche. In truth, he really thought Nietzsche "an abomination" but he reread his works anyway. What Dr. Healy never could seem to reconcile was, first, a consciously avowed lifelong ambivalence toward the works of Nietzsche, and second, the fact that his original mentor and sponsor, the Rev. Salter had written a book on this German philosopher, and Healy had been enthralled by it.

But beyond whatever significance one might allow for this selected memory lapse in Healy's past, it seems quite clear to me that his crucial and critical identification object changed in his twenties to William James—James who wanted to be a physician but gave it up; James who railed loud and long against the sterile "brass instrumentation" of the psychologist (as did Healy); James who wrote one of the most significant works in respect to mental eccentricities and abnormalities in his *Varieties of Religious Experience*; James who tried to teach teachers the proper and healthy methods of educating children; and James who was foremost and forever a philosopher—and forever, too, a liberal in his stands on sociopolitical issues as they affected both children and adults.

It takes an inordinately long time to work out, to one's own inner satisfaction, an earlier identification with such an extraordinary scholar and humanitarian as William James. But Healy accomplished it, and in so doing touched all the bases. (All the bases save one, since he did not make a contribution to formal philosophy as did James. I submit, however, that he did contribute a philosophy of lasting import, namely, a philosophy that the actions of an individual should be judged only upon the collection of *all* of the facts of his past existence—a philosophy that, for the first time, guided the approach of all to the problems of the maladjusted child.)

The long excursion necessary for the fulfillment of an identification becomes apparent in the multiform and multivaried activities *and* contributions of Dr. Healy. Following his graduation from medical school in 1900, Healy spent his first year as physician to the Women's Division of the Mendota State Hospital in Wisconsin. The following five years he spent in general practice in Chicago. While engaged in private practice, he became interested in gynecology and became an instructor in this specialty at Northwestern University. Two years later he had shifted his interest from gynecology to neurology and for three years was an instructor in neurology at the Chicago Polyclinic.

Healy married Mary Sylvia Tenney and in 1902 his only child, a son, Kent Tenney Healy, was born; he was to become a renowned professor at Yale.

In 1906, "after a family conference" (probably following *many* of them), Healy definitely decided that his lifework was to be in neurology and he and his family went abroad for a year's postgraduate training. He followed the usual peripatetic course of trainees at that time and spent various lengths of time in Vienna, Berlin, and, of course, Queen's Square Hospital in London.

Of all of his accomplishments I have selected (for what in this presentation can be at best but summaries), first, his role in the establishment of the child guidance movement and as a teacher and trainer of child mental health professionals; second, his research studies relative to the causes and the treatment of the juvenile delinquent and the adult criminal; and third, his role in the introduction of psychoanalysis in the United States.

In respect to the founding of the first child guidance clinic in Chicago in 1909 and of the Judge Baker Foundation in Boston in 1917, it is best for me to quote Dr. Healy himself:

> In Chicago there was a group that included a number of women who centered their interest very largely around Hull House and Jane Addams (1860–1935). They were the same people, very largely, who led the campaign for a legislative act in Illinois forming the juvenile courts, which was a very important step, because their interest led to the first juvenile court in the world. The first one was established in 1899 in Chicago. These women, Jane Addams and particularly Julia Lathrop (1858–1932), who afterwards

became head of the Federal Children's Bureau, were also interested in the children who, even before they came to the court, were held in jail, and so they started something else. They built a juvenile detention home; a very nice building was erected. They were certainly a glorious and most remarkable set of women. They had observed that the judges in the juvenile court didn't know what to do with the children.

These women had heard about me through statements I had made about what I had seen in the Polyclinic, especially about the youngsters who had disorders that led them to be offenders. They came to me and said that they thought a well-run investigation of children should be made: medical (already they got very good medical examinations), psychological, psychiatric, social. Examinations should be made in important areas of life in which frequently children could be helped. I had recently come from abroad, and they also wanted to know what was done over there, but I had never heard of such a thing in Europe.

It is interesting that the idea for these child guidance clinics, which are now all over this country and abroad, came from three or four lay people, not from medical men or psychiatrists. Miss Lathrop, who through work in mental hygiene had become a friend of Adolf Meyer at Johns Hopkins, consulted him about the matter, and he said that certainly something of this sort ought to be done, studies should be made. Then she went to see William James, who knew me quite well, and he said, "If you're going to start something, why don't you get Healy to do it himself?"

In 1908, I went around the country, to see all kinds of people I thought might have some ideas about beginning, and to see what there was already in clinics. One of the problems was how many feeble-minded children were being sent from the courts to ordinary institutions, and it was already known that there were quite a few. I made quite an extensive tour. I found only two people who were even giving any mental tests: Goddard, a psychologist who was working with the feeble-minded, and Witmer, at the University of Pennsylvania, who again was working with the feeble-minded, and even they didn't give well-rounded studies of the cases. Everybody agreed that *it* should be done. When I went around, they said, "You'd better blaze a trail." A number of them, in just those words, said, "You've got to blaze a trail." So I went back to Chicago with this news and met with the group at Hull House. Mrs. Ethel Dummer, a member of that group, said, "None of us knows what should be done and what to find out. I'll give you funds for five years to pay for the research for a study of the material that comes into juvenile court"—particularly the juvenile court, because we could readily get parents in and get information from them and from probation officers. There were only occasional social workers around. In the early days of our work, there were no such things as psychiatric social workers in this country.

I am only fair to myself when I say that when I gave up my practice for research, I gave up more money than Mrs. Dummer did in financing the five years of research. I was building up a good neurological practice. But the chance to do something like this seemed to me of great public importance and benefit, and being research, besides, which I thought I'd like to do, intrigued me absolutely into giving up my practice and doing this.

As a fair-minded researcher, I don't think I had any idea of what I would find out. I didn't have any preconceived theories. I had never studied children before that, in that sense. I didn't have any theories about them. The only theories I could get were those of people who had published in various volumes. I soon thought that that was pretty poor stuff.

All I hoped to accomplish was to find out what needed to be done by way of treatment, because at that time I already knew that the institutions were very ineffective, even the good ones, the so-called parental schools.

It must be understood—I don't think it has been well enough understood—that those five years were really given up simply to fact finding. We could give a certain amount of advice to the judge in the juvenile court, but there was almost nothing to be done in the way of treatment except to send them to an institution—but we soon found out that most of the institutions didn't do anything for the youngster. He would live there for a while and would come out, and no one had done anything about the main circumstances that had caused him to be delinquent, in the family, the neighborhood, and so on.

One of the reasons that we went to Boston was that the Children's Aid Societies—a number of them were very old, a hundred years old or more—promised to work with us and do something about what we suggested. But in Chicago we couldn't get anything done. There were no agencies to do it.

So we started. Mrs. Dummer gave the money for me and for a psychologist and for a secretary. We were given quarters in the detention home, where the juvenile court was held and where the juvenile offenders were detained. We met with a great deal of warmth.

Jane Addams, of course, gave her blessing, but was too busy ever to do anything. Julia Lathrop formed a board of advisors, and one very able and useful member was Professor James Rowland Angell (1869–1949), professor of psychology at the University of Chicago and afterwards president of Yale. He was very helpful with suggesting mental tests. A number of others were very nice and very good.

One of the people who welcomed us and steered us a great deal was (John) Henry Wigmore (1863–1943) of the Northwestern University Law School, the world's greatest authority on evidence and testimony. He helped us a great deal and became one of our very best friends.

But we did have to meet the question of the heredity of the criminal.

I, like everybody else at that time, thought I knew an awful lot about heredity; from my studies abroad and so on, I knew more about heredity then and later on than I ever imagined. It just shows you how early those studies were.

Doctor Edith Spaulding, who came from New York to help me, wanted to do a thesis, and so she worked on the question of heredity in our cases, and tabulated them very thoroughly to see if we could really show that there was heredity of anything like criminality. By her very careful studies, which she reported to a medical society later on, we determined that we couldn't find any such thing as inheritance of criminality.

By the way, we called our institute the Juvenile Psychopathic Institute. That just goes to show you how much, at that time, I was under the influence of everybody else—there was something the matter with the kid mentally or he wouldn't be an offender. So we called it the Juvenile Psychopathic Institute, which was really a silly name for it, because we didn't find out that most of them were psychopathic. It was called that for a number of years, and then the name was dropped.

Some of the social workers and a judge or two in Boston had heard of our work, and in 1912 I was invited to give a course at the Harvard summer school, and again in 1913. Coming to that course—to my utter surprise—were prominent social workers and a judge or two and doctors. In the case studies that were printed up for use in those summers there were blank pages left for notes and discussion, to save my spending an hour or two describing a case.

In the class of 1913, I found Dr. Augusta Bronner. She had been Thorndike's assistant at Columbia. He advised Dr. Bronner to take the course, since she had presented a thesis for her Ph.D. on the mentality of delinquent girls, following out the idea that existed over many years that people who do wrong are not right mentally. She came, and at that time, the psychologist I had was moving to a permanent position, and so I invited her to come out to Chicago at the minute salary that was offered in those days, and so she joined forces with me. And she has been with me all the time, 1913 to the present [1960].

At that period, we were just beginning to know Binet. Goddard at Vineland and I were the first two users of the Binet test in this country. Our first psychologist had been a student under Professor Angell, but even Angell knew very little about tests.

Serious tests were lacking both here and abroad, with the exception of those first tests by Binet which later on came to be very much developed in this country, especially by Terman. When we first knew them, they were not even under age levels. This was way back in 1911, when we got out that first monograph. I've been looking over it, and I am amused by it. We would think it pretty faulty now. A number of the tests in that monograph were devised by me and by Dr. Bronner. They were useful because they were practical, and by the time this was published were being used in conjunction with the Binet tests.

Dr. Bronner was the first psychologist appointed in the state of Illinois under a new law that called for the verdict of a psychologist to place an individual in an institution for the feeble-minded. It's a serious matter to call a person feeble-minded and put him in an institution.

So these tests were of practical importance at that time. They were not all mine; some were taken from ideas from abroad and so on. Later, I got out a test called the apperception test, which I liked very much. That is the only one that could really be accredited especially to me. So I was a pioneer in the field of mental testing, too.

At the end of five years—1914, that must have been—the judge of the juvenile court, a man I admired very much indeed, said, "Well, now, I cannot get along without your type of studies of cases even though we do very poorly on treatment; still, it gives me some understanding of *youngsters.*" He got the county to appropriate funds for us to continue the work under the same title, the Juvenile Psychopathic Institute. Our offices were still in the Juvenile Detention Home. Whereupon a howl was set up by the politicians. They had never heard of such a thing. They lopped off the psychologist's salary—if I had a psychologist, I had to take somebody from Chicago. At which I went to a fine judge there, Henry Horner (afterwards governor), and told him the story. He put the kibosh on that. And so we kept Dr. Bronner. I stayed on that basis a couple of years.

I think people thought a good deal of our type of work in Chicago, but for the sake of selling the idea, getting it spread, I needed to publish something. I had enough material on hand by 1915 to get a book published —*The Individual Delinquent.* In it you will find the little tables telling the mixture of causes in certain cases. The idea of this book was taken up at once by Dean Wigmore, who got Little Brown and Company to get it out—quite an expensive book, by the way, to publish. They got it out as a legal book and that's one reason it went around to judges so much. Some criminologist made the statement that the book represented a new era in criminology. And in a way it did, I think, because the old criminology dealt with the individual offense, but the individual was considered only very casually. This book went all over the world. Years afterwards I was in Norway—the person I was seeing said, "Oh yes," and he reached up and there was that book. I found the same thing in a good many other places in Europe, too, and I know that it even went to Russia. I never inquired about its sales; the royalties must have gone to the expenses of the Juvenile Psychopathic Institute. I never got any royalties. Most of my books have been published while I was getting a salary and I was paid in that way for doing the work. Yes, that book certainly had a great deal of influence.

Twice a splendid man from Boston, Judge Harvey Baker, had come to Chicago to study with us for a few days, to see cases and how we studied them. He was judge of the juvenile court in Boston, and in his last report, written before he died in 1915, he said that what he wanted done for the children of Boston was to have them studied as we did it so that advice could be given to social agencies and to the court. Interest in such a clinic had also developed in Boston as a result of my Harvard summer school course, which had been attended especially by various social workers.

Dr. Bronner talked with me about going to Boston, and I said that I would be glad to go, provided that there were funds provided for a long enough period of time to accomplish something, and we stipulated, therefore, that ten years would be the minimum.

There were good reasons why we responded favorably to suggestions that we head a clinic in Boston. The lack of adequate facilities for the treatment of delinquents in Chicago was most discouraging, and there was almost nothing that we could do to secure proper treatment. We already knew that a great many of the cases seen by us earlier had, after being released from juvenile correctional institutions, turned to serious criminality.

In contrast, Boston had a number of well-established children's agencies, and it was particularly as a result of the promise of the heads of them to give us full support and cooperation that we were willing to go.

After Dr. Bronner left, a meeting concerning the initiation of a clinic was held. A surprising number of professional and public-spirited citizens attended, and afterward Judge Cabot set about raising the rest of the money that would be required.

In the meantime, Dr. Herman Adler, whom I had known earlier because he was at the Psychopathic Hospital in Boston with my friend, Dr. Southard, was making a study of Chicago for the National Association of Mental Hygiene. I asked him to take my place there, and he proved that he was just the man to do it. He was very much better at outside planning, at persuading people, than I ever would be. He went right to work on the state authorities and convinced them that the type of work that I had set up there should be carried on. They established, at his insistance, an institute for juvenile research, state supported and doing work all over the state.

Then in April, 1917, we opened our clinic in Boston under the name of the Judge Baker Foundation (changed in 1933 to the Judge Baker Guidance Center). We started with a small budget of $14,000 and occupied five rooms in a business building. Our staff consisted of Dr. Bronner, myself, a secretary, and Miss Margaret Fitz, a so-called school visitor, really a social worker. She knew the districts from which many delinquents came, and fortunately spoke Italian well, which recommended her for the position. Judge Cabot became president of our board of trustees.

One of the most interesting features of our work, therefore, was that from the first in Boston the type of services that a good child guidance clinic can offer were sought for, quite aside from juvenile delinquents—problems referred by social agencies, many families independent of organizations, and, very interestingly, private schools.

In the beginning, by far the largest part of our work was diagnostic in nature, undertaken for the juvenile court. By the end of ten years less that half of our cases were referred by the court.

It was particularly the promises of the heads of social agencies in Boston that we would be involved in treatment programs that led us to go there so enthusiastically, since we felt so strongly the treatment limitations in Chicago. But a curious fact about the treatment of young offenders from the court was that Judge Cabot felt very strongly that their treatment was the function of the court. We were to make the diagnosis and recommendations, but he and his probation officers were to carry out the treatment. As we look back on it, we regret very strongly that we did not stoutly insist that this would not work. That it did not was shown by the Gluecks' study of youthful offenders. About 1930, we did get the first of a series of grants from Mr. Godfrey Hyams and the Hyams Fund for entering more into treatment.

Our early efforts to establish ourselves on a professional basis were amply backed up by Dr. Walter Fernald (1859–1954), administrator of a leading institution for the mentally defective, and Dr. James J. Putnam (1846–1918), professor of neurology at Harvard Medical School. They gave us a great deal of advice and attention and served on the board of trustees. They and others made our beginnings extremely well sponsored. I make that point because we advise others interested in establishing a child guidance clinic to do the same.[1]

Such were the beginnings of the child guidance clinic as told by Dr. Healy. The national and worldwide spread of this new institution for child care is commented upon fully in material already published over the years. Suffice it to emphasize here but two important items. The first is that the idea spread through the influence of hundreds and hundreds of students in all disciplines who spent varying amounts of time in observation and training with Dr. Healy and Dr. Bronner, both in Chicago and in Boston in those years from 1909 up to and beyond the 1940s. The roster of those people comprises a portion of the "Who's Who" and "Who Was Who" in the child guidance field, and it was they who contributed much to the eventual emergence of child psychiatry as a medical specialty.

A second, and very important, item is the wholehearted support for this movement on the part of the successive medical directors of the National Committee for Mental Hygiene and the Commonwealth Fund.

Yet I would emphasize the obvious fact that the brilliant and resourceful Dr. Healy and Dr. Bronner were never alone in their work. In the very beginning of it all, they had (and profited by) the thoughts, the inspiration, the help, and the loyal support of a host of dedicated people. It is shortsighted in the extreme to assume that the support that the Chicago group gave to Dr. Healy was purely monetary assistance. They were men and women with innovative ideas aimed at the betterment of childhood; they were liberals in the truest and best meaning of the term, of the same caliber and determination as those who helped in Boston. And Dr. Healy was always a good listener!

The second and a lasting contribution of Dr. Healy was made through his outstanding research publications in the areas of juvenile delinquency and criminality. There is hardly a topic in these two fields to which his intense investigatory drive and his desire to know did not turn his attention.

I have already cited the publication of *The Individual Delinquent: A Textbook of Diagnosis and Prognosis* in 1915. In it he first sounded in initial statements (or perhaps a single sentence) those themes that were to recur again and again in later definitive works resulting from extended particularized research and more detailed discussion: the inestimable value (indeed the *basic* value) of getting the individual's own story (and in depth); the need to utilize in diagnosis all known knowledge from all known disciplines; and the utilization of any person or any group of persons that could help the patient. These three concepts became the structural pillars of the child guidance clinic.

There seems to be little question on the part of those professionals who have evaluated Dr. Healy's work over the years that *The Individual Delinquent* was not only his greatest work but had the greatest influence. It is interesting, and satisfying, that Dr. Healy himself believed this to be a true and just evaluation.

In all, Dr. Healy published ten books, and I shall list the others mainly to indicate the broad scope of his studies dealing with antisocial behavior:

1. *Case Studies of Mentally and Morally Abnormal Types* (1912), his first publication;
2. *Pathological Lying, Accusations, and Swindling* (1915), written in collaboration with his first wife, Mary Tenney Healy;
3. *Honesty* (1915);

4. *Mental Conflicts and Misconduct* (1917);
5. *Judge Baker Foundation Case Studies* (1923);
6. *Delinquents and Criminals: Their Making and Unmaking* (1926), with A.F. Bronner;
7. *Manual of Individual Mental Tests* (1927), with others;
8. *Reconstructing Behavior in Youth* (1929), with others;
9. *The Structure and Meaning of Psychoanalysis* (1930), with others;
10. *Roots of Crime* (1935), with F. Alexander;
11. *New Light on Delinquency and Its Treatment* (1936), with A.F. Bronner;
12. *Personality in Formation and Action* (Salmon Memorial Lectures);
13. *Treatment and What Happened Afterward* (1940), with A.F. Bronner;
14. *Criminal Youth and the Borstal System* (1941), with B.S. Alper.

Few scholars are more productive than this record indicates. It is all the more remarkable when one considers that in addition Dr. Healy carried on the administration of a relatively large clinic, raised money to support it and his research, saw hundreds of patients, taught college courses, lectured here and abroad, worked in professional organizations, and taught clinic trainees week after week through the staff conference method.

His third contribution—and one that up to this moment has never been stressed—was his tremendous influence in the introduction of psychoanalytic thinking to the mental health personnel in this country. This influence emerged through the publication of *The Structure and Meaning of Psychoanalysis* in 1930.

Certain items associated with the publication of this book are quite interesting, including an exchange of letters with Freud and another with Ernest Jones. These letters came to light in 1957, at the time the Judge Baker Center moved its files from the building on Beacon Street to its new building on Longwood Avenue.

But first, what about Healy's interest in and acquaintance with psychoanalysis? That his interest stemmed from his early years at the Institute for Juvenile Research, there can be little doubt. He read Freud thoroughly and wasted no opportunity to apply psychoanalytic concepts and findings in his discussion of cases. In *The Individual Delinquent*, he included a reasonably clear treatment of psychoanalysis and emphasized that "early mental experiences and strange, altogether hidden, mental conflicts have arranged the destinies of many a chronic offender." And he continued to carefully read the psychoanalytic literature and utilize it.

However, Healy's own personal contact with psychoanalysis before his book came out was at best meager. And in respect to this the record becomes hazy; its facts are solely in the minds of those now living who in the 1920s were young psychoanalysts. Healy himself used to refer to "my psychoanalysis" from time to time, and in his interviews in the 1960s with Professor John C. Burnham he refers twice to his "psychoanalysis."

I am indebted to Dr. Ives Hendrick and his excellent memory for the clarification of this question. In a personal communication Dr. Hendrick stated that Healy was analyzed by Franz Alexander in 1931. Alexander came to Boston in September of that year, at the suggestion of Dr. Hendrick, to work with Healy on his research grant that involved the psychoanalysis of criminals. This was after the publication of *Structure and Meaning* and was when Healy was sixty-two years old.

But an exceedingly interesting bit of additional information on this point came to me very recently from Dr. Helene Deutsch. I asked Dr. Deutsch if she could tell me anything about when, where, and by whom Dr. Healy had had an analysis. Dr. Deutsch replied:

> Both Dr. Healy and Dr. Bronner had three months of analytic work with me in 1929. It was not an analysis and both Drs. Healy and Bronner—and I—agreed that this was not our intention. Dr. Healy specifically wished to have enough analytic hours with me to observe the results of the technique of free association. He found it a very profitable and enlightening experience. And I myself was certainly content with the outcome of this interesting "experiment."

But to return to the correspondence that related to Freud's attitude. While engaged in writing the book in July 1929, Healy apparently, through a friend, tried to get an appointment with Freud for the purpose of discussing its contents and its aims. Freud wrote to Healy from Berchtesgaden on July 17, 1929:

> Dear Dr. Healy,
>
> I was prepared to see you in Vienna but here I am eager for some rest, deeply engaged in writing and not anxious to see visitors. As I know your attitude towards psychoanalysis to be a negative one and no influence may be expected from one hour's conversation—I think you are no loser by not coming.
>
> Sincerely yours,
> Freud

Healy was evidently deeply hurt and indeed angry at this obviously untrue last sentence. However, he did not answer Freud's letter but waited till the book was published. And at that point he forwarded a copy and a letter on April 30, 1930. This letter not only contains Healy's attempt to account for and to negate Freud's wrong impression of his attitude toward psychoanalysis, but is additionally interesting in that it reveals some of the angles of the battle that was raging in America over psychoanalysis. Healy's letter was as follows:

April 30, 1930

Professor Sigmund Freud
Berggasse, 19
Vienna IX, Austria
My dear Professor Freud:

We are sending to you one of the first copies of our book, which is just off the press. I think you will see clearly our reasons for producing this work. The immense amount of time that we have had to give to it seemed justified because a more organized presentation of this subject is necessary in order that there may be fairer understandings. Even such a man as McDougall, though he renders splendid tribute to you, has not taken the trouble to read deeply enough into psychoanalytic theory to state it correctly. And others, friendly and unfriendly, have not found time enough to develop appreciation of what we call the "structure" of psychoanalysis. There will be no excuse for this in the future and we look forward to a much sounder knowledge of what psychoanalysis is through the stimulation that this work will give toward reading the original productions in this field, particularly your own works.

Even already, the work has received some excellent reviews. We pushed our work on it very fast recently in order to get the book out for the International Congress of Mental Hygiene and in doing so, we were unable to give a final last reading, I am sorry to say, so that there are a dozen or more typographical errors which appear in it.

You can imagine the irony of the situation when I received your letter, which you kindly sent me here, stating that you knew that I was unfriendly to psychoanalysis. In the light of the fact that Dr. Bronner and I have given this great amount of work in the endeavor to further open up the field that you had first explored, this would seem more than passing strange. Notwithstanding the fact that we are Americans, we do not happen to be "money-making" Americans and stand above everything as being lovers of the truth. With our public duties and our research work, we are not able to be even practicing psychoanalysts, although we have accumulated much data bearing on the validity of psychoanalytic concepts.

I might parenthetically add that we were given a sum of money by someone who was aided by psychoanalysis to help us partially in defraying the expense of this work. Otherwise, it has come entirely out of our own pocket and through our own efforts, nor shall we get any returns from it.

And all this brings up another matter which has some large significances. It makes little difference that I was misrepresented to you, apparently, and that Dr. Bronner was misrepresented to your daughter by a man who had called on us for help frequently in the past and had our advice in some of his own situations—situations in which we thought he was doing good work in connection with a certain institution—and that we supposed that he was our friend. I should not have asked him to have made the first appointment with you if he had not been with us at that time and had not written to me most effusively while I was in Berlin. But it does bring up the whole question that I should have liked much to have talked to you about, namely, whether or not psychoanalysis as a procedure can be expected to alter for the better personality and character.

Now, I agree with you fully that psychoanalysis is primarily to be regarded as a scientific instrument for understanding the human mind and conduct, but there is also the prime question of how a person behaves as a result of being psychoanalyzed or practicing psychoanalysis. To me, it would seem as if the result ought to be the development of really finer qualities and understandings and moderations, but evidently this does not always happen, at least here in America. It is quite beside the mark to say that we are money-mad or that we are crude, because in many respects we are not, and are developing certain very good techniques aimed at a better civilization and culture. And the broad outlook that psychoanalysis should give into human motivations ought to enable the person to stand out against our national defects, if they are national with such a mixed population.

It was just such matters as these and the possibility of developing further lines of research, such as we have shown you by this book that we have begun, that I wanted to discuss with you. I am afraid that the chance to get any funds for such research through the Institute of Human Relations at Yale is lost because the man who had the broadest vision in projecting the work of the Institute, together with his assistant, who was friendly to psychoanalysis, have gone to the University of Chicago—the former person having become the president of that great university. Perhaps they will find some way of doing something out there.

Yes, it was quite ironic that you, whom we respect and admire so much, and for the furtherance of whose ideas we were so earnestly working, should harbor such attitudes about us.

As far as I can ascertain from our files, Freud never replied to Healy's letter nor did he ever comment on the book. (If he did, such items might be in the Freud Archives in London.)

But Healy seemed undaunted by whatever Freud's reaction might be for he sent a copy of the book to Ernest Jones. I doubt if Healy could ever offer a better example of ambivalence than that afforded him in Jones's reply:

81 Harley Street
London, W.1.
8th May, 1930

Dear Dr. Healy,

I wish to thank you and your associates for kindly sending me a copy of your last book "The Structure and Meaning of Psychoanalysis" and also to congratulate you on it. It is, I think, the first book written by a non-analyst on the subject of psychoanalysis which we analysts will find really useful. I have not been through it very carefully as yet, but so far my impression is that the exposition of the subject is a good deal better done than the random selection of quotations from analytical writers.

It is a pity that the latter could not have been read through by someone more versed in the literature before going to press. However, it is very hard for us to induce you non-analytical people to cooperate with us.

Yours sincerely,
Ernest Jones

Such was the exchange between Healy and the two leading psychoanalysts in the world at that time. Nonetheless the book was a tremendous success. It sold in the thousands. It was assigned reading in universities and in schools of social work. Its value in furthering the acceptance of psychoanalysis in America was its timeliness, since it appeared and was a success just prior to the arrival on our shores in the mid-1930s and thereafter of many illustrious training analysts who were fleeing from the scourge of Hitler. Scores of professionals who later became analysts, and countless others in those professions who utilized Freudian concepts in their clinical work, had their first introduction to the field through reading Healy's book.

Healy was also in the forefront of those psychiatrists who welcomed the newly arriving psychoanalysts. He received them at the Judge Baker, and he assisted in their attempts at placement in Boston and in other cities in the United States.

It is significant that his contributions were recognized in that from the first establishment of the Boston Psychoanalytic Society he was made an honorary member. Again, his work as a member of professional organizations was great and it was effective. He was one of the founders of the American Orthopsychiatric Association and its president; he was also president of the Boston Society of Psychiatry and Neurology and of the

American Psychopathological Association. And for nearly a quarter of a century he was chairman of the Board of Trustees of the Boston Psychopathic Hospital and rarely (if ever) was absent from its monthly meetings. He did much to guide the policies and assist personnel that made the Boston Psychopathic Hospital one of the outstanding training research centers in this country—and, indeed, in the world.

Finally, what were the lasting impressions that this great man made upon his students and upon those who were associated with him as members of his staff? What manner of man was he in the everyday affairs of clinical work?

First—and of great significance—was the never ending zest and enthusiasm and optimism with which he listened to (and commented upon) the details of the life history of a child being presented to him for his diagnosis and evaluation, and his suggestions in regard to treatment. He listened with the attentiveness of the newest student of human behavior, and time and again when the thought would occur to all that surely this case must be the absolute repetitive prosaic model in both content and meaning noted by Dr. Healy a thousand times before, his comment would be a zestful "How extraordinary!" Then followed an unfolding of interrelationships in the child's life or an emphasis upon some particular item in it, the significance of which had not seemed to be very great to others in the room. It should be added that he was equally zestful and enthusiastic when colleagues elaborated some significant, important, but perhaps difficult to discern, clinical fact.

Added to the enthusiasm that Dr. Healy brought to any and all outlining of clinical data was his extraordinary memory of the pertinent clinical facts of the hundreds of cases that he had dealt with over the years. If you gave him just the name and a few facts about some child that had been at the clinic years before, he would describe the case in greatest detail—and not infrequently give follow-up data concerning the child that he had gleaned from some source or other in the years since. This gift of clinical memory that Dr. Healy possessed, beyond that given to any other clinician I have ever known, seemed all the more remarkable to me thirty-two years ago, when I would recall that he, even then, was seventy years of age.

A third and lasting significant impression that Dr. Healy made upon all—and that can be checked today in his publications—was his adroitness and deftness in his own interviews with children. He surely had the needed ingredients that immediately activated a sense of trust in a child and that could entice from him a revelation of his deepest feelings. When one remembers that in most instances he was dealing with youngsters who had been severely traumatized by adults (with their questions and doubts) in both the recent and the remote past, the fullness of some of his single interviews is all the more remarkable. It would seem that his concern was for the child's story, told by the child; the story of the child by another was of lesser importance to him.

A fourth major attribute of the man was the comprehensive approach that he followed in arriving at his clinical judgments. He wanted a complete evaluation of the child, and any body of knowledge that aided in effecting this completeness he insisted should be advanced and considered. As he wrote about and applied the latest psychoanalytic concepts, findings, and teachings of Freud (and Freud's colleagues and students), he kept informed about, and commented upon, the work of the biochemists and endocrinologists, whom he numbered among his closest friends and colleagues. He never lost his interest in and his insistence upon the importance of neurology, and he himself did complete informative neurological examinations on all children who came under his care.

What other remembrances and impressions does one recall of Dr. Healy in his clinical work and in those affairs that paralleled his direct work with children?

There was the insatiable curiosity in regard to human behavior that led to his significant publications. Yet one always felt that Dr. Healy was torn somewhat by an old and abiding conflict between his desire to add to knowledge and his love of direct clinical work with children and their parents in his desire to help them. He seemed to leave his research room with a feeling of joy and relief that for an hour or two he would deal with the urgent problems of the patient—to return thereafter with a sense of pressure that the analysis of data and writing was of highest priority in his life. It was perhaps his greatest gift to his students and staff that he never could quite solve, with the firmness of finality, such a constructive and productive, severe and sincere conflict of interests.

One remembers that he was a liberal and a progressive in respect to the affairs of the community and the nation, and he made certain that we in the clinic knew it. He studied the issues of the day seriously and sought in the best tradition of the liberal to determine as exactly as he could that aspect of the issue that called for the rectifying of an inhumanity, a wrong, or an unfairness, and he acted to correct it. It was in this spirit that he welcomed many professional colleagues to the Judge Baker Center who were victims of Nazi terrorism, and he worked to assist others to our shores who did not join the Judge Baker staff.

Surely the captain and the crew of the White Star-Leyland steamship *Colonian* could never have known the eventual immense value to mankind of that nine-year-old immigrant boy that they transported to America in 1878. But we do.

References

[*] Originally presented as a Founders' Memorial Lecture before the American Academy of Child Psychiatry, October 9, 1971; *Journal of the American Academy of Child Psychiatry, 11* (1972), 1–29.

[1] From a recorded interview with Dr. Healy by Dr. John C. Burnham, professor of sociology, Ohio State University.

Early Vicissitudes of Psychoanalysis at the Austen Riggs Center

EDGERTON McC. HOWARD

I have been asked to discuss the early vicissitudes of psychoanalysis at the Austen Riggs Center and I will give also a bit of background and some conclusions from my work in psychotherapy and psychoanalytic psychotherapy. I think that the contents of my short impressionistic report are worthy of a careful, historical, and analytic research, but this report is not that study.

I am bound to be asked how I, an analyst, came to work at Riggs. In 1935 C. Macfie Campbell[1] told me that Dr. Riggs[2] was looking for another staff member and asked me, as a favor, at least to talk with him. I did and was very impressed by Dr. Riggs and his approach to psychiatric problems. However, I was not ready to leave Boston, as I intended to get analytic training. Dr. Riggs approved, said he was anxious to have an analyst on the staff, and asked me to consider joining after I finished my training.

I graduated from the institute in 1938, having been lucky to have Ives Hendrick[3] and Moe Kaufman[4] as my control analysts. I was less than lucky in my timing as it was during the worst of the Depression, and I was unable to earn my living in practice. Because of the tight economic situation, few physicians referred patients to psychiatrists and analysts, and then only to those who were well known. The main sources of referrals for the younger analysts, Drs. Anthonisen,[5] Clothier,[6] d'Elseaux,[7] and I (the most recent graduate), were from the "older" analysts, Drs. Hendrick, Kaufman and Jock Murray,[8] and they were keeping all of the $10 an hour patients, most of the $5 ones, and referring to us only the $2.50 and the occasional $5 patients. I had to borrow heavily and when, after Dr. Rigg's death, in August 1940, I was invited to join the staff at Riggs, I did so. I figured that at a salary of $9,600 a year I could save enough money in two years to set myself up in practice again. Then the war came. My interest in the work at the center and the fact that my leaving would have forced Riggs to close down because of the shortage of staff changed my plans.

I have never regretted my decision to stay, though the burden of keeping Riggs going during the war was almost unbelievable. The potential for the future was exciting and made it worthwhile. I began working with the Board of Trustees to restructure Riggs by putting the staff on salary to better streamline control and solve some economic problems. This was done. After the war, when it became possible to get staff, Dr. Kubie,[9] who was on the board, some of the other members, including Mrs. Riggs, and I laid plans to develop the center into a truly psychoanalytic institution.

In August 1947 Robert P. Knight,[10] a nationally known psychoanalyst, was appointed medical director. Our staff was soon augmented to include Joseph O. Chassell,[11] Margaret Brenman,[12] David Rapaport,[13] Merton Gill,[14] and Erik Erikson.[15] Further, many of the fellows at Riggs were also in training at the Western New England Psychoanalytic Institute (then nicknamed the Stockbridge-New Haven Axis, Route 63 between Stockbridge and New Haven being dubbed the Sigmund Freud Highway). Incidentally, five of the charter members of the Western New England were from Riggs, and the first three presidents were on the Riggs staff. Eight of the early fellows at Riggs were later graduates of the Western New England and several stayed on the staff at Riggs for a number of years. Thus the Riggs staff eventually consisted of twelve analysts.

I have gone into this much detail to emphasize that teaching, study, and therapy at Riggs were based on psychoanalytic psychology. The learning atmosphere, including the staff conferences, was exciting. Erik Erikson has written that staff conferences were the best he has known, and the list of staff publications runs into the hundreds. A training program, psychoanalytic in orientation, was developed for advanced psychiatrists and psychologists. There have been nearly ninety fellows, many receiving their analytic training at the Western New England Institute for Psychoanalysis.

This constitutes the background. I turn now to the fascinating topic of developing a psychoanalytic residential treatment center and the problems we faced and solved in doing so. Developing a center in which the staff running it are not only the therapists, but also closely involved in administrative and social functions with the patients creates unique problems. We knew of no precedents to guide us. Later we learned that Dr. Thomas Main at the Cassel Hospital in London had already established such a center and his experience proved to be most valuable to us. But at the beginning we were truly experimentalists venturing into unknown areas. It is this venture that I am recounting here.

The first and most obvious problem was that the median age of the patient population was dropping, soon to be twenty-one years with a minimum age of eighteen. These adolescents and postadolescents were all individuals who had flunked out of home and school and who were unable to tolerate regulated lives. The old Riggs regime of prescribed schedules and activities had truly proved helpful to older patients who had achieved some success in life. It was an inappropriate atmosphere for younger patients. Earlier, when the majority of patients were older, it always had been that younger patients could order their own lives as they wished without disrupting the social order in the institution. This was impossible with mostly younger patients.

The second problem, and an enhancement of the first, was that the majority of the patients were much sicker, most being borderline schizophrenics, or schizophrenics, some severely so. No usual ordering of society appealed or would be effective.

Our last problem was one that is completely unfamiliar to analysts having office practices—that in a small therapeutic center such as Riggs, situated in a small town, the staff and patients live in close proximity to one another. The patients know all about the staff and their families down to, almost, the most intimate details. The usual analytic blank screen on which transference reactions can be projected and analyzed was impossible.

All patients were in psychoanalytically oriented psychotherapy four or five times a week, many for long periods of time. Only about ten percent of the patients were in "orthodox" psychoanalysis (and its orthodoxy can be questioned, considering the goldfish bowl within which we all lived.)

With our patients entrusted to us for twenty-four hours a day, we analysts were faced with the unique problem of how to develop a hospital milieu that would support individual analytic psychotherapy. We did not know how to do this without instituting rules that would be reminiscent of the patients' family and school environments and that would vitiate our therapeutic roles. This was an exciting challenge. The vicissitudes that we went through make fascinating history. I can only touch the high spots.

Our initial approach was to remove all constraints, since we naïvely believed that if the center provided a wealth of opportunities for active involvement our young patients would somehow become involved and make something of their lives at the center. As we should have expected, this led to unbelieveable chaos: much complete day-night reversal; absenteeism from therapy; many patients returned by the police to the hospital drunk; a few landing in jail; a few serious auto accidents; and a few pregnancies. Stockbridge was up in arms about the change at Riggs, and both staff and patients were distressed by the situation.

After two years of this chaos, the staff was desperate, and uncertain how to correct the situation. Several times we drew up rules and regulations to impose on the patients. But each time we discarded them, knowing that they were inconsistent with our goals and that they would not work. We had to find a way to give the patients (or leave them) a full share and responsibility in the management of their own individual lives and the life of the group in such a way that they would accept it, and at the same time preserve the goal of individual psychoanalytic psychotherapy. In 1949 a consultant in group dynamics was invited to hold a series of seminars with the staff. This initiated regular weekly meetings of the whole staff about the administration of the hospital, meetings that continued through the years. Then in 1950 regular staff meetings that included the entire patient body were inaugurated to deal with shared problems.

Lengthy discussions eventually led to some basic agreements. To put it simply, it was agreed that the staff had the responsibility for psychotherapy and for maintaining an atmosphere that was not antitherapeutic. The patients had the responsibility for conducting their own lives and for maintaining a social atmosphere that maximized individual freedom by setting limits (no more trumpet playing up and down the halls at 2 A.M.).

Various patient committees were formed to deal with various aspects of life. The principal one was the Community Committee, the overall governing committee, which also dealt with any individual behavior that was a problem to the group. Then an Activities Committee was formed which planned and developed various activities. Later, after the patients requested by petition to be allowed to care for their own quarters and to do much of the work around the hospital, a Common Work Committee was formed to supervise this.

There were staff representatives on each of these committees; I myself was the representative on the Community Committee for a number of years. The staff helped to maintain a broad liberal perspective and to prevent narrow demanding attitudes that characterize so many "student governments." Also, in contrast to most "student governments," it was agreed that the patients would *really* have control over their own lives. Many of us, including me, were deeply concerned about giving such sick and "acting-out" individuals almost complete control. Our fears proved groundless. Patients took their responsibilities seriously. In my own experience as staff representative on the Community Committee, I saw many irresponsible patients act responsibly and wisely about community affairs.

The whole process of developing a special community was carefully followed by a group dynamics research team consisting of Stuart Miller,[16] Eugene Talbot,[17] and Robert White,[18] which both guided and studied its growth.

It was not all smooth sailing. As soon as a somewhat orderly society was established, it became the establishment and something to rebel against, and the process of involving, trusting, and building would begin all over again. Actually, this process of working together for a common goal is what I believe was good and beneficial. The goal itself was important as a goal; its achievement was not.

Perhaps even more difficult than developing a group spirit among the patients was creating it within the staff. Most of the staff were analysts, extraordinarily competent and creative. All were prima donnas. I say this approvingly; all were leaders. Bob Knight, our medical director, was a leader who did not direct, but guided through his wisdom and encouraged each person to take an active role. Under his leadership this group of able analysts worked together as a team.

Weekly administrative staff conferences were held to plan and evolve policies. Total staff agreement on issues was never possible, and the meetings were frequently difficult. I say this with feeling, since for several years I chaired them. Yet full support from the staff, not necessarily full agreement, was absolutely essential. There was always some staff turnover, and opinions and values changed. Lack of staff support and interest invariably led to lack of patient interest. A sense of deep interest and support for what Riggs was trying to accomplish, no matter what the shades and variations of opinion were, led to strong patient support and participation—the Stanton and Schwartz phenomena.[19] There were many evidences of the subtle influences of staff cohesiveness, or lack of, on patient involvement. A clear and simple example was the arrival of a strong persuasive leader who sincerely questioned the value of work and the Common Work Program. Many hours were spent debating this. Patient interest in it dropped and the program fell apart. But the ups and downs of particular aspects of the program were not as important as was the sense of all the staff and patients working together to achieve something good.

The dynamics of the group of patients and staff were constantly changing, but the goal remained constant, namely, to create a meaningful atmosphere in which the patients could become involved and gain feelings of self-respect. Essential to the success of this undertaking were that the patients ran their own lives and the social group virtually autonomously *and* that patients and staff worked together. An essential safeguard to preserving the individual one-to-one therapy was a rule that no therapist could be involved in administrative decisions about any patient he had in therapy.

Thus Riggs created an atmosphere that was as unlike as possible that of the demanding and regimenting earlier home and school atmosphere. Individual patients could fit in or not as their needs dictated. However, the overall social atmosphere and expectations that were developed proved to be less noxious and permitted individual patients to try out self-motivation. It is my belief that the involvement of staff in this nondemanding but directed environment enabled immature patients to experiment with incorporation of the do's and don'ts of the staff's superegos. It was an environment that stimulated growth of the individual and supported individual psychoanalytic psychotherapy.

This was an exciting and successful experiment. It must be stressed that its success was due to the extraordinary leadership of the medical director, Bob Knight, as well as to the enthusiasm of the whole staff. After his death in 1966, I wrote this eulogy of Bob Knight: "He created an atmosphere of work, industry, and high scholarliness. He expected the best from everyone—even perfection—but gave each complete freedom to carry out his own endeavors, and to be responsible for his own work. He had a complete, almost naïve, trust in others' ability to do this."

I am going to add here some reflections based on my nearly forty years of practice, most of it at Riggs. Much will be obvious to all, but I want to emphasize one aspect of the therapeutic relationship. In my early years I became impressed with the importance of the patient seeing the therapist as a real person. The importance of the transference relationship is obvious. But I also consistently watched the rapport relationship, the reality relationship, the here and now. Through the years I have seen more and more clearly the importance of this reality relationship, especially in my work with adolescents and with severely sick adults. My greatest successes have been with those patients, but I have done almost no work with clear-cut neurotics.

It was in my work as a psychiatrist at Smith College that I first realized the importance that I, as an individual, played in therapy. I saw young women who had severe anxiety, depression symptoms, or confusion about their identity and goals in life, but had not yet developed neurotic symptoms as solutions to their inner conflicts. It was startling to me that many times their tension, anxiety, or depression cleared up in two or three interviews and, on a year's follow-up, did not return. I was the first person with whom they had completely and frankly discussed their secret sexual and aggressive conflicts. I was a potential parent surrogate, who might or might not be critical and disapproving, whose reactions they were testing out. In those adolescents' value judgments, the do's and don'ts were not yet completely internalized and they needed this test. Because I, as a real person, was not judgmental or disapproving, they became free to adopt a nonjudgmental attitude themselves and could handle their guilt or anxiety.

At Riggs I continued my work with adolescents, though they were much sicker adolescents and required long-term therapy. Here, too, it was clear that the interpersonal real relationship, very tenuous at first and at times tenuous for years, was the medium within which the schizophrenic patient could gradually feel his way toward intimacy. Of course, at Riggs, peers among patients also tested out relationships with one another, but that developing with the therapist was always the crucial one. Dr. Otto Will, now medical director, has written extensively of his work with severely regressed, "back-ward" schizophrenics, and emphasized that it is the relationship with the therapist as a real person that has enabled those patients to overcome their isolation and fear of intimacy and eventually to lead normal lives.

In the early days of the center, under the direction of Dr. Riggs himself, therapy was called reeducation, the therapist playing an active role in teaching and guiding patients. This was successful for many older patients who already had integrated egos. A review of Dr. Riggs's writings and of early patient records convinces me that the patient-therapist real relationship was the crucial factor in that therapy, though this was not recognized at the time.

It seems to me that the interpersonal immediate relationship between therapist and patient is the matrix of therapy with those with immature or damaged egos and possibly, of all therapy. I suggest that this is also true in strictly conducted psychoanalysis. Here, of course, much of the time the therapist is the transference object of a real person in the patient's earlier life, making possible the resolution of conflicts rooted in that earlier life and now deeply ingrained in the personality structure.

Studying and developing a better understanding of the dynamics of the real relationship between patient and therapist, is particularly important today when the therapeutic field is flooded with many different approaches to therapy, each having success, but few taking cognizance of the relationship itself between therapist and patient. The need for this study cannot be too strongly emphasized if we are to understand what is therapeutic in the various differing therapies. Psychoanalytic theory provides the most comprehensive understanding of human relationships, and is a challenge for psychoanalysis.

References

[1] C. Macfie Campbell, M.D. (1876–1943), director, Boston Psychopathic Hospital.

[2] Austen Fox Riggs, M.D. (1876–1940), medical director, Austen Riggs Center.

[3] Ives Hendrick, M.D. (1898–1972), training analyst; professor of psychiatry, Harvard Medical School.

[4] M. Ralph Kaufman, M.D., professor of psychiatry, Mt. Sinai School of Medicine; dean, Page and William Black Postgraduate School of Medicine, New York.

[5] Niels Anthonisen, M.D., chief, Neurological Psychiatric Service, Veterans Administration Hospital, White River Junction, Vermont.

[6] Florence Clothier Wislocki, M.D., chief psychiatrist, Fall River Mental Health Center, Fall River, Massachusetts.

[7] Frank C. d'Elseaux, M.D., Marblehead, Massachusetts.

[8] John M. Murray, M.D., professor of clinical psychiatry, Boston University.

[9] Lawrence S. Kubie, M.D., consultant and senior associate research and training and therapy, Sheppard and Enoch Pratt Hospital, Towson, Maryland.

[10] Robert P. Knight, M.D. (1902–1966), medical director, Austen Riggs Center.

[11] Joseph O. Chassell, M.D., Austen Riggs Center.

[12] Margaret Brenman, Ph.D., Austen Riggs Center.

[13] David Rapaport, Ph.D. (1911–1960), Austen Riggs Center.

[14] Merton C. Gill, M.D., professor, Chicago, Illinois.

[15] Erik Erikson, consultant, Austen Riggs Center.

[16] Stuart C. Miller, M.D., director of admissions, Austen Riggs Center.

[17] Eugene Talbot, Ph.D., clinical psychologist, Williams College, Williamstown, Massachusetts.

[18] Robert B. White, M.D., professor of neuropsychiatry, University of Texas, Galveston, Texas; training analyst, New Orleans Psychoanalytic Institute, New Orleans, Louisiana.

[19] The Stanton and Schwartz phenomena was reported in their book on the phenomena at Chestnut Lodge. What they found was truly startling, but is readily discernible when looked for, namely, that disagreements within the staff of a hospital, however

well covered up, are reflected in the patient body. When one gets restlessness and tensions in the patient body, look first at the staff relationships for the source. Likewise good interpersonal relationships in the staff are reflected in the patient body.

Austen Fox Riggs: Pioneer in the Psychotherapy of the Neuroses

BENJAMIN C. RIGGS

Psychiatry at the turn of the century was in a state of dramatic flux, as all other contributions to this volume have documented. The place of each entry to this field of the new humanistic battle, this awakening to the dignity and needs of people not as "cases" but as people, was deeply determined by the personal backgrounds of the protagonists themselves. Surely the socioeconomic origins of Freud, and his personal history, strongly influenced the development of the operational framework of psychoanalysis, but not, in the end, its scientific contributions to the understanding of human nature. But was this only the frame of the picture, or was it an integral part of developed understanding? From empirical clinical experience come the birth of hypothesis and the tools for generalization. While this is less true in the maturing phases of any science, it is germane to an understanding of its origins. It is therefore relevant to look at the personal determinants of the early contributors to our science, the better to evaluate their contributions.

Austen Riggs was a highly significant, though currently neglected, pioneer in psychotherapy. The neglect is in part due to his intense reluctance to reduce his findings to professional papers for peer review. He wrote mainly to reach his original professional friends in internal medicine and the lay public from whom he drew his patients. He was held in high regard by his colleagues, and was known affectionately to hundreds of them. One can only speculate why so fluent and literate a writer kept his light beneath a bushel. I am told that Lewis Hill would never have produced his classic monograph on *Psychotherapeutic Intervention in Schizophrenia* had not his peers and residents literally forced him to dictate his thoughts for reproduction. There are those who can (or must) crystallize their thoughts for publication, and those who are essentially clinicians, whose lives are bound up in and fed by their clinical relations.

Freud never wished to be considered a "therapist" but unrelentingly used his clinical experience for the scholarly, scientific development of theory. The clinician, conversely, uses whatever is available in both the literature and himself to help his patients. There are rare instances of a combination of the two, perhaps best illustrated by the career of Bertram Lewin, of whom someone once said that he walked about the unconscious of his patients in stocking feet. Riggs did this, but without ever labeling or formulating the process. We shall later examine his divided attitude toward psychoanalysis, whose major principles he came increasingly to apply. In any case, the Riggs bibliography is a short one, addressed either to the lay public (*Play* and *Intelligent Living*) or to rather restricted observations of neurosis, something of its definition, and some sound observations on psychotherapy, but lacking the full scope of his originality or the key to his unique method. At this point, the biographical background becomes important.

The Riggses of Maryland are a very old American family. Austen Riggs's father, Benjamin Clapp Riggs, was the first to move north to New York. He was a scholarly physician of no small artistic talent as well. A graduate of Yale, he had followed medical school with a sojourn in Europe, largely in Vienna doing postgraduate work. He was married by then to a native New Yorker, Rebecca Fox, and was already a deep friend of the later famous surgeon, Charles McBurney, who was also for a time in Vienna. Austen was born in Germany in 1876, the second of three children. His father was already ill with tuberculosis, and after returning to this country spent most of his time at the sanitarium of his friend Trudeau at Saranac Lake. He died in 1883, when Austen was seven.

Dr. McBurney became almost a father figure to the Riggs children, but it was Austen who was thrust far more into the father role both in his dramatic and powerful mother's mind and, especially, in his own. This was of vital importance in his development not only in latency but particularly in adolescence. It is as though his precocious ego development was up to the task, but he paid the price of short-circuiting the normal crises and solutions of these periods. He had a deep, affectionate tie to his father and showed throughout his life the accompanying identification, which was carried on with Dr. McBurney. A further contribution to his character was the strict, upper-class Victorian tradition of the age, with all its moralism, rigidity, and intense discipline. This is not to say that in either family there was any lack of humor or joy in living, but young Austen found little opportunity, and gave himself even less permission, to confront and work through the natural rebellions of adolescence. In both his professional and personal life, perhaps in large part owing to these circumstances, he showed a kaleidoscope of conflicting traits in his personality. In sum, it was a massive personality: he was not so much an intellectual giant, like his contemporary, Freud, as he was a deeply feeling, captivating, creative clinician. But to describe him only in the professional context is to miss much of the secret of his success, and his uniqueness.

His marriage to Alice McBurney might appear to have been simply inevitable, granting the closeness of the two families. His older sister, Rebecca, was close to "Uncle Doctor" McBurney and to Alice, though not without conflict. And Alice was a raven-haired, petite beauty. The depth, the tenderness, and even the passion of their relationship, built upon all the growing years of adolescence and young adulthood, culminating in marriage two years after Austen's graduation from Columbia College of Physicians and Surgeons, lasted undiminished until his death in 1940. Alice's beauty grew with her years until her own death in 1970 at the age of ninety-two. And during almost all those years of widowhood she played a vital, inspiring, and steadying role in the reorganization of the Austen Riggs Center, her husband's dream and his legacy to the profession. The Board of Trustees dedicated Lawrence Kubie's thorough and perceptive study, *The Riggs Story*, to this gallant lady. A whole chapter could be written just about her. There is no question of the profound importance of this marriage not only to Austen's personal life and that of his children, but also to his work. His attitude toward marriage, discussed to some extent in his volume *Intelligent Living*, emphasized his belief in the paramount importance of an underlying partnership of truly shared living.

After graduation from medical school, Austen took a year's surgical internship, planning to follow Dr. McBurney's path. He quickly discovered his total intolerance for the sight of blood, and spent the next year in a fellowship under Sir William Osler. He did not like Osler, nor the trend in medicine he represented: the cold precision of organic diagnosis left out the whole concept of the person as opposed to the "case." Here was the unrecognized beginning of Austen's interest in psychiatry.

He came back to New York, to begin the practice of internal medicine under the guidance of Dr. Walter James. Another thread was weaving into his fabric. Walter James was one of the three sons of Austen's most influential teacher at Harvard, William James, whose philosophy enticed and inspired him increasingly as the years went by. Austen's relationship and work with Dr. James were the happy beginning of fulfillment, but, as though some powerful force were choosing differently, in only two years he sent his own sputum to the laboratory to discover that he had active tuberculosis, like his father. Like his father he went to Dr. Trudeau at Saranac, who advised country living. So it was that Austen found himself in a rocking chair on the porch of Cherry Hill, Dr. McBurney's country house at Stockbridge, Massachusetts. He began to read extensively, to think, and to make notes. This was in 1907.

Now another thread joined the tapestry. It happened that "Uncle Doctor" was gradually retiring, suffering advancing arteriosclerosis and periods of deep depression. For this he made two visits to one Dr. John George Gehring of Bethel, Maine, who ran a residential center for the treatment of neuroses. Alice's aunt was once there also. Austen made a trip to visit Dr. Gehring and was impressed with what he saw. The basis of treatment was a strictly regulated life at "The Inn," and ventilating interviews with Dr. Gehring. These had to be "earned," as it were, by time spent at the woodpile sawing logs. (One can imagine large, Victorian ladies in their layer upon layer of voluminous dresses and vast, elaborate hats, wielding saws at the woodpile under a blistering August sun—a strict propriety of dress for dinner was required.) In any case, the setting of a country inn away from the ordinary stresses of family and work life, and a carefully constructed routine struck Austen as an appropriate setting for what he began to develop as a method of psychotherapy, far beyond Gehring's efforts. He read easily in French and German, and delved into the works of Charcot, Janet, DuBois, and the early papers of Freud, along with James, Santayana, and other philosophers. He began seeing patients. He began rearing a family. He bought an old and lovely yellow-painted brick house on a rise of land above Main Street, "The Knoll."

It may not have been easy growing up with such powerful, talented, colorful, and deeply affectionate parents as Austen and Alice Riggs, but it was never dull. Austen's work permeated his life, including "The Knoll," and his personal life permeated his work. But his life was not all work, by any means. It used to be that leisure belonged only to the privileged, although Austen vehemently objected to this being so. (His volume *Play* describes his philosophy and methods for distinguishing play from work, and making play creative and truly *re*-creational. With increasing egalitarian affluence, the book has taken on a new relevance today.)

By the time I joined the world and The Knoll in May 1914, beloved Uncle Doctor McBurney was gone, an office wing had been added to

The Knoll, and Dr. Henry Douglas Eaton had joined as an associate. Dr. Alvin Klein came soon after, and Dr. Lawrence Lunt replaced Dr. Eaton. The household was big, and from the very start the staff were very much part of it, not only at weekly dinners, but at teatime and on other occasions. There were four children, Anne, Marjorie, Alice, and myself last. Some autobiographical comments seem appropriate not only to specify my inevitably subjective limits, but to give the basis for some interpretive attempts.

As I said, the household was large, but it was closely knit, and very much dominated by the impressive figure of Austen Riggs. To a growing son he was deeply invested in his children and intensely loving, while at the same time equally terrifying and inspiring. My father was filled with humor and an easy, infectious laugh; he was a gay, delightful companion, raconteur, comedian, gourmet, conversationalist, skilled at attracting artists, philosophers, even priests and Buddhist scholars to the house. But he also harbored the somber in himself, and the depressed. He could be filled with anger and given to veritable rages against his children for seemingly small infractions of his olympian ideals for them. Then a truly serious piece of misbehavior would come along and he became quietly supportive and loving.

As I have mentioned, much of his own boyhood had been bypassed in the premature development of his qualities of leadership and responsibility. He never outgrew his boyishness and his inner rebellion, which broke through from time to time. He combined the essence of the true Romantic with that of the Renaissance man. He had grown up in the outdoors and on the sea in summers, and had an abiding love of craftsmanship. He was an accomplished sailor—but always conservative, noncompetitive, and perhaps secretly fearful. He had a string of boats built, some quite sizable, and there was always a subtle feeling that they were like toys to a boy. He was an outstanding ship-model builder, a passable etcher and worker in leather and metal, and he loved the working model in just the magic way that his little son came to absorb its world of miniature and fantasy. He could switch his role from a polished, disciplined, conforming gentleman suddenly to saying "bah and humbug" to all the formalities, and feel more at home in the woods or on a spray-swept deck in old, tattered canvas pants with the salt in his teeth. And all the while he fought recurring illness and profound fatigue. It seemed to me, growing up with this giant, that he held the gleaming moon in one hand, but some mysterious, frightening shadow of night in the other. Then came my own adolescence, with little overt rebellion (who would dare?), but at every chance for some wild exploration or even dangerous adventure he gave his enthusiastic backing and an assignment of full freedom and responsibility. His life was in his work, his work in his life. Was this also in some way the quality of his relation to his patients?

If Austen Riggs failed to achieve a unified, recognized place in psychiatry, it was in large part for the same reasons that he was, in his way, a great pioneer. He revealed himself as a conflicted man who used himself ruthlessly in the exploration of challenging questions, first this way, then that. Perhaps if he had developed and maintained close contact with others in the new field of dynamic psychiatry, he would have crystallized his thoughts and methods. Adolf Meyer, for whom Austen Riggs had great respect, was influential at this time. Developments were proceeding apace both in Worcester and at the Boston Psychopathic Hospital. But Riggs suffered two tendencies that enhanced the country isolation first enforced by his tuberculosis. On the one hand, he was extremely sensitive to rejection or criticism, whether by family, friends, or colleagues. He reacted by withdrawal and turning his attention to other matters. On the other hand, his experience from boyhood on had been concentrated on the role of undisputed responsibility and leadership. He really knew no other role. His charm, talent, and originality made him attract the people he needed like iron filings to a magnet. At one time, partly owing to the influence of a close friend, the neurologist Frederick Tilney in New York, he was offered a clinical professorship in psychiatry at Columbia, and turned it down. Partly he felt too greatly his physical limitations, but partly, I am sure, it would have broken the safer unity of his carefully constructed world in Stockbridge. He *had* to build the structure and the life in which he could reach his optimum, and hold it.

There were so many facets to this man, endlessly warring, always creative. There was the inner man, somewhat revealed in his notebooks begun with his arrival in Stockbridge—the creative answer to a tragic, total blocking of his chosen career; this was an endlessly searching, openminded, thoroughly identified physician. There was the man that only his eternally devoted wife knew. She once said that several years before his death, at the very peak of his success, he remarked, "Alice, I'm afraid I've shot my bolt;" this was the humility he never otherwise showed. There was the public man, who often reviled Freud and Jung, stood out for the Victorian mores, and used closely worded instructional manuals (the famous "Green Books") to guide the lives of the patients at Stockbridge. (The "Green Books" were pamphlets privately printed for distribution to patients. They were five in number, entitled "The Individual," "Sensations and Emotions," "The Problem of Adaptation," "The Technique of Adaptation," and "Rest." These pamphlets came very close to a presentation of ego psychology in lay terms, with a strong theme of making the most of cognitive power (intelligence) to overcome emotional conflicts.) There was the staff leader and clinician, who insisted on a total, thorough medical study of every patient, a painstaking history and personality exploration, a passion for weeding out "the facts," and a demand for immediate, flexible, appropriate intervention. Finally, there was the unique psychotherapist himself, whose methods were never clearly transmitted to anyone, nor ever formulated in a paper.

A few things can be deduced, however. In the first place, Austen Riggs was first and foremost a physician, like his father before him and like his renowned father-in-law. At the very start of his career in medicine, he was struck by what he called the "no man's land" between psychological and organic illness, in short, psychosomatic medicine. He was aware not only of the emotional impact of illness, but of its psychological components as well. He maintained throughout his career the emphasis upon the total psychobiological entity of man.

Second, his reading and experience led him first to a feeling of great confusion in the field of psychiatry, and then imbued him with a resulting challenge to unify the concepts in some clinically validated way. He therefore drew heavily upon Freud, Adler, Meyer, and the philosophers to clear his way. Curiously, he developed an interpersonal kind of ego psychology not vastly different from that of Sullivan, with whom he had no contact. He conceived clearly of the unconscious, of conflict and defense, of the epigenesis of adult neurosis, and of the curative effects of the therapeutic relation. That he studiously avoided the sexual basis of the neuroses was due probably to a misunderstanding of Freud's concept of sexuality, coupled with the same Victorian resistance to the idea of infantile sexuality that confronted Freud. He was intensely conflicted in his own attitudes to sexuality.

A further influence was the impact of early analytic attempts in this country based essentially upon Id-analysis and the removal of repression which dominated Freud's work until the 1920s, when the essay on the Ego and the Id changed the emphasis and ushered in the era of ego psychology. From this atmosphere came many wild analyses and destructive results, especially in New York, from which came many of Riggs's patients. He did reparative work and resented deeply the injury to those occasional people.

It is worthy of note that while Riggs vehemently denied that his charismatic personality was a factor in his therapy, he was really denying both transference and countertransference. Intense transference he handled by changing therapists. Dependence was often never resolved. His efforts could in modern terms be called a form of ego analysis with a heavy assist from behavioral modification and a strong emphasis upon crisis intervention and the forced maintenance of a high degree of autonomy on the part of the patient. At the same time, although probably not aware of Ferenczi's early excursions into role playing, Riggs unconsciously played a very strong parental role, and did his best work with those patients that most needed it.

His combined use of transference, role playing, and suggestion was well illustrated in a case I knew of by accident during my adolescence. I remember certain details vividly. He had given me a record player for Christmas, and one day came boiling out of the office into the house to borrow it, along with some dance records. Later in the day, he remarked, "I've brought everything to a white-hot focus on this." He went on to say that the young woman in question had suffered a hysterical impediment to walking—she was essentially crippled. He had put on the dance records, induced her to dance with him, and finally cured the impediment, after many hours of preparatory exploration and psychotherapy.

An illuminating account of life at Stockbridge and a statement of the Riggs philosophy, methods, and theoretical implications are given not only by Kubie but also by Millet in a paper presented before the American Psychiatric Association in 1969. This is a particularly valuable contribution since it stems directly from Millet's own participation with Riggs at the Foundation for a number of years. In it, there is special emphasis on the "team" approach used at Stockbridge, which was the forerunner of today's reliance on the team in hospital settings, and in community mental health centers. Riggs's magnetic, charismatic qualities mentioned above were cherished by his staff as well as his patients. There was a quality of great closeness, intimacy, and affection among the members, and especially toward their "chief." This kind of leadership no doubt derived largely from that early loss of his father, with his own and his mother's attendant assignment of heavy responsibilities.

The full history of what is now known as the Riggs Center parallels and extends the history of Austen Riggs. Besides the detailed account in Kubie's book, *The Riggs Story*, there is an excellent study by Gaylord P. Coon and Alice F. Raymond, published in 1940, in which are included a large number of retrospective reports by patients. Only a brief outline of the story can be presented here.

A nonprofit corporation was first formed in 1919, with a tiny staff and only what was known as the "Foundation Inn" to accommodate patients. The Board of Trustees included Dr. Felix Adler, Clinton Crane (Riggs's brother-in-law), Mr. Allen Forbes of Boston, Dr. Walter James, Dr. James Alexander Miller of New York, Dr. M. Allen Starr of Philadelphia, Dr. Fredrick Tilney, and others. A medical advisory board was begun in 1921, including Dr. Stanley Cobb of Boston and, interestingly, Dr. George A. Waterman. Later additions during the twenties included Dr. C. Macfie Campbell, Dr. Warfield Longcope of the Johns Hopkins, Dr. Thomas Salmon (an old and valued friend), and Dr. Edward Strecker of Philadelphia.

The staff gradually grew, with the addition of both temporary and long-term affiliates. Lawrence K. Lunt came in 1920, and John A.P. Millet in 1923. Dr. S. Spafford Ackerly was there for a year in 1933. There were a total of twenty-six physicians present at some time or other before 1940, the year of Riggs's death.

There were three basic objectives in Austen Riggs's mind, which gradually found fruition in the growth of the Austen Riggs Foundation. One was the development of the method and the setting for the psychotherapy of the neuroses, available to all regardless of ability to pay. The second was research into the process, which had its modest beginning in Coon and Raymond's work but came to full flower in 1947 under the leadership of Robert P. Knight. The third was teaching, which began soon after the establishment of the corporation and the foundation, with the introduction of fellowships in psychiatry. After 1947, the name was changed to the Austen Riggs Center, and affiliation was made with the Western New England Psychoanalytic Institute, with increased opportunities for fellows and psychoanalytic candidates. What a pity that carcinoma had to take Riggs's life before he could see so much of his dream come true. But at least his widow, his deepest and closest friend, could see it all and rejoice. (And so indeed, but watching from a distance, could his son.)

To conclude: who should speak better for the man, the physician, and the psychiatric pioneer than he himself, from his own notebooks?

In 1913 (speaking of empathy): "To feel every quality from the vilest to the best in one's own individuality—to really and honestly feel the shame of the disgraced, the joy of the happy, the sorrow of the oppressed, is to love and understand humanity. Individual differences are insignificant. The great human likenesses are the all-important and significant battles of life."

In 1932 (speaking of a behavioral science): "The dearest and youngest science of all, the science of human nature and human conduct, has not yet had its say. Nor is it yet steady enough or wise enough to say much. Its strength and wisdom are growing rapidly, however, and soon it will be called on to function not as the youngest child but as the parent science of all the social sciences."

In 1937 (the poet-philosopher speaks in grief): "Night and day, day and night: darkness and light. Light and darkness are but part of the day, the whole day and of the uninterruptible flow of the ages. Birth and Death are darkness and light and darkness again of the individual life. Experience as we know it is confined to the interval of light, to the brief period of consciousness we call Life. But life itself is an uninterrupted and uninterruptible stream, beginning aeons before birth and continuing after death. Only the whole is immortal: and an individual is immortal if in life he expresses all that he has received and in expressing it passes it on to others. Unity and individuality—individuality and unity again."

References

I am particularly indebted to Dr. Lawrence Kubie and his volume, *The Riggs Story*, for the painstaking research on factual details and the quotations from the Notebooks, which are unfortunately no longer available. The reader is referred to this source for thorough exploration of both the man and his work, as well as the events at Stockbridge from 1940 to 1960, the many important leaders in psychiatry and psychoanalysis who have been there, and a complete bibliography of works emanating from the Austen Riggs Foundation and the Austen Riggs Center.

Coon, Gaylord P. and Alice F. Raymond, *A Review of Psychoneuroses at Stockbridge*. Stockbridge, Mass.: Austen Riggs Foundation Inc., 1940.

Kubie, Lawrence S., *The Riggs Story: The Development of the Austen Riggs Center for the Study and Treatment of the Neuroses*. New York: Paul B. Hoeber, 1960.

Millet, John A.P., "Austen Fox Riggs: His Significance to American Psychiatry of Today," *American Journal of Psychiatry, 125* (1969), 7.

Peattie, Donald C., "Dr. Austen Fox Riggs: A Portrait," *The Atlantic* (August 1941), p. 200.

Riggs, Austen F., "Adverse Suggestion," *Medical Record, 73* (1908), 1071.

———, "Treatment of Neurasthenia," *Bulletin of Johns Hopkins Hospital, 27* (1916), 281.

———, "Nervousness: Its Cause and Prevention," *Mental Hygiene, 6* (1922), 263–287.

———, *Just Nerves*. Boston: Houghton Mifflin, 1922.

———, "Psychoneuroses, Their Nature and Treatment," *American Journal of Psychiatry, 3* (1923), 91.

———, "Neurotic Disturbances of Eye Function" (with L.K. Lunt), *Archives of Ophthalmology, 52* (1923), 313.

———, "Psychotherapy," *Boston Medical and Surgical Journal, 189* (1923), 269.

———, "Five Brain Tumors" (with W.B. Terhune), *Boston Medical and Surgical Journal, 190* (1924), 1121.

———, "The Ophthalmologist and the Psychoneuroses" (with L.K. Lunt), *Journal of the American Medical Association, 83* (1924), 1968.

———, "Psychotherapy" (with W.B. Terhune), in Billings-Forchheimer, *Therapeutics of Internal Disease*. New York, D. Appleton, 1924, vol. I, chapter 1.

———, "Psychoneuroses: A Problem in Re-education" (with W.B. Terhune), *American Journal of Psychiatry, 4* (1925), 407.

———, "Uses of Psychotherapy in General Medical Treatment," *New York State Journal of Medicine, 26* (1926), 1.

———, "A Psychoneurosis Case Report" (with W.B. Terhune), *New York State Journal of Medicine, 26* (1926), 185.

———, "The Balanced Life," *Saturday Review of Literature, 5* (November 10, 1928), 338–339.

———, *Intelligent Living*. New York: Doubleday-Doran, 1929, p. 230.

———, "The Relation of Psychiatry to Medicine," *Annals of Internal Medicine, 3* (1929), 360.

———, "The Significance of Illness," in L.E. Emerson, ed., *Physician and Patient*. Cambridge, Mass.: Harvard University Press, 1929, chapter 4.

———, *Play*. New York: Doubleday-Doran, 1935, p. 239.

———, "The Role of the Personality in Psychotherapeutics" (with H.K. Richardson), *Annals of Internal Medicine, 10* (1936), 13.

Fifty Years of Research Contributions*

MILTON GREENBLATT

When the infant Boston Psychopathic Hospital burst into life in 1912, Abraham Flexner had just written his report about the sorry state of medicine throughout the nation. Medicine suffered from its primarily biological orientation, subject to the domination of the autopsy table. Psychiatry was a specialty one did not talk about in polite society—most men practiced as neurologists—and the treatment of the mental patient reflected fears and horrors reminiscent of the Dark Ages. On the streets of Boston, if a man roamed about mad, most likely he would be remanded to a jail or a local place of detention without any medical care, or he would be whisked to the Boston City Hospital where, after perhaps days of delay, he might receive the attentions of an alienist.

Some of our enlightened citizens at that time objected vehemently to this state of affairs, and through their efforts the legislature, surely under divine guidance, authorized the creation of a psychopathic hospital, to provide immediate care and treatment of acute disorders, to promote teaching and training, and to undertake *research* into the causes and cures of mental disease.

It was fitting that the remarkable Elmer Ernest Southard should be the hospital's first leader. He was then professor of neuropathology at Harvard, pathologist to the state, widely known for his brilliance as a philosopher, etymologist, litterateur, and chess champion, and the possessor of extraordinary imagination and indefatigable energy. Still in his thirties, he saw in psychiatry and in the Boston Psychopathic Hospital a magnificent tool appropriate to his talents, and he set out to illuminate the world of thought, feeling, and behavior in a manner not merely to reflect but to transcend his time.

The Southard Period, 1912–1920

With characteristic foresight, the hospital was planned to avoid a merely custodial function. Therapy as well as diagnosis was stressed, and so were broad humanitarian goals and scientific progress. Pathology, psychology, social work, neurology, child development—all sectors of human thought that might impart a new or exciting note or spark research beyond the immediate necessities of an individual case—were encouraged. Despite his skepticism of the Freudian movement and sharp criticism of its "pessimism," Southard had several promising analysts on the staff. He called these men psychopathologists. Eugenics, dietetics, and the study of history were added to the ferment. There was work on childhood maladjustments, epilepsy, feeblemindedness, acquired and congenital syphilis, alcoholism, the family, society, industrial unrest.

Of large scope in those days was the study of neurosyphilis, begun by Southard and Myerson and pursued with determination by Solomon, Raeder, and many others. Funds were provided annually by the State Board of Insanity, supplemented by outside contributions obtained through the efforts of the workers. This department led its field for over three decades, experimenting with every rational form of therapy and providing, along the way, important insights into organic psychiatry, neuropathology, and physiology. It never gave up its dogged fight against neurosyphilis until that quarry eventually succumbed, one might say, to the multitude of wounds inflicted by the incessant scientific probers.

I shall speak of this great adventure later, but it is fitting as part of the report on the Southard period to include a mention of the monograph *Neurosyphilis*[1] by Southard and Solomon, an authoritative casebook presenting the disease in all its protean forms, psycho- and neuropathological; it is still worth reading today for its sparkling clear style, cogent case descriptions, and scholarly commentaries.

In those days many alcoholics were treated in the hospital. A prevalent opinion of the time was that prolonged baths were superior to restraint, drugs, or neglect, as previously practiced with this class of patients. More remarkable, however, was the intensive interest in aftercare manifested by Dr. Warren Stearns, who, as part of the management of alcoholism, inaugurated social evenings for these patients. An alcoholic club was born that for years reduced the relapse rate for these patients and that we now can hail as the forerunner of the modern social therapeutic club for ex-patients and of Alcoholics Anonymous in particular.

In psychology, Yerkes, one of the talented people that Southard attracted, led the team and, during his stay, developed and standardized an early method of rating intellectual abilities that aided in the revision and improvement of the important Binet intelligence test. He also devised a multiple-choice method of psychological examination which was an early contribution to that field.

Southard decried the watchful-waiting type of nursing practiced in the average asylum and groped for a more positive and constructive role for psychiatric nursing. He felt that all nurses should have some training in mental hospitals, and a postgraduate course was attempted in 1914. He was also alive to the value of occupational therapy, and he successfully organized such a program for the hospital.

The restless activity of the institution was felt on a still broader front. As early as 1911, Southard had stressed the importance of social work, linking problems of heredity and eugenics with those of practical social service. When he became chief, his first director of social work was Mary Jarrett, who gave a remarkable impetus to the whole field. In an admirable, systematic study, she found that two-thirds of the patients admitted needed social care of one form or another. Soon students were working at the Boston Psychopathic Hospital in connection with the Boston School of Social Work; and the Social Work School for Psychiatry at Smith College was inaugurated in 1918, stimulated and planned by Southard with Jarrett's help. It was immediately followed by similar schools in New York, Philadelphia, and elsewhere.

The social work interest in aftercare of the individual led naturally to a consideration of employment and employability. Adler, Jarrett, and Southard were some of those who soon opened up conceptually and practically the territory they called "mental hygiene of industry"—the study of job, employer, and circumstances governing the ability of patients to maintain themselves in the occupational sphere. His interest in industrial psychiatry led Southard to an association with the Engineering Foundation, which undertook to support preliminary studies of mental abnormality in industry. For them, Southard wrote three interesting papers before he died: "The Mental Hygiene of Industry,"[2] "Trade-Unionism and Temperament,"[3] and "The Modern Specialist in Unrest."[4] In these papers he attempted to define, in his lucid, epigrammatic style, pregnant with symbolism, the place of psychiatry in the world of work.

At this time, too, Southard recommended the establishment of a halfway house, that is, a convalescent home under supervision where the patients could go under a voluntary arrangement, where occupational training might be part of the rehabilitative pattern. Although this idea was proposed to the Permanent Charity Fund of Boston in 1917 with a request for support, it did not come to fruition until 1952, when Harry Solomon convinced a group of community-minded women that their Rutland Corner House could be suitably reorganized as a halfway house for women who had been mentally ill.

Work on patients in relation to their social environment soon led

Southard to approach the total sphere of life problems and stresses that individuals encounter, in a series of writings, published posthumously by Southard and Jarrett, under the title *The Kingdom of Evils*.[5] Here, Southard's practical philosophy came forth in its boldest form. "Men of good will," he said, "should take arms against a sea of trouble, look evil in the eye, accost it and conquer it. The striving for human betterment lies first in looking fearlessly on the dark side of life, for unless evil be destroyed, good will not remain." Southard's classification[6] of the kingdom of evils is worth presenting as one simple example of his tireless work on categories and nomenclature—always a prelude to intellectual mastery of a new field:

> *Morbi*: Diseases and deficiencies and misinformation.
>
> *Errores*: Educational deficiencies and misinformation; these include the errors of not knowing, of knowing wrong, or of misinterpretation.
>
> *Vitia*: Vices and bad habits; both mental and moral qualities are here involved.
>
> *Litigia*: Legal entanglements.
>
> *Penuriae*: Poverty and other forms of resourcelessness.
>
> Morbi—Cure!
> Errores—Teach!
> Vitia—Train!
> Litigia—Counsel!
> Penuriae—Provide!

One of Southard's fondest ideas formulated in his later years was the establishment of a research foundation or institute. He envisaged "a fit building, perhaps four stories high, consisting largely of scientific laboratories with a ten-bed ward for clinical operation and a man to work on each separate problem."[5] Rockefeller would not bite on this idea. Southard appealed to Harvard, again in vain; finally, he turned to the state, with a "proposal for a department of research under the State Board of Insanity." He furnished plans to make the research institute an integral part of the Boston Psychopathic Hospital; but then he died, and his great dream seemingly died with him. Yet thirty years later his dream came to fruition in the present research building, organized almost precisely along lines that would have fulfilled Southard's brave idea; and it has, in fact, two ten-bed wards where intensive studies can be made, and are being made, on both schizophrenia and manic-depressive psychosis.

It must be clear by now how exciting a place was "Psycho" in those days. "From the OPD, its ward and particularly from its daily noon staff meetings under Southard's leadership, radiated innumerable, enlightening rays that still glow in living men and movements...The research stimulus that he gave to all inquiring minds was indeed education in its highest form."[6]

We know a great deal about Southard because Frederick Gay, his friend and collaborator, assembled a biography[6] of him, which includes discussions and evaluations by many eminent men, together with an analysis of his contributions, field by field, of his personality characteristics, and of his enthusiastic catalysis of individuals and works. Unfortunately, we do not have similar systematic material to tell us about the accomplishments of all the others who were associated with Southard, outlived him, and made singular contributions of their own. His team included the following: Harry Solomon, who altogether gave forty-five memorable years of his life to the development of the "Psycho;" Abraham Myerson—who after his neurosyphilis work became fascinated by heredity—was one of the early popularizers of psychiatry, and wrote extensively and interestingly on such themes as *The Nervous Housewife*,[7] "Anhedonia,"[8] social psychiatry, and social anxiety; and Lowrey, Noyes, Coon, Adler, Stearns, Raeder, Thom, and many others. There was Karl Menninger, on whom the "Psycho" left a lasting impression, reflected in the growth and development of the Menninger Foundation, where he established a memorial to Southard at Topeka in the form of the Southard School for Children and Adolescents, a most fitting monument of warm feelings toward him—as is our own Southard Outpatient Department.

The Campbell Period, 1920–1943

Following a considerable slackening of activities in 1918 and 1919, due to World War I and the many professional people in military service, the "Psycho" resumed them with gusto under the direction of Charles Macfie Campbell. It was now an independent organization, having severed its administrative relations with Boston State Hospital, the condition that had obtained since its beginning in 1912. But it still suffered from a divided authority, for the chief executive officer maintained a liaison with the Department of Mental Health and had major control of the purse strings. Service demands were very high; the admission rate was around 2,000 patients per annum, a load carried essentially by a cadre of only six junior physicians (present residents please note). Hence, it functioned primarily as a rapid diagnostic center.

In his first report, Campbell spoke of plans to upgrade nursing; he asked for expanded recreational and occupational activities and outlined broad new vistas for the hospital as a mental health center serving the district, surveying health needs, attending to school problems, and giving aid and consultation to a variety of community agencies.

If the institution under Southard could be viewed as expanding its horizons, the Campbell period, in contrast, could be characterized as a time of delimiting goals, settling in, a deepening of the stream—in certain specified directions.

Campbell invigorated the staff by some first-class appointments: Karl Bowman as Chief Medical Officer, Frederick Lyman Wells as Chief of Psychology, G. Philip Grabfield as Chief of the Biochemistry Laboratory, and others. These new men, together with Solomon, Chief of Therapeutic Research, and Douglas Thom, Chief of the OPD, who continued to function from the previous era, assured the hospital of a lively intellectual climate in the years immediately ahead.

The story of the Department of Therapeutic Research is exciting drama, as I have mentioned, featuring a variety of ingenious attempts to bring antibiotics in contact with the spirochete or to raise the body's resistance to its invasion. First there was the intraspinal injection of salvarsanized serum, apparently of benefit in tabes but not in other forms of the disease. Then the blood of patients who had received intravenous arsphenamine was injected into the subarachnoid space. This influenced the course of meningovascular lues but did not touch paresis. Then arsphenamine was introduced directly into the ventricles and the cerebral subarachnoid spaces, with apparent benefit. By a roundabout technique, spinal drainage was tried after intravenous injections of active agents. Around 1923, tryparsamide came into use and another great step forward was achieved.

Fever treatment, introduced by Nobel prize winner von Wagner-Jauregg, was quickly adopted in the clinic and systematic experimentation with fever-producing agents was carried on, using milk protein, malaria, typhoid, sodoku, electric blankets, diathermy, and so on. Combinations of fever with arsenicals were investigated, and treatment of patient groups extensively over months and years with various patterns of chemotherapy and fever were explored. A number of patient groups were carefully followed up for their adaptation in the community, the effect of their luetic condition on family, spouse, children, and social life. Such studies, involving careful psychiatric social work investigation, resulted in the informative book *Syphilis of the Innocent*,[9] by Dr. and Mrs. Solomon. Although there were many disappointments and frustrations during these years, success rates in the treatment of neurosyphilis moved steadily upward.

Along with the clinical efforts there were basic studies of the circulation of the spinal fluid, the physiological effects of fever of various types on the human organism, neuropathological investigations of the brains of patients who had succumbed while on different therapeutic regimens, biochemical studies of specific homestatic mechanisms, and, further, the development of diagnostic tools through the specialized use of x-ray (pneumoencephalography), immunological tests (Wasserman and Hinton), and psychological test batteries, the latter research conducted in collaboration with the Department of Psychology. Further, the Department of Therapeutic Research did not limit its explorations to neurosyphilis alone, but epidemic encephalitis, multiple sclerosis, epilepsy, catatonic schizophrenia, alcoholism, and malaria all came under their research purview.

When at length, through mass testing during World War II and the use of penicillin, the problem of luetic infection was quantitatively greatly reduced, the inpatient wards were finally closed and the large OPD load of ambulatory patients gradually faded away. Please remember that research studies conducted at this time were carried on alongside of a massive treatment load; for example, in 1936 some 382 new patients with neurosyphilis were accepted into the hospital, 6,549 visits to the outpatient department were made by ambulatory patients, and 581 fever treatments and well over 1,200 lumbar punctures were performed.

The Biochemical Laboratory, under Dr. Philip Grabfield, began in 1921 to organize its responsibility for clinical-pathological examination of patients. A number of interesting problems of research order also began to occupy Dr. Grabfield and his students, despite a mounting demand for routine tests. For example, the basal metabolism of mentally ill patients was studied and it was found that psychotics, particularly schizophrenics, frequently suffered from a low BMR. The specific dynamic action of foodstuffs and of blood sugar level in the psychoses and in epidemic encephalitis, the effect upon the nitrogen excretion of iodides and other ingested substances, gastric functions in patients with intestinal disturbance, the blood levels of calcium and potassium, were investigated. This, of course, was the period of the widespread search for specific biochemical deviations from the normal in psychotic individuals, a task that had to be done, although the yield was unfortunately small.

In the 1930s Dr. Frank D'Elseaux began to enthusiastically contribute to the department and to enrich the scene methodologically by new techniques. The startling discovery at this time, reported by D'Elseaux,

Solomon, and Kaufman, that the catatonic condition could be dramatically, though transitorily, resolved by a few whiffs of concentrated carbon dioxide, resulted in the immediate launching of new investigations into the regulation of the pH of the blood, the acid-base balance, and the control of respiration. Later, D'Elseaux turned his attention to blood organic phosphorus in depressives, noting that the levels correlated with changes in their mood. D'Elseaux then left the laboratory for full-time clinical work and teaching, and many of the fascinating leads he uncovered still remain to be fully explored by future chemists.

In the Psychological Laboratory, the chief for thirty-seven years was Frederick Lyman Wells, who, together with his staff, carried out the teaching, training, and research that eventually established his department as preeminent in its field. Earlier psychological studies had to do with explorations and revisions of the Stanford-Binet and Army Alpha tests of intelligence and with the reaction of individuals to simple stimuli of light and sound. This progressed to more complicated research on affective processes, problems of psychosexuality of college men, determinants of aesthetic preference, and assessment of musical talents. In 1927, Wells published *Mental Tests in Clinical Practice*,[10] a standard in its field.

Further broadening the scope and range of psychological interests, in 1929 Dr. S.J. Beck brought in his special concerns with the Rorschach tests. His studies resulted in the publication in 1935 of the highly important "handbook" on the Rorschach, in which emphasis is laid on the findings of the psychotic individual.[11] Studies of the preschool child, of his reading difficulties, and, later, of the adopted child and placement problems were undertaken by Miss Viola Jones, a psychologist. Around 1932, Nathan Goldman began to work on the establishment and extinction of conditioned reflexes as related to the IQ in psychotic states. He also became interested in the mental changes of patients undergoing thyroidectomy, a procedure then practiced extensively at the Beth Israel Hospital in an effort to aid patients with cardiac decompensation. Finally, in the latter part of the period with which we are concerned, an interest in the socialization process was evidenced, not only in Wells's study of the behavior of spiders, but in various investigations of socialization in humans and learned discussions of the problems of social adaptation. Although Wells left the department, turning it over to Charles Atwell in 1938, and joined in the study of the college students at Harvard, where he was enormously productive, he returned years later to his beloved "Psycho." After his retirement, in fact, he joined the Russell Sage Project on social psychiatry, and helped us greatly by devising a simple and useful instrument to assess socialization of mental patients on wards of custodial hospitals. I always suspected that he drew heavily on his experience with the socialization of spiders, decades before.

On the clinical side, of course, were Bowman, Campbell, and others. Bowman catalyzed a variety of studies, sometimes in collaboration with metabolic and physiological investigators. Impressed by the finding of hypometabolism in many cases of schizophrenia, he tried glandular feedings on a therapeutic basis. The following substances were fed to mentally ill individuals: whole pituitary, anterior pituitary, posterior pituitary, pineal gland, thymus, thyroid, thyroxin, suprarenal extract, parathormone, and amniotin. Studies in this field, partly financed by the Rockefeller Foundation, were eventually published in 1934 under the title *Schizophrenia*.[12] Anyone now perusing this volume will find in it a wealth of solid information on basic problems in the field, often countering popular mythology about the etiology of schizophrenia. In terms of closer collaboration and firm guidance of the program by top statistical consultants, this project had a modern approach.

Bowman emphasized the importance of junior members of the staff taking on research projects during their period of training; thus, for example, in the 1930s a number of now famous individuals were involved in research, some of them under the aegis of the Commonwealth Fund: Kaufman, recently returned from Vienna, was studying the psychoanalysis of the psychoses; Scott, depression with reference to gastric function; D'Elseaux (working with Solomon), the chemistry of stupor; Coon, studies of dementia praecox; Saul, clinical physiological correlates in psychosis; Kasanin, blood sugar in schizophrenia; Michaels, the relation between calcium and potassium in psychosis; Fleming, alcoholic patients as a group, and the effect of alcoholism on body fluids; Holt, epidemic encephalitis, using air encephalography; Green, psychoses due to bromide; Semrad and Schwab, treatment of alcoholic delirium with dehydration; Semrad, audiometrics in hallucinations; Dyne, progynon B in involutional melancholia; Krinsky (with Coon), personality and psychopathology in DTs; Finley and Brenner, insulin and metrazol effects on the central nervous system; Finley (with Campbell), the use of the EEG in assisting the diagnosis of schizophrenia and related conditions.

Campbell, of course, was directing the destiny of the hospital and giving a great deal to the training of his residents and students. I count it as one of my blessings that for two years I was among those who enjoyed contact with this charming, incisive, and erudite man. Campbell was also busy in research endeavors, assembling vast quantities of notes on patients with schizophrenia and summarizing his thoughts at intervals in highly readable gems such as *Destiny and Disease in Mental Disorders.*[13] At the approach of his retirement in 1943, the year that unfortunately also marked his death, he was looking forward to extensive writing on schizophrenic reactions with a view to a more sensible and comprehensive nosology, based on his vast experience.

The Solomon Period, 1943–1958, and
The Ewalt Period, 1958–1962

In 1943, when Dr. Harry C. Solomon succeeded to the directorship, the hospital was still functioning mainly as a diagnostic center, with upwards of 2,000 patients admitted per annum, and a pattern of patient management prevailed that, by later standards, we must regard as somewhat custodial. It was then two years after Pearl Harbor and, to a considerable extent, the institution had suffered from the general diversion of men and resources to the battlefronts. Nevertheless, it was soon apparent that the hospital was in for a period of intense social reform, which began at once and gained strength and momentum, especially at the cessation of international hostilities.

Emphasis shifted from the custodial or diagnostic function to total treatment; the admission rate in a few years was cut in half; patients stayed longer. "Few were admitted, more treated, more recovered." Many of the then routine methods of patient care, such as seclusion, tubs, packs, and physical and chemical restraints, were cast out in favor of intensified staff-patient relations. The physical environment was spruced up, opportunities for wholesome social interaction and pleasant recreational diversions were multiplied, and staff and patients began to participate in a group experience directed toward mutual understanding and growth. Doors were opened, the public was let in, and the patients were let out. By some Solomonic legerdemain, the staff increased sharply in numbers, as its therapeutic powers were enhanced.

In 1943, research was going on in four fields: neurosyphilis, electroencephalography, biochemistry, and clinical psychiatry. But the number of research workers could be counted on the fingers of one hand. Funds were limited. Many areas that could properly enrich the intellectual climate were uncultivated, and some departments that might have been expected to make a contribution were not being heard from. What is more, the Department of Neurosyphilis, which had been quite active, was looking forward to a diminution of its function due to its great successes and those of other laboratories in conquering paretic infection. However, the social system of the hospital had escaped notice altogether. Psychology was dragging, physiology was neglected. Connections with vigorous intellectual streams elsewhere at Harvard and other universities left something to be desired.

With this critique in mind, Dr. Solomon appointed a Director of Laboratories and Research in 1945, with a mandate to develop investigative activities along a broad front, to mobilize the creative talents of the institution wherever they could be found, to look for the new, the promising, the different. It therefore behooves me to warn the reader that much of the remaining narrative deals with the period of my stewardship as director of the laboratory research program. My point of view is necessarily subjective, and I hope that whatever biases I display are corrected in other presentations.

As new openings became available or were created, men with a potential for investigative work were attracted; thus, Funkenstein, Hyde, Holt, Rinkel, and Bockoven were some of the early crew that contributed so richly to the excitement of that period. Patient care was greatly aided by the appointment of two remarkably effective teachers—Dr. Ives Hendrick and Dr. Elvin V. Semrad—who not only introduced the psychoanalytic point of view, with its almost revolutionary effect upon the teaching climate of the hospital, but also helped make the detailed study of every aspect of the patient's inner life and reaction to his total environment a more legitimate area of inquiry. Intensive studies began immediately on methods of treatment as they were introduced—electric shock, insulin treatment, lobotomy, ether treatment, amytal narcosis, to mention the biological area. Lobotomy studies assumed very large proportions, indeed, as multidisciplinary teams began to cooperate, from surgery, pathology, sociology, psychology, and physiology, and a concerted effort was made to evaluate changes that frontal surgery produced in formerly hopeless cases, and to allay our ignorance concerning frontal-lobe functioning.

Lobotomy was the first procedure pointing dramatically to the potential for improvement that was still latent in patients with chronic psychosis, and, despite its controversial nature, it excited both research and treatment staffs and evoked interest, dedication, and a sense of accomplishment. The research efforts paid off, not only in definitive knowledge about this debatable treatment, but in a host of methodological innovations in the study of the mentally ill patient that later were applied to the many studies that radiated from this one point.

The social reforms of which I have spoken in themselves constituted a fascinating experiment in the reorganization of a total institution. Ideas stemming from our experiences were introduced into other state and federal hospitals. Social psychiatry burst upon our scene and, aided by support from the Russell Sage Foundation, whatever we learned from action, from experiment, and from theory eventually found its way into publications such as *From Custodial to Therapeutic Patient Care in Mental Hospitals,*[14] *The Patient and the Mental Hospital,*[15] *Experiencing the Patient's Day,*[16] *Rehabilitation of the Mentally Ill,*[17] *As the Psychiatric Aide Sees His Work and Problems.*[18]

It was Robert Hyde who helped put into operation the mass of social reforms and rationalized the changes at the theoretical level. It was Jerome Bruner from the Social Relations Department who set up the bridge, so well-traveled now, between social relations and the "Psycho." It was Levinson who anchored that bridge at the hospital by establishing a Department of Sociopsychological Studies, which, in the course of training its Ph.D.s, enlightened all of us about the social structure of the mental hospital, custodial ideology, patienthood, nursehood, residenthood —yes, even administratorhood.

Bockoven participated in many studies but perhaps became most identified with historical investigations into the remarkable moral treatment era, its rise, decline, and late resurgence in some of the best attitudes of our day. Thus Bockoven gave us a sense of continuity between past and present, and instructed us in the lessons to be drawn from the successes of our forefathers, unaided though they were by shock treatments, drugs, or psychoanalytical principles.

Our physiological foundation stemmed from the fascination of Ax and others with multiple simultaneous recordings of physiological parameters related to emotion—a welcome addition, I might say, to electroencephalography, which, though it recorded from the brain, nevertheless had less to say about the emotions than did the peripheral measures. Shakespeare's query, "Tell me where is fancy bred, Or in the heart or in the head?"[19] rang strangely true for that particular problem.

Studies of the physiological concomitants of evoked emotional states by both Ax and Funkenstein showed that different emotions could be physiologically identified, a finding that laid low Cannon's postulates to the contrary. Polygraphic methods were later extended to the study of the psychiatrist-patient dyad during psychotherapy, which demonstrated an elaborate interplay between the two parties, paralleling psychological interaction, and resulted in new terminology: "physiological empathy" or "physiological concordance and disconcordance." Funkenstein's correlations of physiological reaction type with personality and social measures led eventually to the publication in 1957 of his inspired *Mastery of Stress.*[20] Through a succession of engineering developments, the Polygraph Laboratory, which early was hampered by technical difficulties, was finally set on a firm footing, and then duplicated, so that now we possess one of the largest and best equipped such laboratories in the country.

In the 1950s, psychiatry was flourishing as it had not been for decades. Never before had it been so fully accepted as a basic element in the medical curriculum, equal, in fact, with medicine and surgery. A growing number of students opened their minds to careers in psychiatry, and most of the disciplines that could shed light on human behavior joined the family of sciences that could work together under the mental health banner.

The hospital's philosophy of treatment had earlier emphasized the creation of a therapeutic community within its walls. In the 1950s the dominant theme was to break down the barriers between hospital and community, to create a group of surrounding facilities that could serve as stepping stones from the hospital to the outside, soften the blow of discharge, prevent relapses, and eventually handle new cases as a way of circumventing hospitalization altogether. Thus, the aftercare clinic, specifically the Community Clinic, was formalized under separate management; the Day Hospital and halfway house came into being; the ex-patient club was organized; and rehabilitation became a strong motif.

As the hospital began to step outside of itself in this manner, research, too, developed expanded vistas. In the 1950s, foundation support increased by rapid increments and the "Psycho," which had worked hard and early in a number of fields, was able to win its share of support. By the late 1950s and early 1960s the research endeavors had grown too large and varied to be encompassed under any one heading; administratively they are now subdivided into a number of areas of inquiry, each under a responsible scientist. Here I can discuss only selected developments illustrative of special trends.

Research consonant with the "community mental hospital" trend has been reported in a series of publications on employer receptivity,[21] occupational adjustment,[22] analysis of structure and function of the Day Hospital,[23] the halfway house,[24] and the ex-patient club.[25] A special variation of the rehabilitation theme, showing how much volunteers can contribute, is the noble experiment of Harvard and Radcliffe undergraduates at Metropolitan State Hospital, developed in collaboration with the Massachusetts Mental Health Center.[26] They now have three well-established service-research areas: ward work, case aide, and Wellmet, a unique halfway house where students and ex-patients live together in a cooperative arrangement so intense that it sears the souls of the students while it raises the rehabilitation level of the patients. The student program within the hospital has been so dramatic that there are already some fifty to seventy strong counterparts throughout the nation; the Wellmet experiment outside the hospital is so bold that the public needs at least two more years to assimilate its full impact.

In 1957 we started the Community Extension, or Emergency, Service[27] specifically to prevent hospitalization of patients referred for admission, whenever possible and indicated. This service demonstrated that at least fifty percent of cases so referred could be prevented from hospitalization, at least for a year, by judicious mobilization of family and community resources and by crisis management by the psychiatrist-psychiatric social worker-nurse team. Following this demonstration, emergency services have become an established hospital function for both adult and adolescent cases.

The Anti-Depression Project illustrates our reaching out into coordinated multihospital research with Metropolitan, Medfield, and Westborough, demanded by the necessity of obtaining large numbers of patients for certain types of investigations. Apart from what we are learning about the efficacy of antidepressant drugs and placebos in relation to EST, we are bringing together hospitals desirous of expanding their research activities into a mutually enlightening arrangement.

Two metabolic wards—one for the study of depression, emphasizing catecholamines and collaborating with the Peter Bent Brigham Hospital Pharmacology Department and the other a Clinical Research Center for the multidisciplinary study of chronic schizophrenia—illustrate the trend toward highly controlled, integrated, long-term work on refractory problems.

At the basic science level, a laboratory of neurophysiology was established in 1961 and this year [1962] we expect to build a biochemistry division. We are very well-equipped for psychophysiological and psychopharmacological activities, and psychoendocrine research will receive additional scope and emphasis in the immediate future.

At the training level there has been initiated a more orderly sequence of research training and practice, starting with first- and second-year residency courses and seminars from which are eventually selected promising candidates for a formal two-year research training program run by an interdisciplinary faculty from the hospital and Harvard, representing both basic and behavioral sciences. Psychiatrists preparing for a career in research also can rub elbows with Ph.D. contemporaries while they pursue an arbeit under scientists of senior rank. This development helps bridge the gap between basic and applied science, brings the hospital closer to Harvard Medical School, and, we hope, prepares a cadre of future workers in mental health much better prepared to do the job than were those of us who ventured forth untrained and inexperienced.

Members of the research staff have, of course, been recognized by their being widely sought as consultants at all levels, including national committees, foundations, and industry, as well as visiting lecturers and professors, editors of books and journals, and officers of societies. I think we can be proud of what has been accomplished, yet never satisfied or complacent, for we are painfully conscious of the big unsolved problems before us and of the fact that nature will not give up her secrets without exacting a hard sacrifice.

This brief account of where we came from and where we stand now purposely leaves out any attempt to evaluate the significance of the burgeoning Ewalt period, partly because in the historical sense it has only just begun, and partly because we are too close and too involved to have objective perspective. Let me merely express my deep personal admiration for Dr. Ewalt's leadership and venture the prediction, paraphrasing Adolf Meyer, that in his regime "many vital things will happen."[28]

I conclude with this reflection. Much that Southard dreamed about has come true in our time. We have had an adequate opportunity to demonstrate the soundness of belief in the "fecundity of aggregates" that he stressed, the stimulation of thought and work by the freest interchange among excellent minds of varying creative bents. It is now for us, this generation, to dream even greater dreams and to pursue them with courage and vigor that will be equal to those of the earliest "Psycho" men of science.

References

* Presented at the semicentenary of the Massachusetts Mental Health Center (Boston Psychopathic Hospital); symposium: The Psychiatric Teaching Hospital, October 11–13, 1962, in the session, "Research Contributions," on October 11, 1962.

1 E.E. Southard and H.C. Solomon, *Neurosyphilis* (Boston: William Leonard, 1917).

2 Southard, "The Mental Hygiene of Industry: A Movement that Particularly Concerns Employment Managers," *Industrial Management, 59* (1920), 100–106.

3 "Trade-Unionism and Temperament: The Psychiatric Point of View in Industry," *Industrial Management, 59* (1920), 265–270.

4 "The Modern Specialist in Unrest: Place of the Psychiatrist in Industry," *Industrial Management, 59* (1920), 462–466.

5 Southard and Mary C. Jarrett, *The Kingdom of Evils* (New York: MacMillan, 1922).

6 Frederick P. Gay, *Open Mind* (Chicago: Normandie House, 1938).

7 Abraham Myerson, *The Nervous Housewife* (Boston: Little, Brown, 1920).

8 Myerson, "The Constitutional Anhedonia Personality," *American Journal of Psychiatry, 102* (1945–46), 774–779.

9 Harry C. Solomon and Maida H. Solomon, *Syphilis of the Innocent* (Washington, D.C.: U.S. Interdepartmental Social Hygiene Board, 1922).

10 F.L. Wells, *Mental Tests in Clinical Practice* (Yonkers-on-Hudson, N.Y.: World Book, 1927).

11 S.J. Beck, "Problems of Further Research in the Rorschach Test," *American Journal of Orthopsychiatry, 5* (1935), 100–115.

12 *Schizophrenia*. Publications from the Clinical Service and Laboratories. Statistical Studies from the Boston Psychopathic Hospital (collected reprints), 1925–1934.

13 C.M. Campbell, *Destiny and Disease in Mental Disorders* (New York: W.W. Norton, 1935).

14 M. Greenblatt, R.H. York, and E.L. Brown, *From Custodial to Therapeutic Patient Care in Mental Hospitals* (New York: Russell Sage Foundation, 1955).

15 M. Greenblatt, D.J. Levinson, and R.H. Williams, eds., *The Patient and the Mental Hospital* (Glencoe, Il.: The Free Press, 1957).

16 R.W. Hyde in collaboration with the attendants of the Boston Psychopathic Hospital, *Experiencing the Patient's Day: A Manual for Psychiatric Hospital Personnel* (New York: Putnam, 1955).

17 M. Greenblatt and B. Simon, eds., *Rehabilitation of the Mentally Ill: Social and Economic Aspects* (Washington, D.C.: American Association for the Advancement of Science, 1959), publication no. 58.

18 F.L. Wells, M. Greenblatt, and R.W. Hyde, "As the Psychiatric Aide Sees His Work and Problems," *Genetic Psychology Monographs, 53* (1956), 3–37.

19 William Shakespeare, *Merchant of Venice*, III, 2.

20 D.H. Funkenstein, S.H. King, and M.E. Drolette, *Mastery of Stress* (Cambridge, Mass.: Harvard University Press, 1957).

21 D. Landy and W.D. Griffith, "Employer Receptivity Toward Hiring Psychiatric Patients," *Mental Hygiene, 43* (1958), 383–390.

22 M.P. Linder and D. Landy, "Post-Discharge Experience and Vocational Rehabilitation Needs of Psychiatric Patients," *Mental Hygiene, 42* (1958), 29–44.

23 Bernard M. Kramer, *Day Hospital* (New York: Grune and Stratton, 1962).

24 D. Landy and M. Greenblatt, in collaboration with Bertram S. Brown, Ralph Colp,

Jr., Mary Scanlan, and Sara E. Singer, *Halfway House. A Sociocultural and Clinical Study of Rutland Corner House. A Transitional Aftercare Residence for Female Psychiatric Patients* (Washington, D.C.: Vocational Rehabilitation Administration, 1965).

25 Henry Wechsler, "The Expatient Organization: A Survey," *The Journal of Social Issues, New Pathways from the Mental Hospital, 16* (1960), 47–53.

26 Carter C. Umbarger, Andrew P. Morrison, James S. Dalsimer, and Peter R. Breggin, prepared with the assistance and supervision of David Kantor and Milton Greenblatt, *College Students in a Mental Hospital* (New York: Grune and Stratton, 1962).

27 Milton Greenblatt, Robert F. Moore, Robert S. Albert, Maida H. Solomon, with Margaret H. Anderson, Lenore A. Boling, Bertram S. Brown, F.W. James, Betty Ann Glasser, and Mary Jane Manning, *The Prevention of Hospitalization* (New York: Grune and Stratton, 1963).

28 Adolph Meyer, "Psycho-Biology in the First Year of Medical School," *Journal of the Association of American Medical Colleges, 10* (1935), 365–372.

DISCUSSION

William Malamud, Sr., presiding

G. COLKET CANER: Dr. Gifford's paper has taught me more than I knew about Dr. Waterman, although I worked with him for twenty years. He was a fine sort of person, I thought. I liked him very much and so did most of his patients. It is true that many of them became dependent on him and followed him around from Maine to Palm Beach, but he also cured many patients in only one or two interviews. I think he was an effective psychotherapist.

He used suggestion mainly to help people. At first he termed it hypnosis, but later he called it suggestion and relaxation. In a sort of hypnotic voice he would tell his patient to relax his feet and legs and later his arms and eyes and face, and then he would give the suggestion that he thought would help.

This was particularly effective in the case of General Patton, who had developed severe pain in his leg and hip, which had lasted for over a year. Dr. Waterman soon found that this pain was due to a fear of cancer which the general had had pretty much all of his life because his father had died of cancer after a long illness and much suffering. Dr. Waterman treated the general by suggestion, and at the end he said, "Now that you know what the cause of this pain is, you'll be able to face it just as you faced all the threats that you encountered during the war." Later the general wrote Waterman that he felt like a damned fool to have been cured in one treatment of a pain that he had had for a year, but he was glad to report that the pain had entirely gone away.

EVEOLEEN REXFORD: I am delighted to have the opportunity to speak as a Judge Baker alumna and as one who has worked for a long time in the field of child psychiatry. It is impossible to overestimate the importance of William Healy's contribution to the field of child guidance and child psychiatry, and his investment in children in general. His patterns of working with children made a tremendous difference in our field. Dr. Healy was the one who institutionalized the team approach, the practice of bringing together psychiatrists, psychologists, social workers, and pediatricians; he thought that each specialist should work with the child and the family in accordance with his skill, and then together they should evaluate the total situation.

Some of his basic teachings now seem to us so commonplace that it is difficult to understand how revolutionary they were. I find that few people who have come into training in the last twenty years or so have even read his book, *The Individual Delinquent.* It is full of facts and theories, and wisdom, and I commend it to every person in our field who has not read it thus far. The basic idea of the book is the importance of trying to understand the particular child before you. When I first came to the Judge Baker, I was told that I must dictate my interview with the child under the heading "Child's Own Story." This was symbolic of Dr. Healy's teachings; he wanted to find out a great deal about the child, and of key importance was to listen to the child and find out what he thought, what he could say, what he was feeling.

I came to the Judge Baker after the chiefs had retired. Shortly after I arrived, Dr. Gardner and Dr. Rosenheim, the young chiefs, took off for the military service and so Dr. Healy and Dr. Bronner came back to the corner offices to lend some support and, I think, a note of respectability to various of the young fry, many of us women, who were trying to keep the Judge Baker going. Dr. Healy and Dr. Bronner wanted to see each new trainee and I remember very well my first talk with them. Dr. Healy was extremely serious, courteous, a rather slim, gray-haired man, wanting to know what my interests were, what I planned to do, and talking a good bit about the work he and Dr. Bronner had done. I was impressed by his courtesy because he spent a good bit of time talking about what seemed to him the future of this kind of work and what I might expect if I remained in the children's field. His assumption that I could converse with him as though we were indeed equals was quite striking, and that same basic courtesy came across when one listened to him interviewing youngsters. This was an amazing experience. People have criticized various of his clinical materials by saying that they were diagnostic studies and that there was little therapeutic in them. But if one had the opportunity to watch and to listen to him interviewing youngsters, one was struck by the rapport and understanding that came so quickly; within two or three seconds there was no one else in the room besides the child and Dr. Healy. That three or four such interviews were often highly therapeutic, one could see. His understanding, his compassion, his humor came out in such interviews. But his expectation that so far as possible the youngster would try to live up to certain standards also came across and I think did not interfere with his therapeutic effectiveness.

The research on delinquency that Dr. Healy and Dr. Bronner did is still far and away the most important body of work in this area that has ever been done. Many of the questions they raised remain to be studied, if we are to advance from what they were doing in the twenties into the fifties.

S. SPAFFORD ACKERLY: I had the good fortune to work on a research project with Dr. Healy for two years, 1930 to 1932, at the Yale Institute of Human Relations—the first attempt to study the nondelinquent sibling as a control. Dr. Healy and Dr. Bronner had been past masters at digging out the long array of etiological factors in a given delinquent, social and family pressures in particular. Up to the time of this research, however, it had not been clearly shown that the delinquent, not his sibling, suffered in the main from fractured human relations, especially within the family. The many other pressures were common to both delinquent and nondelinquent sibling. Therefore, treating the family became important.

Nor had the special meaningfulness of acting-out behavior for the delinquent's intrapsychic equilibrium been clearly brought out previously. Delinquency was often the lesser of two evils. The delinquent was faced with a complete mental breakdown on the one hand, or rebellious delinquent behavior on the other, with gradations of emotional turmoil and acting out in between. It all helped to make treatment more specific and individualized, which showed up clearly in the percentage of cases in which cessation of delinquency occurred.

I feel sure that if this research project into therapy in the three centers (Boston, Detroit, and New Haven) had not been curtailed after three years, an even greater contrast in results would have been shown between the Healy studies and the depressing findings earlier from Sheldon Glueck's follow-up study of one thousand delinquents.

JOHN A.P. MILLET: When the Riggs staff painfully learned that in regulating the lives of patients, therapy is by no means enough, we looked for some sort of group dynamics expert to be a kind of dean of patients who would somehow do the regulating, while the therapist pursued therapy without participating in any other intervention in the patients' lives. We could not find one and the joint patient-staff experiment in patient government began. Before that, while the therapy staff was trying to be an administrative body as well as a group of individual therapists, we frustrated not only ourselves but many other people too. Troubled by a number of recurrent problems in occupational therapy, the OT staff sent the therapy staff some questions. Here, from the notes of a staff conference, are some of the attempts to give answers.

On the problem of patients not leaving the shop at closing hour, it was felt that, in general, patients should definitely be asked to leave at closing time and that no special dispensation should be made for those who arrived late, but that flexibility was desirable and there might be occasions when one of the teachers should remain longer.

In regard to some form of daily physical exercise, it was agreed that this should not be required. On the other hand, it did seem to be the consensus that in general such physical exercise is therapeutic and that all patients should be encouraged or induced to try some such physical activity to give themselves a chance to judge whether it might be really helpful. Regarding the therapeutic value of some form of constructive daily activity, it seemed that no unequivocal answer could be given. Some patients appear to get better if they are left strictly alone until they get ready to plan some activity for themselves, whereas others need a great deal of planning and direction. In regard to the desirability of patients' carrying out responsibilities undertaken and whether this is a therapeutic issue, it seemed agreed that it certainly was a therapeutic hope that patients would carry through such responsibilities, even though some might be too sick at a particular time to be expected to show responsibility; the doctors wanted to be informed of instances of success or failure.

Reading these paragraphs several years later, one gets the impression of a parody, though nobody had that impression at the time. It looks like a skillful exercise in the technique of making unresponsive responses, of boldly stating a mild position and then retracting it because there are some factors on the other hand. It took many years for the psychotherapists to realize that the principles guiding psychoanalytic treatment seldom are appropriate guidelines for hospital administration. Without such a realization, replies like those above were inevitable.

As Dr. Howard has said, most of the psychotherapists, and I think most if not all of the nurses—important figures in the community—had serious doubts about giving much responsibility to patients. So did the patients. When the Community Committee was first formed, there was of course a decision to be made about its chairmanship. One of the committee's first acts was to pass a resolution that there would be no chairman, "because the committee is made up of sick people, and hence it is not possible for any member always to be able to act as chairman." There are also early statements that no group of patients should have any authority over another patient. About a year after that, the patients and staff voted to set up an *ad hoc* committee to draft a set of rules. This group, the Community Code Committee, was composed of six patients elected at large by the whole patient group and two patients, two nurses, and two therapists appointed by the medical director. One of those was Dr. Howard. Every patient on the committee began work with the conviction that the patient members would end up rubber-stamping a set of rules already secretly worked out by the staff. Much time and effort and persuasive power, with an occasional interpretation, were needed before this master-plot fantasy could be cut through and patients could believe that they were really quite important and respected contributors to the work of the group. Then, from that point on, they were just that.

What the Community Code Committee eventually produced was not a set of rules, but a more general code of behavior, with clear statements of areas of responsibility and lines of communication. At about the same time that the committee's report was accepted, with a few modifications after a series of patient-staff meetings, the medical director invited the whole committee to present its work as a part of the semiannual meeting of the Riggs Board of Trustees. The committee accepted the invitation, but with so much apprehension that at one point there was an anxious two-hour discussion about seating arrangements. The meeting was to be held in the staff conference room, a place ordinarily entered by patients only at the time of their presentations at clinical conferences. Hence the room, and especially the table, heavily emphasized both the usual patient role and the departure from it that this meeting would require. Who would actually sit at the table and who, so to speak, in the bleachers? One patient finally said, "Hah, let's forget we're neurotic for one night and sit at the conference table."

When the time came, all the members participated actively and well in the presentation. Everybody concerned, patients and staff as well as trustees, found this innovation welcome. The patients felt that presenting some of their own active and creative contributions to the Riggs community was highly preferable to some of their earlier experiences at the semiannual meetings of trustees. Then they had been looked at by touring trustees as they worked in the shop or sat around the Inn, the building where our patients live, just passively being patients. Now they were actively presenting their work and were being given a chance to trade questions and answers with interested and very much impressed visitors.

Dr. Howard mentioned the common work program. It got that name somewhat by accident. When patients proposed a program of paid work, with the money going to a patient-aid fund to help provide reductions of fees for some patients, a study group of patients and staff incorporated the proposal into part of a plan in which each patient would work at an assigned job each weekday morning from 8:30 to 9:30. Everybody would be working at the same time, with a number of envisioned advantages, among them a boost in morale, a simplified means of keeping track of work done, high visibility of any patient doing anything else at that hour, and high invisibility of patients still in bed. It was the time that was common, not the work. Eventually, however, common work came to mean something like scut work and under the conditions Dr. Howard noted it was discontinued.

A later attempt to reinstate it was entirely staff initiated and failed totally. Finally, through the last quarter century of Riggs history, we, patients and staff, have tried, as Dr. Howard said, to create an atmosphere that was as unlike as possible that of the demanding and regimenting earlier home and school atmosphere. "As unlike as possible" clearly does not mean "directly opposite." We sought and usually found a milieu that provided sanctuary from excessive pressure but enough social demand to forestall unnecessary regression. I shall close with a quotation from Freud: "Any analyst who out of the fullness of his heart, perhaps, and his readiness to help, extends to the patient all that one human being may hope to receive from another, commits the same economic error as that of which our nonanalytic institutions for nervous patients are guilty. Their one aim is to make everything as pleasant as possible for the patient, so that he may feel well there and be glad to take refuge there again from the trials of life. In so doing they make no attempt to give him more strength for facing life and more capacity for carrying out his actual tasks in it."

JOHN A.P. MILLET*: I happened to join "The Team," as Austen called it, in the role of physician to the foundation, in 1923, at a time when the success and reputation of Austen's work was approaching its peak. He felt that there was a growing need for a good clinical laboratory and for an internist to look after the general health of staff and patients. The invitation came at a most opportune time in my life, when I had to make a new connection and was considering an offer to work with Alan Gregg in the medical education field, in which the Rockefeller Foundation was then actively engaged. My old friend and medical school roommate, Lawrence Kirby Lunt, was at the time Riggs's office manager and team leader. My decision was greatly influenced by this old friendship, as well as by the magnetism of Austen's personality and the delightful prospect of doing creative work in such stimulating company and in such an ideal setting.

I became extremely busy with my work there, and it was not many weeks before Austen called me in to say that since the laboratory was now in good order and my technician could attend to the necessary routines, I should begin to learn the subtle skills of the psychotherapist. Already the other members of the staff were working on a ten-hour-a-day schedule. Accordingly I was apprenticed as an observer during hours of patient interviews conducted by either Austen or Lawrence. I sat quietly in a dark corner of their consulting rooms, drinking in the atmosphere of the psychotherapeutic encounter. This was a whole new approach to the practice of medicine for which I felt an immediate sympathy. Thus began a career in this field, which came later to encompass the education of psychoanalysts and of psychiatric residents, as well as the organization of community mental health services at the county level.

The seven years I spent at Stockbridge with my growing family were among the most rewarding of any consecutive seven years that I can think of. What is not generally known is that Austen had developed a full-fledged ego psychology based on his own ruminative experiences during a period when he was confined to bed with a tubercular infection. During these long months of confinement he read widely in the writings of Freud and the other psychoanalysts, as well as other European therapists such as Déjerine, DuBois, and Janet. Significant influences also came from the psychology of William James and William McDougall, the physiological discoveries of Walter Cannon at Harvard, the research into the behavior of anthropoids by Yerkes at Yale, and the studies of brain physiology conducted at the Neurological Institute in New York under the leadership of Tilney.

Austen Riggs entered psychotherapy by internal medicine, as had both Lawrence Lunt and myself. A most gifted craftsman in wood, he emphasized manual crafts as significant additions to the daily life of his patients. He termed his therapeutic method the reeducational approach to the therapy of the neuroses. He had been a good neurologist in his time, a great admirer of the British, especially Hughlings Jackson and Sherrington. The direction of therapy was toward clarification of goals, especially those consonant with the ethical outlook and objectives of the patient, as described in the first "Green Book" (see Benjamin Riggs, "Austen Fox Riggs: Pioneer in the Psychotherapy of the Neuroses"). He saw the neurotic patient not as one whose adaptive integration had broken down under some stress of emotion or misfortune, but as one endowed with a higher degree of sensitivity than the average and therefore more likely to overreact with the self-protective emotions of fear, anger, and hurt pride. He saw the human being as an organism endowed with a complicated adaptive system in which the emotions provided the thrust, the intelligence, the power of understanding, the control of expression, the choice of action, and the ideals provided a direction finder. Although he drew much of his insight from his wide reading and his personal frustrations, he was stoutly opposed to the Freudian insistence on the primary role of sexuality in the etiology of the neuroses. He preferred the phenomenological summary of instinctual drives as devoted either to self-preservation or to the continuation of the race, with sexual instinct on the same level of importance as all the rest.

The second "Green Book" covered the important field of disturbances in sensory registration and the anxieties that it occasions. The third goes into the most common mistakes in the management of emotional responses, with the occasional disturbances of body function that can follow. The later pamphlets deal with sleep and the causes of insomnia, and with the basic laws of successful living, emphasizing the skillful use of trained observation, and the power of choice in the service of a more genuinely adaptive posture.

Every day was scheduled, the details set by the psychiatrist who took the history and made the original physical and neurological examination. The schedule ran about like this:

7: up, exercises, bath, dress;
8: breakfast; 8:30: bowels, newspaper, mail, etc.;
9–12: one hour exercise (walk, ride, golf, etc.), one hour occupational therapy, one hour conference with doctor, or personal errands;
12–1: relaxation, read mail, etc.;
1: lunch; 2–3: rest; 3–5: exercise and occupational therapy;
5–6: social hour; 6–7: relax; 7: dinner;
8–9:30: social activities; 9:30: bed; 10: lights out.

In addition to the reeducational conferences with the doctor, the patient was usually seen three or four times during his or her stay by Austen himself, and on Sunday afternoons at four Austen gave talks, with a question box, on the general principles of Darwinian evolutionary theory and adaptation and on questions that might be raised concerning the points made in the little green books.

The foundation operated a child guidance and adult mental hygiene clinic for the inhabitants of Berkshire County in Pittsfield. A good deal of consultation work was done with the schools in the area as well as with Vassar and Williams colleges.

From this fragmentary account it will be seen that most of the current practices in the field of institutional and outpatient care were adumbrated in the many services given by Riggs and his staff. During the period I was there the foundation had achieved a high reputation for effective therapy and a medically scientific approach to the understanding of the neuroses. Stockbridge was recognized as the premier center for modern psychotherapy. There were annual meetings of the advisory committee, which included many of those best known in the field: Adolf Meyer, Edward Willy Taylor, George Waterman, Frederick Tilney, Thomas Salmon, and Macfie Campbell. The staff met weekly after dining at the Riggs's house, where Alice Riggs was always the warmest and most welcoming of hostesses.

The Austen Riggs Foundation then in its heyday (from 1924 to 1935), when Riggs was still very much in command, led the way to a clearer understanding of the neuroses and of at least one psychotherapeutic method that showed good results. The work of the foundation included community mental health services and consultations with educational institutions, as well as intensive individual therapy. The team idea represented the essence of what has since been called the therapeutic community. It is amazing that Riggs's name as the founder of this successful method should be so little known to the informed public today. In 1968, I read a paper ("Austen Fox Riggs: his significance to American psychiatry of today," *American Journal of Psychiatry, 125* (1968), 120) before the American Psychiatric Association in Boston, outlining what I considered to be the principal features of his ego psychology as applied to his Stockbridge work. On this occasion a young psychiatrist stopped me in the room where the exhibits were housed, saying; "Oh, Dr. Millet, I see you are giving a paper on Austen Riggs this afternoon. I did not realize he was a psychiatrist. I thought he was some rich industrialist who had founded a center for the study and care of the neuroses!" Such is fame!

Reference

* This was a solicited contribution.

Illustrations

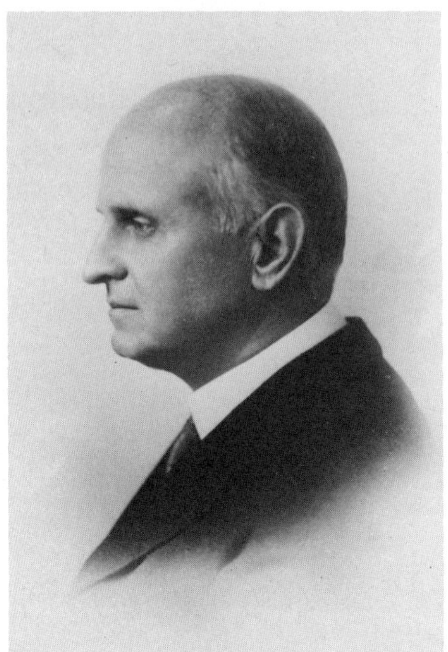

28. George A. Waterman.
Countway Library.

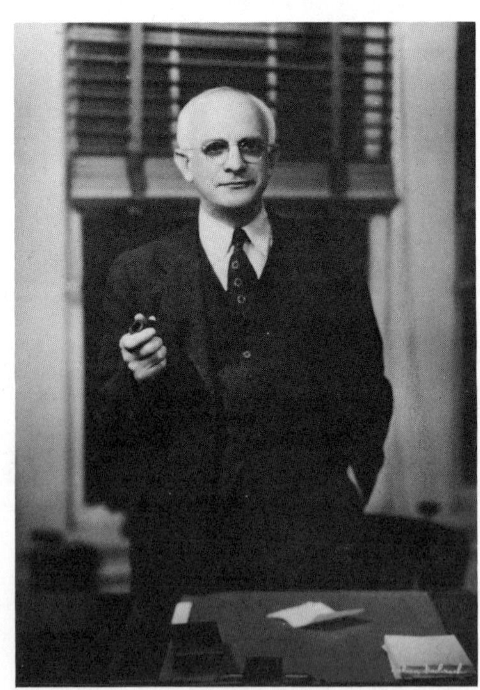

29. Abraham Myerson.
Courtesy of David Myerson.

30. Augusta Bronner and William Healy at the Judge Baker Guidance Center, 1957. *Courtesy Nancy Staver, Judge Baker Guidance Center.*

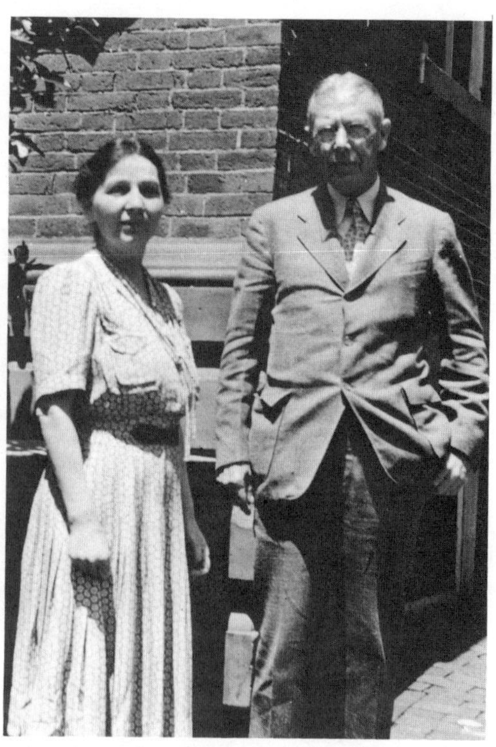

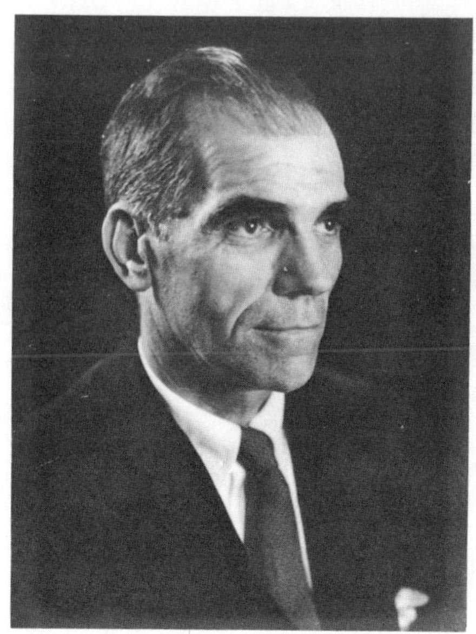

31. Austen F. Riggs, founder of the Austen Riggs Center, Stockbridge, Massachusetts. *Austen Riggs Center.*

32. *a & b.* Harry Solomon was professor of psychiatry at the Harvard Medical School and superintendent of the Massachusetts Mental Health Center. His wife Maida H. Solomon was professor of social economy at Simmons College School of Social Work. Her service to the Boston Psychopathic Hospital began almost at its founding and continued to her role as consultant in psychiatric social work research. *Greenblatt Collection, Countway Library.*

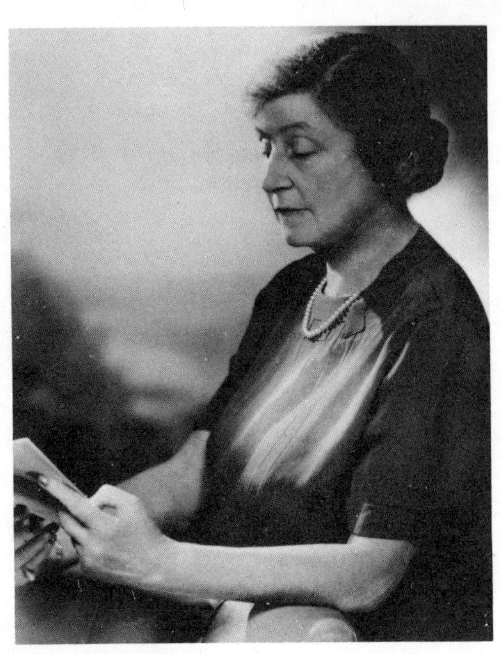

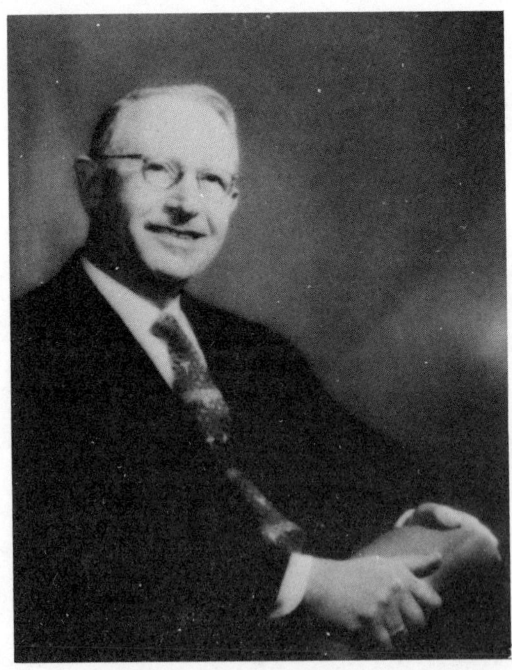

Early Psychoanalysis in Boston

Psychoanalysis in Boston: Innocence and Experience Introduction to the Panel Discussion—April 14, 1973

SANFORD GIFFORD

Until very recently, the average American analyst had a hazy picture of our origins. A dim photograph of Freud at Clark University in 1909 was familiar as a shadowy ancestral tableau, "a fadograph of a yestern scene." Even in Boston, James Jackson Putnam was remembered, if at all, for his friendship with William James, his Adirondack camp and the visit of Freud, Jung, and Ferenczi, with their quaint impressions of our native customs. For the average analyst, these hazy notions of our past, along with some awareness of A.A. Brill as a founding father, and of the ubiquitous presence of Ernest Jones, were probably derived from Jones's monumental biography of Freud.[1] Of course, for the more curious student, there were a few specialized histories, by Oberndorf,[2] Ives Hendrick,[3] and Lewin and Ross,[4] who wrote as participants in the events they described, each with the limitations of his time and place in the analytic movement. The curious reader might learn that Freud called Putnam "the first American to interest himself in analysis,"[5] that analysis was "cradled in Boston [but] raised and grew up in New York,"[2] or that Putnam was the first president of the American Psychoanalytic Association, founded in 1911. But even the most inquisitive student might still wonder why Jones, an Englishman, was secretary to the American Association, or why Brill had founded the New York Psychoanalytic Society four months before the American, and which only joined the American in 1914.

All this has been changed by our professional historians, by the work of Burnham,[6] Ellenberger,[7] and Hale,[8,9] who have contributed to our symposium. But I would like to emphasize how recently these new studies have appeared, all but Burnham's monograph still unpublished or in press when we began, in 1969, to plan these meetings. Our aim has been to give a clearer picture of the preanalytic psychotherapy movement in this country, which reached its peak at the turn of the century, just as the ideas and writings of Freud were beginning to touch these shores. We also hoped to provide a more detailed, less parochial view of the interrelations between psychotherapy and analysis, and to sketch some characteristic features that still distinguish analysis in America from its European counterpart.

Having considered some major figures in the preceding papers, we come now to the history of New England psychoanalysis proper, and to the recollections of colleagues who created this history. Some were "at the hot gates fighting" in 1933, when our third Boston Psychoanalytic Society and Institute was founded, while others are no longer here. To make these informal, eyewitness accounts of our early days more understandable, a brief historical outline will be useful. We must acknowledge our omission of some significant figures, like Adolf Meyer and Boris Sidis, who were not discussed in individual papers, and the absence of several colleagues, like the late Molly Putnam and Ives Hendrick, with whom we discussed our symposium and who would have made important contributions to it.

As we have already learned in part, the advent of psychoanalysis in America presented several historical accidents, or ironies, that helped determine some distinctive differences between analytic developments here and abroad, and particularly between Boston and New York. First, there was the coincidence that analytic theories arrived here at the height of the psychotherapy movement, derived, like analysis itself, from the hypnotic methods of Charcot and other French neurologists. In 1902 William James had hailed "the mind cure movement,"[10] for its "practical fruits," as a typically "American" contribution to psychotherapy, eminently befitting our "practical," optimistic national character. Thus analysis was first welcomed as an addition to psychotherapy, and some American neurologists like Morton Prince began calling their hypnotic studies "psychoanalysis." But Ernest Jones emphasized the differences: psychoanalysis depended on the patient's own free associations, rather than the commands of a charismatic hypnotist, and he insisted that the term should be restricted to the methods of Freud. Instead of being assimilated by the psychotherapy movement, analysis superseded the popular psychotherapies of suggestion and eventually permeated the theoretical foundations of many later psychotherapies, up to the present day.

A second, more subtle irony was the contrast between American therapeutic optimism and Freud's worldly, deeply pessimistic view of human nature. Even in 1909 at Worcester, which may be seen as one of many encounters between American innocence and European experience, Freud expressed his forebodings about the American predilection for eclecticism, religious enthusiasms, and excessive therapeutic zeal. He feared that our passion for popularization would dilute psychoanalysis with the baser metals of psychotherapy, and that our strong medical orientation would reduce analysis to a mere therapeutic technique. Freud's forebodings were partially confirmed by later events, in our antipathy to lay analysis, our insistence that only physicians could become analysts, and the continuing close relation of analysis to clinical psychiatry and general medicine.

Finally, Freud lived long enough to witness a third historical irony, that the analytic movement was to flourish more luxuriantly in this country, which Freud had never loved, than anywhere else in the world.

As a background for our panel discussion, the analytic movement in Boston and its environs can be outlined in a few well-marked periods, by sketching in some principal figures and events of each period.

The Prehistory of New England Analysis, 1894–1909

This period begins with the first published reference to Freud's theories in American journals and concludes with the Clark University lectures in September 1909. The earliest was William James's review[11] of Breuer and Freud's preliminary communication on the treatment of hysteria by "abreaction" or the "cathartic method." This was followed by Robert Edes's discussion in his Shattuck Lecture of 1895, "The New England Invalid."[12] This has a special interest because Edes represented a local tradition of "medical psychotherapy" using hypnosis and suggestion as techniques carried out by internists and general surgeons. Edes saw some value in the cathartic method, but he expressed more interest in the conscious inhibition of aggression than in unconscious sexual impulses. He concluded that the method of Breuer and Freud "was not far removed from the common-sense observation that it is much better to 'get mad' and be done with it than to cherish the grievance in silence."

In 1906 Putnam published his observations on the treatment of hysteria, conducted over several years in a special ward on the neurological service of the Massachusetts General Hospital.[13] In this paper, which appeared in the first issue of Morton Prince's *Journal of Abnormal Psychology*, Putnam reported on three cases treated by "Freud's method of 'psychoanalysis.'" In Ernest Jones's obituary of Putnam,[14] Jones called this paper "the *first* one on psychoanalysis in English," but he later withdrew this honor[1] and conferred it upon himself, for his own paper of 1909.[15] How much Putnam's paper represented psychoanalysis, and how much a form of abreaction, can be debated, but there is a refreshing sincerity about Putnam's self-taught approach to analysis, by applying its methods and subjecting it to empirical proof.

In 1909 Ernest Jones paid his first visit to the weekly meetings at Morton Prince's house (Appendix A), where Putnam, William James, E.W. Taylor, Isador Coriat, and other enthusiasts of the psychotherapy movement often gathered. Here Jones discussed psychoanalysis, as he did at innumerable scientific meetings throughout this country and Canada. (During the following five years Jones was, in effect, an American, residing in Toronto.) Jones also met and encouraged Putnam in his growing sympathy for Freudian theory. He described Putnam's "absurd deference," as an eminent professor of sixty-two, toward himself, a brash young man of twenty-eight.[16]

A major event in New England analysis before the Clark University lectures was a meeting of the American Therapeutic Society at New Haven, in May 1909. This was an intermingling of the preanalytic psychotherapies and the beginnings of analysis, reflecting the most advanced psychiatric thinking of those years. The meeting was organized by Dr. Frederic H. Gerrish,[16] an elderly general surgeon who had become an enthusiastic practitioner of hypnosis in the late 1880s. (He had greatly influenced Dr. George Gehring,[17] also a medical psychotherapist who established a treatment center for the neuroses at Bethel, Maine, which became the model for the Austen Riggs Foundation.) In the first address, Morton Prince reviewed the successes of the psychotherapy movement, and there were papers by E.W. Taylor, George Waterman, and other neurologists belonging to Prince's circle. Putnam's essay on "Character Formation" reflected his background in the psychotherapy of suggestion, his new admiration for "the genius of Freud" in discovering the childhood determinants of adult personality development, and his mildly euphemistic view of the sexual etiology of hysteria. Jones's paper contained a ringing declaration of analytic independence from psychotherapy, as well as a crude but skillful popularization of analytic theories for the general physician, and compared the uncovering of repressed conflicts to the drainage of a surgical abscess. Boris Sidis gave the last paper. Best known as a clinical psychologist and pupil of William James, he was said to have transmitted Freud's theories to the staff of Manhattan State Hospital, during the years 1898 to 1905, but he later repudiated analysis. He now proposed his own method of treatment by the "hypnoid state," or "waking suggestion." Proclaiming its superiority to hypnosis, Sidis stated that the therapeutic successes of Weir Mitchell's rest cures were caused by waking suggestion, and that Freud's results in the treatment of hysteria were "not so much due to 'psycho-analysis' as to the unconscious use of the hypnoidal state."

The Age of Putnam, 1909–1918

Many aspects of Freud's visit to Clark University in September 1909 have been discussed in previous papers, but some aspects may be reemphasized here. The meeting between Freud and Putnam established a lasting friendship that continued through correspondence until Putnam's death in 1918.[8] The strong mutual respect between these two dignified, rather reserved scientists, at a time when Putnam was ten years older than Freud and our most eminent neurologist, swept away Putnam's lingering doubts about Freud and soon enabled him to write about analysis as "our cause." This relationship, mediated by the ubiquitous Jones, who already saw himself as Freud's emissary *in partibus infidelium*, was the basis for a new era, in which we can speak of an organized psychoanalytic movement in the United States and Canada. Jones, in his role as agile go-between, persuaded the modest Putnam to accept the presidency of the American Psychoanalytic Association in 1911. Putnam was reluctant, but he acquiesced to Freud's wishes for an American branch of the international association. Freud regarded Putnam as a shield and protector of analysis, believing that "all important intellectual movements in America have originated in Boston."[8] Jones was, in fact, the chief architect of the American Psychoanalytic Association, and the history of analysis in the country might have been very different if Putnam had succeeded in getting Jones appointed to the faculty of Harvard Medical School. But when Putnam's efforts failed, Jones returned to England in 1913, to found the British Analytic Society and to remain the master diplomat of the international movement.

Another aspect of the Worcester meetings was the presence of Ferenczi and Jung, at a time when Freud and Jung were still close collaborators, thus linking them in the minds of Americans. Jung's analytic studies of schizophrenia and his word association test had already been influential in attracting Americans to psychoanalysis. Frederick Peterson's advice to Brill in 1907, to leave Paris and study with Jung in Zurich, was a turning point in Brill's career and in the future history of analysis in New York. Having met Jones in Zurich and accompanied him to visit Freud, Brill returned to New York in 1908, with a translation of Jung's book and Freud's permission to translate his books and papers. Brill was the first American to proclaim himself a full-time psychoanalyst, with an office practice in New York. He was soon followed by Oberndorf, Karpas, Frink, and others, and with them founded the New York Psychoanalytic Society in 1911.

The New York Society had twenty-eight members in 1914, compared to the eight founding members of the American Psychoanalytic Society, and always showed certain characteristics that differed from the American as well as the Boston analytic group. A majority of the New York group became interested in analysis at Manhattan State Hospital, on Ward's Island. The study of analysis was encouraged there by Adolf Meyer (1902 to 1910) and August Hoch (1910 to 1919), both of whom had previous relations with Worcester State Hospital and McLean Hospital. Nearly all the New York analysts began as psychiatrists rather than neurologists, and were accustomed to working with psychotic patients at Manhattan State or, like Brill and William A. White, at other state institutions. All were physicians, unlike the psychotherapy movement in Boston, which was equally shared between neurologists like Prince and Putnam and clinical psychologists like James and Münsterberg.

These characteristics of the New York Society increased the differences between American and European patterns of analytic practice, and also differed from certain features of the Boston analytic group. First, the institutional background of the New York analysts favored an interest in the treatment of psychoses, which they shared with the Swiss but not with Freud and the Vienna circle. Second, the leap from a hospital setting to the office treatment of neuroses favored full-time analytic practice. Most Boston analysts, however, were neurologists who had no experience with psychoses and were accustomed to office practices that facilitated part-time analysis, part-time psychotherapy and academic positions. Finally, and most important of all, Brill and the New York group insisted from the beginning that only physicians could become analysts, a rule that the American Psychoanalytic Association adopted only in 1924. This medical orthodoxy strengthened the tendency of American analysts to remain within the field of psychiatry and general medicine, and of analysis to become a subspecialty within it.

Returning to Boston itself during the years of Putnam's leadership, the group remained quite small and heterogeneous. Putnam founded the first Boston Psychoanalytic Society in 1914, with Dr. Isador Coriat as secretary; he announced this in the International *Zeitschrift*. But Putnam described the society very modestly to Freud as "a small group that meets at my house every Friday afternoon, and although we are not geniuses, yet we do fair work and, I think, keep our heads level."[8] Its most regular member was L.E. Emerson, a clinical psychologist and pupil of Royce, whom Putnam had appointed to the neurology department of the Massachusetts General Hospital. He was known as "Red-Necktie" Emerson[18] and continued to represent analysis until his death in 1939. A colorful but elusive member was Dr. James S. Van Teslaar, a Roumanian with a Dutch name, who claimed a medical degree from the University of California that could never be confirmed.[19] Though he disappeared from the scientific scene in the mid-1920s and may have been a charlatan,[20] he wrote fluent popularizations of analytic theories and edited the Modern Library *Outline of Psychoanalysis*.[21] This book, reissued for several decades, reprinted early papers of Freud, Putnam, and Brill and influenced many a later schoolboy in his first discovery of analytic literature. According to George Wilbur, these meetings were sometimes attended by Morton Prince and E.W. Taylor, who had become estranged from analysis after 1911 but remained personally loyal to Putnam.[20] Visiting New York analysts like Hoch, Clark, and MacCurdy attended occasionally. Another probable member was the philosopher and clinical psychologist, E.B. Holt, a pupil of William James, who wrote the first popular American book on analysis,[22] which Putnam sent to Freud.

Putnam himself, however, was not a charismatic leader like Brill, and though he was an equally prolific writer and indefatigable speaker in the cause of analysis, he left few followers and no organized Boston "school." In spite of his influential role in the American acceptance of analysis, he seems to have had a genuine aversion to the personal uses of political power. Putnam's Puritan background—though he denied any formal religious belief—and his youthful Emersonian Transcendentalism, as well as his devotion to the defense of unpopular causes, may have attracted him to analysis. And it certainly sustained his persistent efforts to persuade Jones and Freud that an American form of neo-Hegelian idealism should find a place in psychoanalytic theory. They remained skeptical, and an exchange of letters[8] illustrated the encounter between European experience and American innocence. In answer to Putnam's questions about sublimation and ethical ideals, Freud gently rebuked him: "The unworthiness of human beings, including the analysts, has always impressed me deeply, but why *should* analyzed men and women in fact be better. Analysis makes for integration but does not of itself make for goodness. I do not believe, as do Socrates and Putnam, that all vices originate in a sort of obscurity and ignorance. I feel that one puts too great a burden on analysis when one asks that it realize each of one's dearest ideals." Putnam was undaunted, however, and insisted that Freud's "sense of freedom and your love of truth *is* a religion," and that the ideal analysis "would leave one, theoretically, a perfect person."

The Dark Ages of Boston Analysis, 1918–1930

After Putnam's death, just before the Armistice, "the light of analysis in Boston flickered out," according to Dr. John Abbott.[18] This left Dr. Isador Coriat as our sole Freudian analyst, whose remarkable career, as we know from Professor Sicherman's paper, spanned so many phases of New England psychiatry. In 1899 Coriat had studied the biochemistry of schizophrenia under Adolf Meyer at Worcester State, attended the meetings at Prince's house from 1906 to 1912, and collaborated with the Rev. Worcester in the Emmanuel Movement from 1906 to 1913, at which point he joined the American Psychoanalytic Association. Like Putnam, Coriat was reserved about seeking followers, but around 1924 he reestablished the kind of informal analytic meetings that Putnam had held. In 1928 this group was organized as the second Boston Psychoanalytic Society, with Coriat as president and Dr. Martin Peck as secretary (Appendix B).

Its membership was lively and diverse, made up of three principal study groups that had developed independently. The largest and most active were the Rankians: Peck, Dr. George B. Wilbur, Dr. John H. Taylor and his sister Martha, and Dr. Leolia Dalrymple. Peck had been analyzed by Otto Rank in 1921, during one of Rank's many visits to New York but before his break with Freud. Dr. Dalrymple had been analyzed by Peck, and Wilbur and Taylor by Rank at later times. Wilbur was later told that his analysis, conducted in both Paris and New York during 1926, had been "a year of peculiarly bad vintage."[20] The Rankian group also met periodically in New York, at the house of Dr. Frankwood Williams, a prominent figure in the mental health movement and a leader of Rankian analysis in this country.

A second sizable group were analysands of Jung, led by Dr. Henry A. Murray, the well-known professor of psychology at Harvard. They included Dr. Irmarita Putnam and her husband Tracy the neuropathologist, Dr. Christiana Morgan and her husband the anthropologist, and Dr. William Herman, a brilliant young pupil of Dr. Stanley Cobb, who died prematurely in the early thirties. Their meetings were originally held in the Harvard Psychological Clinic, where Wilbur had first met this group and invited them to join the Coriat group. A third, smaller group comprised the analysands of Paul Schilder, still in Vienna and popular with Americans for his swift summer vacation analyses. These were: Dr. S. Spafford Ackerly, Dr. David Rothschild, and Dr. William Malamud. Whatever the theoretical differences among these three groups and Coriat, or between psychiatrists, psychologists and other nonphysicians, they all "got along quite well together," according to Hendrick. "Indeed, if the truth be told, they got along much better together than Freudians got along with Freudians, as soon as there was more than one lone Freudian in the Society!"[3]

Reorganization and Reform, 1930–1935

In the summer of 1930, Coriat proposed a more formal reorganization of the Boston Psychoanalytic Society, with a written constitution, elected officers, and annual dues of $2.50. He was elected president, Peck secretary-treasurer, and with twenty members, they represented "a strange conglomeration of varying inflammable ideas as to what analysis was or should be."[3] The requirements for membership were, for the first time, a medical degree, a personal "training analysis" (as yet undefined), two years of analytic practice, and the publication (or presentation) of a paper on an analytic topic. Although full membership was limited to physicians, following the 1926 rule of the New York Psychoanalytic Society, nonmedical "associate members" were admitted if they signed a pledge not to practice analysis or represent themselves as analysts. In the membership list (Appendix C), the three original groups of Rankians, Jungians, and Schilderians can still be recognized, as well as a new contingent of young American analysts who had just completed their analytic training in Europe. These included Ives Hendrick, M. Ralph Kaufman, and John Murray; Dalrymple again (who had left Boston to be analyzed by Franz Alexander in Berlin); and Margaret Ribble, an early child analyst who later settled in New York.

This new group of Americans trained abroad, who had arrived in Boston during the fall and winter of 1930 and 1931, initiated a new and tumultuous era. Inspired by their European experiences, they struggled to create an analytic institute, modeled on the Berlin Psychoanalytic Institute, that would provide full training, with didactic analyses by a recognized "training analyst," a faculty and curriculum of seminars, and supervised "control analyses" for low-fee patients. The leader of this group seems to have been Ives Hendrick, who had completed two years of training at the Berlin Institute, where he was analyzed by Franz Alexander. He began by organizing the "Freud Seminar" of 1930 to 1932, which met in his office, at 250 Commonwealth Avenue, and formed the nucleus of our present institute. Since there were no training analysts in Boston, the seminars were taught by four instructors from the New York Psychoanalytic Society, Bertram Lewin, Abram Kardiner, Gregory Zilboorg, and Dorian Feigenbaum, who commuted to Boston for one day every few weeks, while the Boston group commuted to New York for alternate meetings.

In 1931, the Boston Psychoanalytic Society imported its first training analyst, Franz Alexander, who had emigrated from Berlin in 1930 to be a visiting professor at the University of Chicago, and who returned, after a year in Boston, to found the Chicago Psychoanalytic Institute. Alexander's appointment was arranged by Hendrick, with the help of Dr. William Healy, director of the Judge Baker Guidance Center. Healy offered Alexander a half-time research position and then, at sixty-two, began his own training analysis with Alexander. The rest of Alexander's time was quickly filled by eight training analysands, some of whom followed him to Chicago to complete their analyses, like Karl Menninger and Henry A. Murray. Although Alexander also found time, during his academic year in Boston, to write a book,[23] he refused to take part in the constitutional battles over reorganization of the new society-institute.

During this stormy period of reformation, there were inevitable conflicts between members of the old 1928 Coriat society and the new European-trained members. Even many years later, John Taylor refused to recall these "personal squabbles and hurt feelings" because he "would only be digging up old bones, some of which might prove to be incompletely decayed."[24] The details of the painful process were complex, fierce, and exhausting to its participants, but reassuringly similar to quarrels among later generations of analysts. To summarize the principal issues briefly, the general aim was to establish uniform standards for analytic training, modeled on European procedures but conforming to the new regulations of the New York Society and the American Psychoanalytic Association. The immediate goal was to obtain recognition as a constituent society of the American, and eventually of the International Psychoanalytic Association, but there were also special local problems. One was the status of members in the old society, many of whom were self-taught, inadequately trained, or analyzed by Rank, Schilder, and Jung.

Some had eagerly sought an approved training analysis with Alexander, or later with Hanns Sachs, but others experienced their second analysis as a forced conversion, a baptism by the sword, which George Wilbur called "getting regularized." At a society meeting in 1933, ten older members agreed to resign temporarily, in order to allow the ten remaining members, who did meet the revised training standards, to be recognized by the American Psychoanalytic Association. These ten founding members became our third Boston Psychoanalytic Society (Appendix D). At a previous meeting in May 1932, however, there had been "nine sets of convictions among the nine members actively engaged" in the discussion.[3]

Another issue was the perennial one of medical orthodoxy, or the requirement that only physicians should be eligible for full membership, so characteristic of American rather than European analysis. A few nonphysicians were accepted for theoretical training, as associate members, but there were frequent controversies about whom and how many to accept. A third issue, which Hendrick regarded as the cornerstone of the reform movement, was the "faculty principle." This meant that applicants for analytic training could only be approved by the Education Committee of the institute, and not by the individual decision of a training analyst, as many European analysts were accustomed to doing.

All of these controversies were intensified in September 1932, by the arrival of our second training analyst, Dr. Hanns Sachs, who was neither a physician nor a believer in the faculty principle. As a member of Freud's original Vienna circle and the first training analyst at the newly founded Berlin Institute in 1920, Sachs's appointment in Boston had been arranged by Dr. Irmarita Putnam with the approval of Freud himself. In Sachs's letter of acceptance, he had refused to submit to the requirements of the new Education Committee, and he continued to accept candidates for training as he saw fit. Nevertheless he was a brilliant theoretical teacher, known for his wit and erudition, and the first nonphysician appointed to a lectureship in psychoanalysis at Harvard Medical School.

The new Boston Psychoanalytic Society had been accepted as a constituent society by the American Psychoanalytic Association in December 1933. Recognition by the American was reaffirmed *de jure* as well as *de facto*, in 1935, after the technical requirements had been fulfilled of acceptance by the International Psychoanalytic Association, at its biennial congress in August 1934. In the same year the Education Committee was incorporated as the Boston Psychoanalytic Institute, which shared the same membership as the society, unlike some analytic training centers. The two overlapping groups were combined, in 1947, as the Boston Psychoanalytic Society and Institute. Permanent quarters were at 82 Marlborough Street, a few blocks from Dr. Putnam's office at Number 106, where the first society was organized in 1914.

The European Migration and the War Years, 1935–1946

The superficial wounds of the five year reformation had healed by 1935, just as the first analytic émigrés from the Nazi persecutions began to arrive. But some internal injuries and conflicts were still palpable, and there had been a few casualties and departures. After several difficult years as chairman of the Education Committee, Dr. Irmarita Putnam and her husband moved to New York. Professor Henry A. Murray, who had followed her as chairman, withdrew from institute affairs, although he remained a member, because he found "an atmosphere too charged with humorless hostility...an assemblage of cultists, rigid in thought, armored against new ideas, and (in the case of two or three overly ambitious ones) ruthlessly rivalrous for power."[25] Dr. Stanley Cobb became inactive in society affairs but continued as a strong supporter of analysis, in the new psychiatric department he established at the Massachusetts General Hospital in 1934, and in later collaboration with European analysts. Dr. Karl Menninger and Dr. Jacob Kasanin departed for Chicago and eventually for Topeka and San Francisco, respectively, where they contributed to the westward propagation of analysis.

The leaders of the reformation supported Martin Peck as president of the new Boston Psychoanalytic Society and Institute in 1935, for his nonpartisan, peace-making abilities. Always called "the gentle Peck" by Hendrick, he was a man without enemies, who had some of Putnam's integrity and innocence, and great optimism about the medical orientation of American analysis. Since the early 1920s he had also taught psychiatry and psychoanalysis at the Boston Psychopathic Hospital, under MacFie Campbell, establishing a characteristic pattern of part-time analysis and part-time academic teaching. On Peck's visit to Freud in the summer of 1937,[26] he was enthusiastic about our unified society-institute. Freud replied with a witty but stern warning against our "medical fixation," offering "a few drops of European spirit" to temper "American self-sufficiency." In 1940, during one of his recurrent depressions, Peck committed suicide.

Among the new leaders themselves, Dr. Kaufman was chairman of the Education Committee from 1934 to 1942, when he joined the military service and later settled in New York. During his years in Boston, he had also held academic positions, teaching analysis at McLean Hospital and establishing a psychiatry service at Beth Israel Hospital, where he collaborated in psychosomatic research with Dr. Felix Deutsch. Dr. John Murray taught a seminar at the institute on adolescence that was open to social workers as well as candidates, recalling Putnam's teaching at the Smith College School of Social Work in 1918 and foreshadowing our later extension course program. Hendrick taught the first seminars in metapsychology, which continued for many years, and he initiated a popular teaching program for Harvard medical students at the Boston Psychopathic Hospital, enhancing its longstanding reputation as the seedbed of analysis in New England. On the committees of the institute, however, Hendrick took a temporarily inactive role, which he called a "seven-year sabbatical," as if the messianic zeal and stubborn determination with which he pursued his reforms had exhausted him and alienated some of his colleagues. In retrospect, Hendrick's letters as a young candidate in Berlin[27] suggest that he exaggerated the procedural rigidities of the Berlin Institute, in accordance with his own exacting standards. He seemed to create a model of efficiency more German than the German analysts themselves, and this personal model, of strict, impersonal regulations and a complex committee structure, was imposed on the Boston analytic community. Hendrick's unswerving pursuit of this ideal may also have influenced the procedural apparatus of the American Psychoanalytic Association, through his indefatigable work on its committees.

Felix and Helene Deutsch were among the first European analysts to arrive as refugees from the Nazi threat, Helene in September 1935. Felix Deutsch followed in January 1936, at the invitation of Dr. Stanley Cobb, to continue his psychosomatic research at the Massachusetts General Hospital. Erik Erikson had already come in 1934, creating a transient problem for the Education Committee, as an analyst, trained by Anna Freud, but lacking any academic degrees. He taught our first seminar on child analysis, before moving on to San Francisco and returning to Harvard many years later as a full professor. In 1935 Mrs. Beata Rank came from Paris, where she had been practicing child analysis since 1926, separated from her husband and remaining loyal to Freud after Otto Rank's break with orthodox analysis. Mrs. Rank became co-director of the Judge Baker Guidance Center, with Dr. Frederick Rosenheim, and she joined Dr. Marian C. Putnam in founding the James Jackson Putnam Children's Center, the first center devoted to preschool age children, normal infant development, and the autistic ("atypical") child.

Jenny and Robert Waelder were the next to arrive, in 1938; she was a child analyst who later moved to Washington, D.C. and he was a non-physician and a brilliant theoretician who settled in Philadelphia. Dr. Lucie Jessner and Dr. Eleanor Pavenstedt came shortly afterward, both child analysts who established child psychiatry units at the Massachusetts General Hospital and Boston City Hospital, respectively. Edouard Hitschmann and his wife Hedwig arrived in 1940; he was the oldest survivor of Freud's early Vienna circle and she was a gifted speech therapist. In the same year, after a sojourn in England, Edward and Grete Bibring arrived. He became our foremost teacher of metapsychology and analytic technique and the author of many important theoretical papers. Dr. Grete Bibring reestablished a psychiatric service at the Beth Israel Hospital, and later became the first woman professor of psychiatry at Harvard. Erich Lindemann had already come to Boston in 1937, having originally emigrated from Germany in 1929.

Although the number of European analysts who settled in Boston was small and not all remained here, their influence was disproportionately large. Most of the émigrés arrived with established reputations, at the height of their creative powers, and many had been the analysts and teachers of our younger members, during their training in Vienna. These reunions in Boston were important on both sides, for the Europeans in creating a hospitable atmosphere during their adjustment to new surroundings, and for the Americans in recalling their best years abroad. In the eyes of early American analysts, the Europeans brought a richer, more elegant cultural patina to the professional life of Boston and Cambridge. Many of us were internal refugees ourselves, from the small towns of rural New England, the Midwest, and the South, part of the reverse migration to the big cities and universities of the East. The European analysts also belonged to a much larger intellectual *Diaspora* from the Nazi occupation, of whom analysts, nuclear physicists, and architects from the *Bauhaus* seemed the most prominent locally. As the American country-mouse became accustomed to *Vanillakipferln*, multiple handshaking, and Austrian ski technique, he was also assimilating other, deeper cultural values, in an intellectual atmosphere where analysis occupied an increasingly respected position.

The Europeans' most important influence, of course, was on analytic theory and technique, creating, by the early 1940s, an astounding renaissance in ego psychology, child analysis, and developmental research on early infancy. Although these new developments in analytic thought were already under way in Europe, evolving from Freud's late papers and the work of Anna Freud, the new wine found old bottles ready to receive it, in American institutions like the Senn Child-Study Group at Yale, the Institute for Juvenile Research in Chicago, the Menninger Foundation in Topeka, and the Judge Baker Guidance Center in Boston. Just as the Europeans stimulated American analysis, the Europeans were influenced in turn by their American milieu. Many seemed to flourish, expanding in new directions and adopting American patterns of analytic practice, as if they had found a wider scope for abilities that had been restrained in their native countries. Notable examples include Franz Alexander, whose meteoric career in Chicago and Los Angeles merely touched Boston in passing, René Spitz and Margaret Mahler, and the metapsychological "school" of Hartmann, Kris, and Loewenstein that found such favorable conditions and enthusiastic acceptance in New York.

New England nourished its share, many of them child analysts like Mrs. Rank, Dr. Jenny Waelder, Dr. Jessner, and Dr. Pavenstedt. The early work of Dr. Felix Deutsch in psychosomatic medicine had never found the wide audience in Vienna that he obtained here, first with Dr. Cobb at the Massachusetts General Hospital and Dr. Kaufman at the Beth Israel Hospital, and finally in the distinctive teaching rounds he developed at the Veterans Administration Hospital, in collaboration with Dr. William Murphy. In 1946 Dr. Grete Bibring was invited by Dr. Herrman Blumgart to reestablish a psychiatric service at the Beth Israel Hospital, left vacant by Dr. Kaufman's departure. Although she accepted with some hesitation, lacking previous administrative experience, she soon developed her own methods of applying psychoanalytic understanding to medical and surgical problems. Over many years she taught applied analysis to medical students and house officers, maintaining such good relations with medical and surgical colleagues that her service was much envied among other psychiatric units in general hospitals.

Dr. Erich Lindemann joined Dr. Cobb's flourishing department at the Massachusetts General Hospital, and continued as director after Dr. Cobb's retirement. But Lindemann also expanded in new directions, from his early psychosomatic research to the study of normal grief in survivors of the Coconut Grove fire and the applied psychoanalysis of family interactions. Always interested in collaboration with sociologists and anthropologists, Lindemann established the first community mental health center in Wellesley, which studied and treated the normal problems of everyday family life, as well as the more severe mental illnesses. We have already heard about another example, in which two traditional American institutions were transformed by European analysts into a unique hybrid: the Austen Riggs Foundation, which evolved from the oldest traditions of New England medical psychotherapy and later acquired a new analytic staff from the Menninger Foundation. This created an unusual treatment center where David Rapaport, Erik Erikson, and other European analysts found the auspicious conditions that shaped their very best work.

While the mutual influences of European and American traditions seemed to encourage some European analysts to new and different achievement modalities, two other features of the New England analytic scene were also emerging in the early 1940s. One was the tendency for European analysts to adopt American patterns of part-time analytic practice, as they accepted academic and administrative responsibilities and became the chiefs of psychiatric departments in medical schools, hospitals, and schools of social work. Of course a substantial number of both Europeans and Americans continued to practice analysis full time, and to limit their teaching and administrative activities to the faculty of the Boston Psychoanalytic Society and Institute. But the tendency toward applied analysis in psychiatry and general medicine was a strong one, going back to Peck's Harvard Medical School teaching in the early 1920s. The pattern was more widespread in Boston than in New York, perhaps encouraged by our high per capita proportion of academic institutions and teaching hospitals. By 1949, Levin and Michaels[28] reported that ninety percent of Boston analysts held academic or institutional posts of some kind. Hendrick, who had expressed his surprise at this figure,[3] in fact, had been an example of this pattern since 1930, when he returned from Europe to teach at the Boston Psychopathic Hospital, succeeding to the position of Martin Peck, his former teacher.

Another feature of the Boston analytic scene was the development of certain regional specialties, which had their origins in past traditions, but were greatly enhanced by the European migration. Principal areas of specialization in analytic psychiatry in Boston have already been indicated: child analysis, psychosomatic research, general hospital psychiatry, and the analytic teaching of psychiatric social work. The practice of child psychiatry dates from the founding of the Judge Baker Guidance Center in 1917; social work teaching began with the collaboration of Richard C. Cabot, Ida Cannon, and Putnam at the Massachusetts General Hospital from 1906 to 1918. The first psychiatric teaching in a general hospital took place in 1920, when Dr. Donald MacPherson, a medical psychotherapist, conducted weekly rounds on the medical wards of the Peter Bent

Brigham Hospital.[29] Interestingly enough, the pioneer department of Dr. Cobb at the Massachusetts General Hospital, and the general hospital psychiatry units of Dr. John Romano in 1940, and of Dr. Henry M. Fox in 1946 at the Peter Bent Brigham Hospital, and of Dr. William Malamud and Dr. Bernard Bandler at Boston University, seem to have evolved independently of each other, as if the impetus were generally in the air.

Postscript: The Years that Were Fat, 1946–1968

The year 1944 was chosen as the end of our symposium, a convenient date to round off the first five decades. Some later events have already been touched on, and we hope that our discussants will not be limited by this arbitrary end point. The year 1946 might have been more suitable, to mark the end of the war years, the return of our members from military service, and the beginning of a new postwar period of rapid expansion. Nevertheless the year 1944 makes a significant point about the early history of psychoanalysis: the essential ingredients for later growth were already present before the postwar influx of new members. The local traditions, institutions, and patterns of practice, and the particular selection of European analysts, predominantly from Vienna, had already given the New England analytic scene its special character, compared to other training institutes that were proliferating throughout the country. Some of these local characteristics have been discussed—our special prominence in child analysis, psychosomatic research, and the development of general hospital psychiatry, and our propensity for academic involvement, and the part-time practice of analysis. But a few closing remarks are in order about our present character, and a brief look ahead at the effects of our expansion.

A comparison of membership lists for 1933 and 1943 illustrates our transition to a mature, unified society-institute, training candidates according to the highest accepted standards. It also illustrates the Europeanization of our society, from ten founding members in 1933, all of whom were American and seven of whom had some or all of their training abroad, to twenty-seven members in 1943, of whom thirteen were American and fourteen European. The handful of native American analysts in the 1920s were an unusual, heterogeneous group of men and women, drawn to analysis as a new radical system of thought, as a potential answer to their dissatisfaction with conventional methods of psychiatric treatment. The next two decades seemed to represent a progressive Americanization, or homogenization, of analysis, including the phenomenally increased acceptance of both psychiatry and psychoanalysis.

After the war, in 1953, we had sixty-six members and one affiliate member; in 1963, 133 active and eleven affiliate members; and in 1973, 227 active and twenty-three affiliate members. Although our criteria for the selection of candidates were presumably as uniform as possible, there was a gradual change in the kind of young psychiatrists who were attracted to analysis, and in what psychoanalytic training represented to them. Many later applicants still resembled their forebears, seeking a radical solution in analytic theory. But, for increasing numbers of young psychiatric residents, psychoanalytic training became simply the next step in their professional education, an ultimate credential in a psychiatric career. The novelty of analysis had also diminished, as its concepts were assimilated into the prevailing *Zeitgeist* and permeated the conventional dynamic psychotherapy that was practiced by many psychiatrists.

For both psychiatry and analysis, the fat years increasingly relied on government grants and private research foundations. This development began with veterans' stipends for analytic training (the G.I. Bill), and continued with grants for research projects and psychiatric residencies, ultimately supporting whole departments largely staffed by psychoanalysts. The modest beginnings of this trend had already been noticeable in Boston before, during the 1920s, when MacFie Campbell distributed Commonwealth Fund stipends for analytic training abroad, and in 1934, with the creation of Dr. Cobb's department at the Massachusetts General Hospital by Alan Gregg of the Rockefeller Foundation. Since, for better or worse, analysis in Boston had entered into a close union with psychiatry and general medicine, the end of an era in government support, toward the end of the 1960s, was probably felt more keenly here than in other analytic communities. At the same time, for other, complex reasons, analysis was passing its period of maximum expansion. We seemed to be entering a silver age of theoretical revision and refinement, or, according to Kuhn's paradigm of scientific revolutions,[30] a phase of "normal scientific activity," after the great wave of creative innovation in analysis during the 1940s and 1950s.

Among the effects of these changes on the Boston Psychoanalytic Society and Institute was a yearning to bring the clinical and research activities of our members back within its sheltering walls, from the hospitals and laboratories where we had worked in collaboration with nonanalysts. There was also a more liberal attitude toward nonmedical affiliate members and candidates, whose numbers had increased over the years, as the early, drastic restrictions on their acceptance for training gradually softened. At our twenty-fifth anniversary in 1958, at the peak of our growth spurt, Freud might have deplored our medical fixation, as he did to Peck in 1937, concluding that analysis in Boston had indeed become "a mere housemaid of psychiatry." But by our fortieth anniversary, in December 1973, Freud might have welcomed these changes, as foreshadowing our return to a smaller, more select minority—to his earliest ideal of an independent discipline, open to all interested persons, physicians and nonphysicians alike.

References

1 Ernest Jones, *The Life and Work of Sigmund Freud, Volumes I–III* (New York: Basic Books, 1953–1957).

2 C.P. Oberndorf, *A History of Psychoanalysis in America* (New York: Grune and Stratton, 1953).

3 Ives Hendrick, *The Birth of an Institute: 25th Anniversary of the Boston Psychoanalytic Institute, November 30, 1958* (Freeport, Me.: Bond Wheelwright, 1961).

4 B.D. Lewin and H. Ross, *Psychoanalytic Education in the United States* (New York: Norton, 1960).

5 Sigmund Freud, Preface in *Addresses in Psycho-Analysis* by J.J. Putnam (London: Hogarth Press, 1921).

6 John C. Burnham, *Psychoanalysis and American Medicine: 1894–1918:* Medicine, Science, and Culture, Psychological Issues, Monograph 20 (New York: International Universities Press, 1967).

7 Henri F. Ellenberger, *The Discovery of the Unconscious* (New York: Basic Books, 1970).

8 Nathan G. Hale, Jr., ed., *James Jackson Putnam and Psychoanalysis. Letters between Putnam and Sigmund Freud, Ernest Jones* (Cambridge, Mass.: Harvard University Press, 1971).

9 ———, *Freud and the Americans. The Beginnings of Psychoanalysis in the United States, 1876–1917* (New York: Oxford University Press, 1971).

10 William James, *The Varieties of Religious Experience* (1902) (New York: Modern Library, 1929).

11 ———, "Review of Breuer and Freud, Über den Psychischen Mechanismus Hysterischer Phänomene," *Psychological Review, 1* (1894), 199.

12 Robert T. Edes, "The New England Invalid," *Boston Medical and Surgical Journal, 133* (1895), 53–57, 77–81, 101–107.

13 James J. Putnam, "Recent Experiences in the Treatment and Study of Hysteria at the Massachusetts General Hospital; with remarks on Freud's method of treatment by 'Psycho-Analysis,'" *Journal of Abnormal Psychology, 1* (1906), 26–41.

14 Jones, "Dr. James Jackson Putnam," *International Journal of Psychoanalysis, 1* (1920), 6–16.

15 Frederick H. Gerrish, ed., *Psychotherapeutics* (Boston: Badger, 1909).

16 Jones, *Free Associations. Memories of a Psycho-analyst* (New York: Basic Books, 1959).

17 Lawrence S. Kubie, *The Riggs Story: The development of the Austen Riggs Center for the study and treatment of the neuroses* (New York: Hoeber, 1960).

18 John Abbott, personal communications, 1971–1973.

19 Hale, personal communication, 1973.

20 George B. Wilbur, personal communications, 1969–1973.

21 James S. Van Teslaar, *An Outline of Psychoanalysis* (New York: Modern Library Books, 1924).

22 E.B. Holt, *The Freudian Wish and Its Place in Ethics* (New York: Holt, 1915).

23 Franz Alexander, *The Medical Value of Psychoanalysis*, revised ed. (New York: Norton, 1936).

24 John Taylor, letter to J.J. Michaels, February 8, 1949, Boston Psychoanalytic Society and Institute Archives.

25 Henry A. Murray, letter to Sanford Gifford, September 14, 1971, Boston Psychoanalytic Society and Institute Archives.

26 Martin W. Peck, "A Brief Visit with Freud," *Psychoanalytic Quarterly, 9* (1940), 205–206.

27 Hendrick, Ives Hendrick Archives, 1918–1971, Boston Psychoanalytic Society and Institute Archives.

28 S. Levin and J.J. Michaels, "The participation of psychoanalysis in the medical institutions of Boston," *International Journal of Psychoanalysis, 42* (1961), 271–283.

29 Donald MacPherson, interview with Sanford Gifford, February 28, 1973.

30 T.S. Kuhn, *The Structure of Scientific Revolutions* (Chicago: University of Chicago Press, 1962).

APPENDIX A

Meetings at the house of Dr. Morton Prince, 1906–1908

Morton Prince
James Jackson Putnam
Ernest Jones
Hugo Münsterberg
Boris Sidis
G. Stanley Hall
William James
E.B. Holt
George Waterman
E.W. Taylor
Elmer Southard

APPENDIX B

The Boston Psychoanalytic Society, 1928–1930

Isador H. Coriat
Martin W. Peck
George Wilbur
John Taylor
Leolia Dalrymple
Henry A. Murray
William Herman
Irmarita Putnam
S. Spafford Ackerly
David Rothschild
William Malamud
Jacob Kasanin
Julia Deming
G. Colket Caner
Stanley Cobb

APPENDIX C

The Boston Psychoanalytic Society, 1930–1932

Isador H. Coriat, *president*
Martin W. Peck, *secretary-treasurer*
S. Spafford Ackerly
George E. Clark
Stanley Cobb
Leolia Dalrymple
Julia Deming
William Healy
Ives Hendrick
William Herman
Jacob Kasanin
M. Ralph Kaufman
Henry A. Murray
John Murray
Irmarita Putnam
Margaret A. Ribble
David Rothschild
Harvey Sanborn
John Taylor
George Wilbur

APPENDIX D

Charter Members of the Boston Psychoanalytic Society

Isador H. Coriat
Leolia A. Dalrymple
William Healy
Ives Hendrick
William Herman
M. Ralph Kaufman
Henry A. Murray
John M. Murray
Martin W. Peck
Irmarita Putnam

Panel Discussion:
Psychoanalysis in Boston, 1918–1944

GEORGE E. GARDNER

CHAIRMAN

DR. GARDNER: Although we are about to discuss early psychoanalysis in Boston, I want to emphasize the fact that our symposium is not confined to the years before 1944, and we hope, throughout the session, for all historical material that anyone can bring forward. I suppose we should begin with a classical allusion, with Virgil's "Forsan et haec olim meminisse iuvabit"—"Perhaps it will be pleasurable to remember these things." To help us start remembering, we have called upon Dr. M. Ralph Kaufman to open our discussion.

Dr. Kaufman's accomplishments, in an organizational, professional, and research sense, are well known to most of you. However, for the record, he served for ten years on the American Medical Association Mental Health Council and was a member of the Joint Commission on Mental Health. He was a colonel in the army, from 1942 to 1946, and it is true that Colonel Kaufman, in landing from a personnel landing craft in the Pacific, had his cartridge belt stuffed with cigars rather than bullets. It is also true that he was decorated for his service under enemy fire. Dr. Kaufman's first love, his first professional love, has always been medicine, medicine's integrity in its proper and most effective practice. His second love has been the practice, and particularly the teaching, of psychoanalysis, psychoanalytic concepts as well as organizational and professional affairs. No man has been a better companion on the barricades than Dr. Kaufman.

DR. KAUFMAN: This symposium has presented me with a tremendous number of problems. It's essentially a historical review of what has gone on in relation to psychotherapy and psychoanalysis in Boston and the New England area, so for analysts, candidates, and so on, I want to remind you of one thing. As you listen to us, go back to Freud and remember, it took him some time to discover that fantasy was perhaps a little bit more important than reality.

Some time ago, when Dr. Gifford first began to talk with me and others at this meeting, I was under the illusion that a couple of us old-timers would get together, sit around, and reminisce. When I finally got the program, I realized that he had intended all along to do more than that. Actually what you have participated in is a tremendously important symposium of psychoanalysis, psychotherapy and the medical scene in Boston and New England. As I look around this group it strikes me that we are like the remnants of a battalion, getting together ten years later to discuss how we survived. I've been puzzled as to how I was going to handle my part of this. Should I just reminisce? Two individuals upset me within the last forty-eight hours, because they both said one and the same thing: shall we gloss it over or shall we tell it as it was? This is the problem, not so much for the older analysts, because they're fixed in their ways and nothing can change them, but for some of you who are candidates. So I think we'll do this, at least I will, in a combination of ways; all contacts particularly of analysts and other people should be psychotherapeutic. I decided several weeks ago, actually, to approach the problem from this point of view. Very few of us on this panel have any documents or notes that would lead to formal presentations, which is an old analytic tradition. I would like to recreate the climate relating to psychoanalysis in Boston and the New England area. What I will have to say will be through a haze of a narcissistically tinged neuralgia. I think that slip both indicates Freud was right and you know where the pain is.

So let me say it again, as if I hadn't made the slip. What I have to say will be through the haze of a narcissistically tinged nostalgia, as I now remember it. Unfortunately, with one or two exceptions, I am not in a position to document most of what I am going to discuss. We've heard a good deal about when and where analysis really came into being. What I'm going to tell you now is through my own experiences, and as I saw things at the time.

I entered McGill Medical School in 1919, and at that time the medical school curriculum, which led to a degree of M.D.C.M., was six years. The first two years were devoted to what we now call basic sciences, in addition to which there were several courses in the "humanities and social sciences." One such area was called psychology, and this was the first time that I had been exposed to a systematic discussion of the subject. As it happened, I was probably one of three members of my class who, at the time of entry into medical school, had already made a decision as to what kind of specialty we wished to practice. Fortunately, among my classmates were two individuals who played a key role in furthering my interest in psychiatry. One was Otto Klineberg, who already had graduated from McGill with a major in anthropology and considered himself an anthropologist. Actually he went into medicine to forward his own career as an anthropologist and ended up, as some of you may know, as a psychologist. The other was John Levy, who was interested in becoming a psychiatrist, particularly a child psychiatrist. This led to the organization of a small group, which continued throughout the six years of medical school, as a kind of seminar in psychiatry and particularly psychoanalysis.

The course in psychiatry at McGill Medical School was not what we'd consider—even then—a very dynamic one. There were about six formal lectures, with a clinic in Verdun, which was the local hospital, and demonstrations of various kinds of patients. I do remember that the lectures consisted essentially of the professor, who wore his hat throughout, reading from parts of Bleuler. The small study circle led by Klineberg and Levy served the function of introducing me to Freud's writings. At McGill, in Montreal in 1919, this was an isolated phenomenon that did not appear to have any effect whatsoever on the rest of the medical students. There were no real facilities for education and training in psychiatry in Canada at that time. There were no residencies, as such, although there was some sort of quasi-tradition in Montreal that if you wanted to become a psychiatrist, you went to a hospital like the Manhattan State for about a year. Small groups of McGill graduates, among them Dr. William Malamud, Senior, David Rothschild, and Baruch Silverman took this route. Fortunately, upon graduation, I became an intern at Manhattan State on Ward's Island. At that time the psychiatric institute was housed on the island. In the institute were George Kirby, Dunlop, and a number of others. It was there that I first met A.A. Brill and Phil Lehrman, both practicing psychoanalysts who were consultants at Manhattan State and who participated, to some extent, in the functioning of the hospital. Since there was no systematic educational program for the house staff, a small group of us took advantage of the presence of the psychoanalysts and the psychiatric institute in organizing our own training and education program. Because Brill and Lehrman were definite Freudian psychoanalysts, our education, therefore, had a Freudian psychoanalytic aura.

After some fourteen months at Manhattan State, I became a member of the residency staff in neurology at Montefiore, which had a distinguished group of neuropsychiatrists on its staff. Dr. Israel Wechsler was one of them. And, when I made plans for the continuation of my education as a psychiatrist interested in psychoanalysis, it was in part through his good offices that I obtained an appointment at the Boston Psychopathic Hospital in 1927. At that time, the Boston Psychopathic was one of the few major psychiatric educational institutions in the country. C. MacFie Campbell, the chief, had been Adolf Meyer's assistant before he was appointed professor of psychiatry at Harvard. He was one of the individual psychiatrists who became interested in analysis early in his career, and had published several papers in the field. Therefore he was, and here the word I use is equivocal, *rather* sympathetic with those of the house officers who were interested in analysis and psychoanalytic psychiatry.

Within the Boston community there were already a number of private practitioners of psychiatry who were either known as psychoanalysts or practiced what was later known as psychoanalytically oriented psychotherapy. In relation to various aspects of the psychoanalytic scene in Boston which eventually led to the formation of the Boston Psychoanalytic Institute and Society, Hendrick's "The Birth of an Institute" is probably the best source of data, and it would serve no really useful purpose, particularly after the last two days, to go into any greater detail. I should like only to reemphasize the fact that the atmosphere in Boston, by and large, was somewhat favorable to psychoanalysis, as Freudians understood it. This perhaps is the key to what happened in the Boston area, for they had the tolerance for various deviations, which permitted all those interested to work together. A number of events in the late twenties were particularly significant for the development of psychoanalysis. Professor Campbell received a grant from the Commonwealth Fund of fifteen three-year Harvard Fellowships, with fairly generous stipends for those times. These fellowships were primarily for the purpose of rounding out the education and training of the recipients and to enable them to make final career choices.

I was fortunate enough to be one of the first recipients, and it is of interest, historically, that one of the conditions that Dr. Campbell agreed to was that I could use the fellowship for psychoanalytic training in Europe. I think there were nine or ten of us, out of the fifteen, who eventually ended up with psychoanalytic training. Most of them actually form the—I was going to say hard core—at least the core of the Boston Psychoanalytic Society and Institute.

By way of digression, another matter of interest in regard to the status of psychoanalysis in the 1920s was the fact that I was also a recipient of an Emmanuel Libman Fellowship, which was a thousand dollars, for the specific purpose of psychoanalytic training. Dr. Libman was one of the outstanding internists connected with Mt. Sinai Hospital in New York. I believe that Dr. William Malamud and David Rothschild were also recipients of Libman Fellowships, which were utilized, in part, for psychoanalytic education in Europe.

I was to leave for Vienna in 1928. Unfortunately, a series of events, precipitated by rather severe medical and physical problems, made it necessary for me to postpone my European study period. When I did go abroad in 1929, I registered with the Vienna Institute, where I first met Helene Deutsch who was very gracious to me. She was either the secretary or, at any rate, the person I had to go to, and I ended up with Wilhelm Reich as my training analyst. I was going to tell you about Schilder and a number of other things I think are relevant. Perhaps I should, because I think it is important. I had made arrangements for my so-called training analysis to go to Paul Schilder in Vienna because I knew that Malamud, and to a certain extent Rothschild, had gone to him. To us in America, Paul Schilder in Vienna was *the* training analyst, but I finally realized that this was so only for Americans and Canadians who didn't have a long time to stay.

Well, when Betty and I got to the Oxford Congress, it turned out that the congress centered around who this fellow Mo Kaufman should go to for his training analysis. Ferenczi offered to take me, and I remember Mrs. Ferenczi talking with my wife Betty, telling her that things weren't too expensive in Budapest. I wrote to Campbell and asked him what I should do. The message I got back was, "So what else are you going to do, learn Hungarian?" Outside of telling you the story, the point I really wanted to make, is a rather simple one, namely, it was the first time we had met the European group. Although they probably didn't even know who I was, I believe they wanted to help me, as an American, to go to a recognized analyst. To me, this is the essential part. I don't know whether they passed an official resolution at the Oxford Congress, but eventually I did end up with Reich, although I had started with Schilder. The important thing is that in 1929 it seemed to be almost the unanimous opinion of the European analysts we talked to that Reich was the man to go to. In the light of what has happened subsequently, I think this is also of some importance.

When I returned to Boston in 1930, I continued my psychoanalytic education and training, which included supervision and attendance at the New York Society on a regular basis. Hendrick and I made regular trips to New York, a good many of them on the Owl. The control analyses were under Bert Lewin, Gregory Zilboorg, and Franz Alexander. The role of these individuals, amongst others in the founding of the Psychoanalytic Institute in Boston, is already well known to you. With the termination of my Commonwealth Fund Fellowship coming up in 1931, I was fortunate enough to be recommended by Dr. Campbell for the new position of clinical director at McLean Hospital. Campbell's recommendation of one of his own fellows to a senior position was an event in itself. Usually he called us in and stated that there was an assistant professorship, let's say, in Colorado, to take the most unlikely place, and asked if we could recommend anybody. Twenty years later I first realized that maybe he was saying, "Would you be interested in going?"

However, its significance was that a relatively young psychoanalyst, about to begin his academic career, was recommended for a major post in a rather conservative institution like McLean. The year before, in 1930, Ives Hendrick had already been appointed to the hospital as consulting psychoanalyst. During my two-year period as clinical director, a number of events of significance to analysis took place. In addition to the responsibility for the clinical professional work of the hospital, I was able to work with psychotics and work as an analyst.

As with me, the experience of the analytic group was that external pressures and situations played a relatively small role in keeping any one of us from being psychoanalysts and using the psychoanalytic point of view. The difficulties that the analytic group in Boston and I had, which I was going to candycoat a little bit, were primarily internal and I hope that during the course of the day we will get to some of those.

When I said "internal," I dropped my voice so you couldn't hear it. There was a definite change in the psychiatric climate at the hospital, for which psychoanalysis had a definite responsibility. John Whitehorn, the biochemist of the hospital, became more interested in psychotherapy and psychoanalysis and, eventually, received some partial analytic training. Since McLean and the Massachusetts General Hospital were intimately related, there was a revival of psychiatry at the Massachusetts General in various ways, again influenced by a psychoanalytic point of view.

Unfortunately, for various personal reasons, I resigned from the position of clinical director at McLean in 1933 but continued as consultant to the hospital for a number of years, almost until the time I left Boston. During this period there was the Marshall Field Grant for the City Study of Suicide, under the direction of Gregory Zilboorg, and I was one of the psychoanalysts who was actually involved. For the most part, this was a psychoanalytic study of various individuals who had attempted unsuccessfully to commit suicide, or were involved with suicidal ideas. Dr. Jessner and I formed a team for patients who were receiving insulin treatment through Dr. Sakel. My role was to study these patients as a psychoanalyst.

In 1933, after my resignation from McLean, I was asked by Dr. Harry Solomon to take over the department of psychiatry at Beth Israel which was headed by Solomon and Abe Myerson. I was given a free hand in this organization, and when I finally left, the staff included twenty-eight members, most of whom were psychoanalysts. An inpatient division and an outpatient division were set up. Since there were no psychiatric beds as such, the department functioned within the departments of medicine and surgery, particularly in relation to Dr. Herman Blumgart's department of medicine. It was during the early 1930s that Dr. Felix Deutsch became a member of the department of psychiatry, and a teaching program for medical students, house officers, and attending staff was set up. This program was unique at the time, and a source of many subsequent liaison programs set up throughout the country.

As already indicated, most of the attending staff in this department of psychiatry were psychiatrists who were psychoanalysts at some level of training. Both Solomon and Myerson deserve a tremendous amount of credit in developing psychoanalysis in Boston.

We heard the magnificent talk by Paul Myerson about his father. To most of us who were so bound up in analysis at that time, he seemed to be essentially a man who gained his reputation because he was anti-Freud. I reread his book *Psychology of Mental Illness*, which was sort of a copy of Hart's book. In it, he discusses analysis, and does it very well. No matter whether you believe in what he said or not, it's incontrovertible that he made a major contribution to the field. I think that behind his own, what we might call, ambivalence, he was interested. The reason I'm presenting his name and Harry Solomon's was simply that they turned over the department to a group of psychoanalysts. At no time, during the whole period that I was there, was there any question as to why we were analysts, why were we talking this, that, and the other thing. They gave us complete freedom. And here again, as I look back with hindsight, this is one aspect of Boston that perhaps was most significant. Because earlier the decision to become a psychoanalyst, whether in Boston or elsewhere, particularly if you were interested in an academic career, was laying your career on the line. With very few exceptions, this never happened in Boston. During the thirties, as you know, Massachusetts General developed an inpatient department of psychiatry under Dr. Stanley Cobb, and there, too, members of the psychoanalytic group were on its attending staff.

I will leave to other members of the panel the detailed discussion of our colleagues who came to Boston from Europe. They were welcomed in Boston with a minimal amount of ambivalence and early became a valuable part of the psychiatric and psychoanalytic scene. Thus they continued to contribute greatly to American medicine, particularly in psychosomatic medicine. The very style of American psychiatry was enriched by their presence. The role of Franz Alexander specifically, who came to Boston in 1931, has already been indicated in previous discussions. In addition, he became the training analyst of a number of individuals who were already in private practice as psychoanalysts in Boston and perhaps this, too, is significant.

I had a rather curious reaction that, when the time came for Alexander to go back to Europe for his vacation, there were three categories of candidates: those who couldn't go over with him were declared finished; those that could go went on with their analytic training; and there was one rather vague category in between. This is not pertinent only to Alexander; at that time, the standards for what constituted psychoanalytic training were rather diffuse. Hanns Sachs, in a sense, was Alexander's replacement, when Alexander became the first professor of psychoanalysis in Chicago, actually in the world. Sachs functioned originally as a sort of director of psychoanalysis. Essentially he was a training analyst, control analyst, and a teacher, and he had a limited number of private patients. Some problems arose which led to difficulties and differences of opinion about the operational extent of his function within the program formulated by the society. That's as euphemistically as I can put it.

The thirties were busy years for psychoanalysis in Boston. Formal organization of the society and institute involved internal and external problems: curriculum, choice of candidates, setting of standards, criteria for the selection of candidates and teachers, both as training and control analysts. In addition were the problems of accreditation, relation to the American and the International Psychoanalytic societies, and the education and training of individuals from related professional groups. Take each one of these problems, raise them to the nth degree, and you can understand the kind of battles that went on. Everything became highly personalized, and there wasn't a single item that was not subject to conflict and controversy. Essentially, however, the principles of psychoanalysis in Boston have always been of an extremely high standard. The path to that attainment was something else again.

The Boston psychoanalytic group, as already indicated by other speakers, participated actively in the education of related professions. Individual members were on the faculties of Smith, Simmons, the medical schools, hospitals, and so on—this has always been a characteristic of Boston psychoanalysis. As some of you remember, the study of Michaels and Levin indicated that some ninety percent of the members of the society and institute were active participants in such programs. The thirties were perhaps a little evangelical, but certainly exciting. Psychoanalysis in Boston, and to a greater or lesser extent in the United States, made its impact on psychiatry and demonstrated its essential validity and its importance in many ways, as analysts began to use the description "dynamic psychiatry" and "psychoanalytically-oriented psychiatry." I want to mention, with a certain amount of immodesty, that there were three people at least, Ives Hendrick, John Murray, and Mo Kaufman, who were young enough, committed enough, converted enough, and had the necessary *chutzpah*, to say what we thought needed to be said. We were responsible for a great deal of what happened, both positive and negative, and it wasn't all transference. So the rest of the panel will now go on and discuss some other details.

DR. GARDNER: Thank you very much for the important background that you've outlined for us, Mo. At this time I would like to call upon one person on this panel who needs no introduction at all to any group of psychoanalysts anywhere in the world, and that's Dr. Helene Deutsch.

DR. DEUTSCH: I was embarrassed how to start. But this is a beginning. Children not only want to be seen, they also want to be heard. I not only want to be heard but also to be seen. I assure you it is not the vanity of a woman. I lost that already twenty years ago. But it is so comfortable when you are old: "You have to excuse me but I am old." When we speak as analysts, we are used to speaking of family members, a son-figure, a father-figure. I am a mother-figure, I am very proud to say.

I am old, and I have many deficiencies, but I am really the oldest pupil of Freud still alive. That makes me very proud. When I left Vienna to go to America—and now comes what you may call my vanity or narcissism—Freud answered my farewell letter, in which I excused myself for leaving Vienna to go to America. He wrote to me, "I hope and trust that you will do for America what you have done here for us in Europe." If there were a life after death, I would ask to be written on my grave that Freud had so much confidence in me that he believed I would conquer America, which, as you know, he never loved.

Since I cannot hide that next year I will be ninety, I am now more interested in old age than before. I have heard that ninety is the maximum in which a person begins to lose hold—comes into the power of regression. I wanted not to be old, but either I am dead or I am old; there is no other choice. I am glad that I have chosen the second alternative, because I would not know all of you and see the success of these meetings.

Perhaps you will be curious how Freud started his analyses. When I came to him, Freud was not taking more pupils; I was really the last. He had great family obligations. Freud was never interested in money for himself, only in the money which he absolutely needed for the education of his six children. I came to Freud in 1918. I dared to come to Freud. At this time, I was working in one of the outpatient clinics, where Grete Bibring also worked. Wagner-Jauregg was the personification of hostility and devaluation of analysis. He was not an aggressive, hostile person, but his aggressiveness against Freud consisted of devaluating jokes. I started at the clinic in 1912, and in 1918 I was still there when I turned to Freud for analysis. Freud warned me: "I think, Dr. Deutsch, you will have to make a choice. Either you have analysis or you stay with Wagner-Jauregg." I did not understand what he meant, but at the beginning of my analysis, I saw it would be impossible to remain at the clinic. When Wagner-Jauregg heard that I was in analysis, all his hostility against Freud came out. Well, you know how I decided. I left the clinic, which was really a sacrifice, because I was interested in psychosis.

Many colleagues who had not elected to go to Freud to be analyzed asked me about the procedure, how he started the analysis, where he gave interpretations. Freud was extremely passive. When something was absolutely right to tell the person, he told it. He left the activity to the patient. I remember that in the second hour of the analysis, after the analytic hour, I went out and started to cry on the street. In one of the streets leading to Freud's office, there was a shop with shirts, men's shirts, and this green shirt has accompanied me throughout my whole life. I started to cry, and the cry was "What will poor Frau-Professor Freud do," because I was so convinced that Freud was falling in love with me. It must have been an agreeable surprise for Frau-Professor that he did not. I wanted to tell you something about my analysis with Freud but it is impossible. If I started, I would never finish. He was passive, that's all, I mean during analysis. I am telling you that because so often these younger analysts ask how Freud was during analysis. I have not yet told you that twice he fell asleep, maybe more often, but twice I knew of it because the cigar fell from his mouth. It's a true story. You see now my old age comes out because I do not know what else I wanted to say. Perhaps I might finish here. I will finish with something I wanted to say at the beginning, which is my great thankfulness to Dr. Sanford Gifford because of what he has done for us. I am astonished that we are such intimate friends because, although I am an excellent clinician and I understood Freud and his teachings very well, I am not historically minded as he is. One of the bridges between us was the great devotion that he had for my husband. Now, since old people like to complain, I will complain. Not once in this meeting was the name of my husband mentioned. My husband really sacrificed a great career to become an analyst and I think that probably some of you know that the whole conception of psychosomatic medicine (including the name) came from Felix Deutsch. I feel a little bit hurt that his name, as an important figure in the history of analysis, was not mentioned. So I mention it. And I finish my speech.

DR. JOHN MURRAY: To stick to the facts of what was really involved is a tough assignment. I think all I can do is to fit in some of the *lacunae*, gaps, that Mo, of necessity, left out concerning the early developmental years in Boston, and some important little vignettes of what went on.

The troika, as Dr. Gardner said, had one essential thesis and that was, we will develop psychoanalysis here in Boston along the lines of the finest of the European tradition. We will set our standards so that when our society and institute becomes viable, it will be a well-oriented and properly established educational institution. Of course, it was quite an undertaking at this time, as Mo has indicated. In the early 1930s psychoanalytic education was still uncertain, still unformulated, still unformed. It was a dream, and I think that the dream worked out pretty well for us. I think Mo is pretty happy about what happened. I know I am. As I look back on my life and my career, I am very happy with what happened and I am quite certain that Dr. Hendrick was fulfilled by his role in what happened in Boston. I'll come back to that later.

When we began our small group, as Mo indicated, Bert Lewin and Gregory Zilboorg came over from New York on alternate evenings to give us seminars. This went on for several years in our developmental phase, until the people from Europe began to come to Boston. The first was Dr. Hanns Sachs who, as Mo said, was not an unalloyed blessing to us. Then came the Deutsches, the Bibrings, the Waelders, and others who played an important role in the progressive development of psychoanalysis in Boston. In those early years, when Drs. Lewin and Zilboorg were coming from New York, we were a devoted, closely knit, very happy little band. It was Dr. Sachs who introduced a note of discontent at that time, because he was a unique individual. He was anti-administrative from every angle. The troika felt it most important that standards be formulated and adhered to, that candidates be scrupulously examined and, when accepted, that their course of training should follow the style the institute had established. But Dr. Sachs felt that he was above these things, and that if he wanted to take a candidate, that made the candidate perfectly acceptable. This was something we had to thrash out, and this we finally did, and after a bit everything went merrily along.

I want to pay particular attention to one other aspect of the early years, that is the contributions made in those years by Ives Hendrick. Ives was, shall we say, a unique individual. He was talented, he was gifted, he was devoted, but he was a bit unsteady and sometimes unpredictable. But those are the things that happen to all of God's children. We all have our uniqueness, our peculiarities, so, as we look back on them, we forget those things and we look at the blessedness that we're endowed with. This Ives Hendrick was truly endowed. The utter devotion he had toward what psychoanalysis was, and what it stood for, and what he wanted it to be in the psychiatric and in the medical community, was expressed almost as Freud himself expressed it. I know of no other person whose life reflected the intensity of this devotion as Ives's did. This was particularly so in his early activities as a training analyst, and also in his work at the Psychopathic Hospital, in his undergraduate teaching, in the residency training program and in the introduction of psychoanalytic principles into their training. Boston psychiatry and psychoanalysis owe a tremendous debt to Dr. Hendrick that we must recognize.

Upon the advent of our colleagues from Europe, the movement took a new impetus. Its foundation and cornerstone were a devotion to emulating the European training centers. Despite some battling here and there between the various groups in those early years, the principles which the troika originally formulated were carried out beautifully with the help of our European colleagues. The institute really attained a maturity and a sense of fulfillment in those years.

Mo spoke of the ambivalence that psychoanalysis encountered. This was true, but, by and large it was all surmounted. This brings me back to an experience I had as a consultant to the United States Public Health Service. Marion Kenworthy and I were the members from the American Psychoanalytic Association, and we made proposals that the psychoanalytic institute should get grants from the government for the excellent work it was carrying on in its training. I can remember very definitely the meeting we had in Washington at which it was turned down, on the grounds that psychoanalysis was not related to the general body of psychiatry, but was an isolated phenomenon. There was controversy about Jung and Adler and Freud, and who was to be the recipient, and we were turned down.

I can also remember a memorable dinner that I had in Dr. Kenworthy's apartment with Allan Gregg. Marion and I were convinced that there was a great misrepresentation of the role of psychoanalysis in the community. We had brought along a copy of what Mo referred to, the paper by Joe Michaels describing the ninety-odd percent of analysts who were engaged in activities in the community. The dinner went on for four or five hours, and that night Allan Gregg became a convert. Marion and I had completely sold him. The next year when he went back to the meeting at the Public Health Committee, he said, "It isn't very often I have to do this, but we came to a decision a year ago that I want to reverse one hundred percent." He gave a very fine positive description of what he thought was the role in psychiatry of psychoanalytic institutes and stated that they were deserving of the support of the government. His evaluation was accepted, and from then on the institutes were given grants from Public Health funds.

So as I say, we went through our childhood and our adolescence and we grew to maturity. As we look back on it, it has been a very pleasant and pleasing journey.

DR. GARDNER: Thank you very much, Dr. Murray. Among the joys of being a chairman at this particular symposium is that one does not have to go into extended introductions of the participants. So the next speaker I'll merely introduce as one of our greatest teachers, Dr. Grete Bibring.

DR. BIBRING: You know I cannot go into what I wanted to say without mentioning what this meeting did for me and to me. It stirred up innumerable things and was a delightful experience first of all, because I really learned to know these pioneering figures so much better than from any books. Second, I learned something which really gave me thought, namely, how admirable these people were. You know, as psychoanalysts, we usually only accept full-fledged classical psychoanalysts, but I was really deeply impressed by these men who struggled, tried to find their way, found it to a large extent, and were so important for analysis. My respect grew immensely. The third thing that happened—you wouldn't believe it—is that I could look at ourselves through the eyes of the historians and I found that we are very important, we psychoanalysts. It was a delicious feeling. You know you don't usually think about yourself like that.

I didn't have the privilege of an early professional development in Boston, though Vienna wasn't bad either. I was a late-comer; we came only in 1941. But I was involved in the Boston analytic scene a long time before we came here, because Vienna was crowded with people who became the analytic flower of Boston. If you consider the time when I was teaching in Vienna, we had as candidates many people who are here on the panel, starting with the main speakers, Dr. Kaufman, Dr. Murray . . . By the way, Dr. Kaufman was known to us because, I was told, he ruled the group of American postgraduate doctors with an iron hand, from his imperial seat at the Café Alserhof, true? Did you?

DR. KAUFMAN: In the Edison, yes, it's true.

DR. BIBRING: Edison, okay. That's one thing I want Dr. Kaufman to hear. The other thing is that I won a bet on him, and I'll tell you how that was. I worked at the Wagner-Jauregg clinic, and you could see through the window to the street which led up to the clinic, the Spital-Gasse. We were once standing there, the different doctors eating our Gabel-frühstück, and a little figure moved up the street and I said, "This is an American." My colleagues said, "How do you know? You can't judge that." He was two inches high at the time because he was very far away. Now, as usual, I made my diagnosis on little side issues and what I saw was the tilt of the hat. I saw the hands were in his pockets and I saw this odd, ambling gait of the American which was so different from the Austrian walk; the Austrians walked straight and he jumped a little, as if he had springs in his soles. The Americans walked like sailors. I got a bottle of champagne because of this man who we found out later was Mo Kaufman.

There were many more—Helen Tartakoff, Joe Michaels, Gibby and Dan Dawes, Mary O'Neil Hawkins, and Molly Putnam. There were many others. Bill Menninger, I think, was there; I know that Dr. Malamud was. We knew so many—Hy Lippman, Margaret Gerard, and Helen Ross, Edith Jackson, Roy Grinker, and Jake Finesinger, Irmarita Putnam, Ruth Mack Brunswick, and George Mohr. We knew them all somehow, but we didn't get involved with them much, because we didn't want to interfere with their training analyses. However, the American—we called them "Little America"—the American candidates moved in packs, and especially when Grinker was among them, or Finesinger. They had a favorite party game to interfere with each other's analyses. Usually they played on transference-figures, so that when our students came to analysis the next morning, you had to disentangle what they were told, that I had a hole in my stocking yesterday, or that somebody was smooching, probably with my husband, at the Cabaret Simplicissimus. It was a hard time for those of us who had them in analysis and were trying to train them.

However, it was also a very interesting time then. Now when we came here, Edward and I, we had one advantage. It was a kind of a cultural cross-section to compare the three institutes, Vienna, London, and Boston. Boston was very close to Vienna, I would say, and it was an enormous relief after the blitz in London, the blitz with Hitler, the blitz with Melanie Klein. When we came here it was a rather well-established institute of very high standards, which had enormous advantages and disadvantages. The advantages really made Boston, even today, what it still is. Its very high standards, and its exclusiveness, made it one of the institutes that kept out a lot of crackpots and fringe-figures. The negative part of it was the rigidity of the institute rules. This was different from Vienna where we were not rigid. We were what we would call *schlampig*; *schlampig* is sloppy. In contrast to our German friends, we were the sloppy ones, which meant you became a training analyst when somebody wanted to have training with you. You first went to the institute, which we established ourselves, with Dr. Helene Deutsch as chairman, and told her that Dr. So-and-so, from Amsterdam or from London or from wherever, wants to have a training analysis with me. And so you became, officially, a training analyst, if your reputation justified it.

Now I don't know whether Dr. Helene Deutsch still remembers, but I have an enormously important document. In our juvenile enthusiasm, we set up an institute in a week. Helene Deutsch came from Berlin and told us about the institute there. I remember I was in the Ambulatorium listening to her story, and we decided that this was a good thing for us, too, and that Helene Deutsch was naturally the right person to be its first chairman, because she knew all about it. And do you know, Helene, you had some certificates printed, for the Bibrings, the Sterbas, the Waelders, for six people, I believe. We had certificates signed by Freud; I don't know how Helene Deutsch persuaded him into doing that. They were signed by Freud and by Helene Deutsch and stated that we had graduated from the Vienna Institute, which hadn't quite existed yet. Now whether they have destroyed the other certificates, mine is still in my safe-deposit box. So there were six certificates for the first graduates of the Vienna Institute, which we almost wrote ourselves because we thought we couldn't be teachers in an institute if we hadn't graduated from one. That is as far as the fun goes.

However I saw problems here in Boston which I found rather perplexing. What impressed me here was the rigidity, which was, by the way, really responsible for the standards. At the same time it introduced elements which I could never quite agree with. I am still irritated about them in the present institute, by the way. I couldn't make peace with it and I'll tell you what it was. I was always called an orthodox psychoanalyst; so was my husband. I always tried to replace this by calling myself a classic psychoanalyst, but people didn't take to that. Now, I am not orthodox because otherwise I couldn't have done what I did with my analytic background at the Beth Israel Hospital, which wasn't analysis, but rather was applied analysis. But I had, and have still, the absolute conviction that training in an institute should be psychoanalytic. First of all that is only fair, since people come to us to have analytic training and not derivatives of psychoanalytic training. And second, I strongly felt that analytic training is the best foundation for taking off in any other psychological or therapeutic direction whatever. I never had any grievance about people developing in all kinds of different directions. This sometimes led to friction with the American psychoanalyists, as I remember. I was frequently involved with people who branched off quite successfully but—and this was very American and quite in contrast to Vienna—they insisted that their actions were proper analysis. In Vienna, if somebody introduced parameters into his field or into his technique, he made a point of it openly and was usually glad to split off. This was not so in the United States. I wondered whether it was because in the States we had such standing already as psychoanalysts that people didn't want to leave the fold, although they did not practice psychoanalysis, but whatever they thought was good and right for them.

I can remember one intense discussion on a panel with Franz Alexander. Those of you who knew him know that he was an extraordinarily brilliant and very charming person, and he could talk you up and out into whatever he wanted. We had a panel on training techniques at the Chicago institute, because it had become an issue by then in the American Psychoanalytic Association, and I was one of the discussants. At that time the Chicago institute had introduced what Alexander called the "Time Axis." This meant that he avoided making candidates overdependent by interrupting analysis the moment their transference became very intense. I insisted that this was bad analysis, because you use the transference, you resolve it, you do all kinds of things with it, but you don't interrupt until it simmers down and goes underground again. At this point Alexander said to me, "Dr. Bibring, we are not a corner drugstore any longer. We are a streamlined institute." I got angry and said "Dr. Alexander, if you were a candidate today and had the choice of going to the Chicago institute or to the old institute in Vienna, where would you go?" You know what he said? He said "To Boston."

This was one thing I minded here. The other was the rigidity of structure in the institutes, which introduced some quite unwarranted procedures. I felt, and I still feel, that there is a tendency to break the contract with the candidates by expecting them to be in a completely trusting relationship with the analyst, while the analysts get more and more used to institute procedures to hide behind. I personally insist an analyst has the difficult task of returning his candidate's trust by telling him what he thinks of him. Whether the candidate is fit or ready, and should or shouldn't become an analyst. This is painful, but it is part of our daily work with analysands. I think if an analyst can't come to this point, but turns to the Students' Committee, or whichever else committee and says "Write a letter to tell this to the candidate," this is improper, and a breach of mutual trust I fight wherever possible.

Otherwise, I must say, I was really very happy to come here. I have never found difficulties; neither my classic or orthodox background interfered with anything connected with my professional work and I am most grateful. I am most grateful to Boston and most grateful to the United States to have accepted me. And I want you to know that the very same feelings prevailed in my late husband. Thank you.

DR. GARDNER: At this point in our program I wish to change direction somewhat. I want to turn to the field of child analysis in Boston, and to call upon Dr. Eveoleen Rexford.

DR. EVEOLEEN REXFORD: It seems to me fitting that this session began with a talk by Mo Kaufman. I came to Boston in November 1942, and within a few months, since I had come to the Judge Baker and Mrs. Rank, I came to know the analytic group. I heard a great deal about Mo and Jock, who were enlisted men at the time. Now I had my fantasies about those gentlemen. There were certain facts that I was told repeatedly. Mo and Jock owned 82 Marlborough Street, and the analytic meetings were held in the basement there. I heard about what astute businessmen they were, and I heard Ives Hendrick speak in a somewhat envious way of their financial astuteness. I had heard him comment that he had to provide the intellectual standards of that troika.

I've been remembering very well the first time I saw Mo Kaufman. Mo had just come back from the service, and he, his wife, and son came down to Bayview where we were summering at Mrs. Rank's and we had a lobster picnic. I remember him very well; with a great deal of admiration I noticed how he seemed to manage all of those various difficult interpersonal situations. He obviously was very tired, but I thought that it was a kind of homecoming to family and friends that the Mo Kaufman I had visualized would certainly enjoy.

I came to Boston to train at the Judge Baker. When I arrived there, Dr. Gardner and Dr. Rosenheim, the young chiefs, were either senior candidates or already graduates of the institute. The two principal supervisors were Mrs. Rank and Dr. [Lydia] Dawes. Mrs. Rank was a short, slim, red-haired woman who always wore smart black suits and white blouses with a little frill. I always thought she was very much a Frenchwoman in her appearance in those days. She decided very early that I should wear hats, and we went over to the shops across from the Judge Baker at the noon hour, looking for hats. It took four or five years before she gave up on my wearing hats.

There were two very pragmatic issues in those days which we then young people at the Judge Baker will remember. One was the recurrent problem of parking Tola's car. She had a large Buick, and parking on the hill was no simpler in 1943 than it is today. We worked out a schedule so that when Mrs. Rank would drive up, one of us would come out to park the car and she would go in to the conference. The other practical item that I've always remembered about Gibby Dawes was her remarkable cocker spaniel, Patsy. Gibby brought her to the Judge Baker and the dog participated in supervisory sessions, treatment sessions, and so on. There were various times when the dog needed attention. Here again, a group of grateful trainees took care of Gibby's dog.

I'm sure that nostalgia and idealization enter into all of these recollections, but in those days the atmosphere of the Judge Baker was a heady milieu. We learned a great deal about children very rapidly. My introduction to the idea of going into analytic training took place a few months after I had arrived. I had gone off to an Ortho meeting and, since the men were in the service, there were plenty of jobs for women. I was offered half a dozen or so directorships as soon as I finished at the various child guidance clinics. When I went for my first supervisory hour with Mrs. Rank, I arrived on the second floor and there, sitting beside her at a card table, was Dr. Gardner, looking his most official. Even in those days he could look quite stern and official. I wondered, of course, what I had done, what sin I had committed, because the brass was obviously there. Dr. Gardner asked me if I had been offered any positions for next year. When I said yes, he wanted to know where and also what I thought about them. Mrs. Rank said softly, in her inimitable accent, "The question is, when are you going into analytic training?" Dr. Gardner cleared his throat and said, "Yes, when, Dr. Rexford?" So I squirmed and said hastily that of course I was going to go into analytic training. They asked when and, to make a long story short, first one and then the other put me into a corner. I was anxious about going into analytic training, but I wanted to put it off. I wasn't ready, I didn't have the money, and you know all the rationalizations. I realized later that these two people dealt with me very skillfully; they didn't leave me an inch in which to move. At the end of this supervisory hour, I agreed that perhaps, if I could find the money and if I could find an analyst, I might consider it rather than going off.

Mrs. Rank said she thought I might talk with Dr. Deutsch, and Dr. Gardner said he understood Dr. Pavenstedt was leaving Wellesley, where she had been the school psychiatrist. So my future was settled for me within a relatively short time. I've been grateful to both of them, but I must say that was a stress interview if ever I had one.

I talked with Dr. Deutsch, and a few days later with Dr. Pavenstedt who, indeed, was leaving Wellesley. I had two half-time jobs lined up, one at the Putnam Center and one at the Judge Baker, and we felt that a third half-time job at Wellesley would take care of the cost of my analysis.

A few days later Dr. Deutsch called me up with a certain perturbation and said, "Make an appointment to see Ives Hendrick right away. We have to do this right. It's the Admissions Committee." So, a little puzzled, I made my appointment and saw Dr. Hendrick. Apparently, in some mysterious way, it had been decided that I could come into the institute, and so I became a candidate. I have the impression that, in those days, there wasn't quite the formality I became accustomed to in later years, in relation to the Education Committee and the various committees and committees and committees.

There are many amusing and heart-warming recollections that I've had of those early days. Dr. Grete and I were recalling an adventure in a blizzard when the Bibrings, Helen Tartakoff, and I were at the institute, and I drove them home. It took us three or four hours and it left us feeling like pioneers. Another incident was the matter of the analytic eggs. I began to hear comments made among various friends about whether the analytic eggs had arrived. Finally, after getting so curious I couldn't stand it, I sat my friend Harriet Robey down and said, "Now what are the analytic eggs?" I then heard about the farm in New Hampshire which the Deutsches and Molly Putnam owned and farmed. I heard that Molly Putnam and Felix Deutsch pitched hay and carried out all of their farming activities with great aplomb. They had chickens and the chickens laid eggs and, every weekend, the surplus eggs were brought to town and left at the back doors of some highly selected homes in Cambridge.

For a moment now, I'll be a little serious and speak about the seminars at the institute in those days. When I started, the seminars were small. Toward the last year or so as the boys began coming back from the service, the seminars grew somewhat in size. One of the most memorable was one on theory that we had with Ives Hendrick, Greg Rochlin, Bill Murphy, and Jake Finesinger's brother, Abe. They were the liveliest sessions. I didn't have to do anything but be admiring and try to keep up with all the pyrotechnics. Indeed, Dr. Hendrick's style of teaching was remarkably effective. He didn't say much but he had everyone going as if it were a championship tennis game. The other seminar that I remember particularly was the one on child analysis. This seminar continued for some years following my graduation and I still look back with a great deal of nostalgia. Every time the Child Analysis Committee gets together to plan courses for the next year, either Sam Kaplan or I begin to talk about the child analysis seminar that we had in the forties and early fifties. Mrs. Rank chaired a good bit of the time. Lucie Jessner and Gibby Dawes shared in the remainder of the chairing. Molly Putnam, Eleanor Pavenstedt, Greg Rochlin, and I attended regularly; and most of the people in child work, and a number of people from the adult field attended frequently. They were really exciting and marvelous occasions. George Gardner and I were working with a pair of twins at one point and we had to present the vicissitudes of our activities. Greg Rochlin wanted to prove that with the proper technique, one could have a psychotic child in treatment in an office on the second floor of 82 Marlborough Street. That was a lively experiment that didn't last many months.

Into this seminar we brought experiences and ideas from the various clinics, as well as the child analytic work that we were actually carrying on. The close relationship of child analysis to child psychiatry here in Boston has been extremely important in the development of child psychiatry in the hospital clinic. In the early fifties there were seven training clinics in child psychiatry, each one headed by a child analyst. The senior psychiatrists were all either graduates or senior candidates; there were no child facilities in the country that could boast of a comparable group of child analysts.

I think this situation in child psychiatry was part of the general situation of analysis here in Boston. When Dr. Lewin and Miss Ross were doing a survey of psychoanalytic education in 1958, they came to Boston. They were much impressed that so many analysts worked in hospitals and clinics, but I don't think they ever recovered from their ambivalence about this finding. On the one hand, they thought it an admirable investment in the community, in general psychiatry, psychology, social work, and so on. On the other hand, they worried a great deal about the effect on the development of psychoanalysis itself. This is probably a question that we're never going to be able to answer, particularly those who have lived through so much of this particular history. I think some of the papers we have heard about the scene in Boston offer an explanation, for it seemed natural to the founders and first teachers of analysis here, in adult work as well as child work, to develop services in hospitals and medical schools, to set up clinics, and to be interested in staffing these activities. When we think about the development of psychoanalysis in Boston, there have been outstanding characteristics of medicine here over perhaps two hundred years: first, a tolerance for deviant ideas and a willingness to let people work who had some far-out notions. No matter how different it seemed from the traditional activity, people in various medical fields have almost always had the freedom to do their work. As long as they worked hard and were people of integrity, places have always been found in the Boston community. There is a second element that obviously appealed to the analytic community and had something to do with the pattern of our development. That is a tradition of service to the community. There is no medical community in the world with so much highly specialized, expensive service given to clinics and to teaching, for which the financial remuneration is modest indeed. When Dr. Michaels did his study in the mid-fifties of the fifty-odd members of the Boston

Psychoanalytic Society, there were only three who were not giving from a third to half time in hospitals or clinics. One person was quite elderly, and two had recently had coronaries. At the present time, when our membership has grown to such an extent, the proportion of members who are giving that amount of time to community and teaching activities may have declined, but it is still a major feature of the Boston scene.

We've been talking implicitly about American history. I know much more about English and American history than that of other countries. But I have the strong impression that from time to time there are significant social, economic, intellectual changes which affect the way lives are lived in a country. If one follows the history of America, one finds that by the third generation of the Puritan fathers, there were important changes in the pattern of living. The little New England town wasn't adequate to the changes that were occurring. There were eloquent people who were unhappy about the deterioration of the family, education, morals, and the church. At intervals throughout our history, there have been concerns each time we've been faced with considerable changes in our society. In some ways the new institutions, the new ways, have often been creative and progressive. Sometimes, in the upheaval, we have lost something precious.

It is my feeling that here in Boston, in Boston medicine, Boston psychiatry, Boston psychoanalysis, we are again in a situation, at a time, reflecting the great tempo of change in our country and, indeed, throughout the world. There are certain institutions, traditions, patterns of reacting, that recur over and over again as one studies our history carefully. I want to refer to one particular point that delighted me in my studies this last year. What I came across was that in the 1830s and 40s there was a considerable upheaval, and a great literature on progressive versus orthodox education, with many articles that could be read at PTA meetings today. The cycles which we've experienced in this country are fascinating indeed. What we would be talking about at a meeting like this even ten years from now is difficult to say. But the enterprise of psychoanalysis in Boston has been an exciting, worthwhile, complex one, and it is one from which a great deal has been given. Those of us who have been part of it have gained a great deal, and I am delighted with this opportunity to have remembered so much, to express my gratitude to my teachers and my friends, those who are here and those who are not. Thank you.

DR. GARDNER: Thank you very much, Rexie, for those nostalgic reminiscences. And now I would like to call upon Dr. Helen Tartakoff.

DR. HELEN TARTAKOFF: I was in the dreadful position of being halfway through my medical studies, and about two-thirds of the way through my analytic training in Vienna, when I came to this country. I couldn't get into any medical school without waiting for a year, unless I had some pull. Well, Joseph Michaels happened to know Warren Stearns, dean of Tufts Medical College, and spoke to him. Joe had been in Vienna with me. He told Stearns that he would like very much to have me considered as a possible exchange student, without having to wait for the regular admission period. I arrived in Boston, went to Tufts Medical School, which was then on Huntington Avenue, and there was Dean Warren Stearns, all dressed for a fishing trip. He looked at me and said, "Oh, I hear you're from Vienna, that you've had some medical training, and would like to enter our school." I said, "Yes, very much." "Well," he said, "I'll tell you what I'll do. If you'll promise to take the National Boards and pass them next year, I'll let you come into Tufts in the fall. But if you don't get through the National Boards, we will have to reconsider it." He left me with his assistant, Dean O'Hare, I remember, to go through the complicated business of finding what courses I had or hadn't taken.

I was equally warmly received, I thought, by Douglas Macfie Campbell when I applied for a psychiatric residency. He asked me very few questions. However, I wanted to make a special appeal. I had been married recently and I didn't fancy having to be on duty weekends and evenings. So, without knowing that I was in advance of my time, I asked if he couldn't make some special concession for married women and let me do all the work the men did, but do it on my own time and not have to sleep in. And he agreed. I didn't ask his permission to get pregnant, and I miscarried a little bit—I don't mean the baby but the residency—in that I had figured that I'd be able to work the whole year and get full credit. Actually my due-date was at the end of the eleventh month, so I went to him rather timidly and told him that I was in quite a dilemma. I'd had ten months and I could see that I was going to have to leave the hospital at the end of one more month, what should I do about it? And he said "Well you haven't had a month's vacation, have you?" So he gave me full credit.

My reception at the Boston Psychoanalytic Institute was not very warm. I think they must have been in transition, perhaps still a bit influenced by Hanns Sachs, and not administratively organized when I first turned to them. I spoke to Mo Kaufman, told him my story, and asked if

I could attend courses and seminars. I had been carrying two control cases in Vienna, and another control case here, He agreed. All was fine until they must have had a meeting, and about six months later, when I was on the way to finishing my candidacy, I was told that my credentials were not orthodox. I hadn't completed my medical school training, and this was essential in America. So I signed off but, fortunately within a period of about a year I completed all my requirements and was permitted to become a member.

I would like to speak briefly of a colleague whose career paralleled mine, in terms of time, but in another country. Dr. Elizabeth Zetzel went to London just about the same time I went to Vienna, without any medical training. She entered analysis with Ernest Jones, and as she wished to become an analyst, she decided she would both study medicine at the University of London and also apply for candidacy, all of which she accomplished. In addition, she accomplished many other things. She stayed there through the war period. She became a major in the British army and was always very proud of that. As you know, she wrote about the war neuroses, as a result of this experience. She was recently made a Fellow of the Royal College of Physicians in London. Now Elizabeth Zetzel's career really—and it's a great loss that she's not with us today—covered the international scene. She not only became a training analyst here, she was active in the affairs of the American, too. She became secretary of the International Psychoanalytic Association and later vice president. As you know, she wrote a book which well documents her intellectual and emotional journey through psychoanalysis. The book is called *The Capacity for Emotional Growth*. She was a uniquely gifted teacher, gifted both in her ability to understand and to use her clinical experience to write constructively about her patients. I think it's very much in keeping with what she contributed that under the auspices of Harvard, there has been a psychotherapy center established in her name, as a memorial. I'm sorry she isn't with us. I would like to mention, among the other people who also went abroad, that several of my colleagues came here to Boston, which made my arrival really pleasant. Among them were Julia Deming, Molly Putnam, both Lydia and Daniel Dawes, the Michaels, and the Waelders. It was not until a couple of years later, that the Bibrings arrived. Thank you.

DR. GARDNER: Thank you very much, Helen. At this time I want to recall to your minds that there was another analyst in the early years who is not able to be with us today but who did send us her recollections. I will call on Dr. Sanford Gifford to read an excerpt from Dr. Leolia Dalrymple.

DR. SANFORD GIFFORD: Dr. Dalrymple offered to write a short and unpretentious account of what she remembered about the early years. It takes us back chronologically to the period before the institute was founded and gives a glimpse of the so-called Dark Ages of the 1920s when there were, in 1930, only three analysts listed in Boston as belonging to the American Psychoanalytic Association. One was Isador Coriat, one was Martin Peck, and the third was Donald MacPherson, who also hoped to be here today.

Dr. Dalrymple writes as follows. "In 1928 following a Rankian analysis with Dr. Martin Peck, I was invited to attend meetings held by Dr. Coriat at his home on Marlborough Street and later, on presenting a paper, I became a member of his group. This was a small group, anywhere from six to ten people, open to anyone interested in psychoanalysis, which met perhaps once or twice a month. The meetings were held in the Coriats' small living room. He was a man of small stature and sat in a highbacked Spanish chair; the members sat in a circle at his feet. Papers were read and discussed, mostly by Dr. Coriat, who was noted for talking at great length. Some in the group were seriously interested while others treated the discussions rather lightly. Some of the members of the group were Drs. Peck, John Taylor, Wilbur, Sanborn, and Kasanin. There were always a few residents from the Psychopathic who dropped in, Julia Deming, George Eliot, Rothschild, and others. At the close of the meeting, Mrs. Coriat joined the group with refreshments. Then occasionally Dr. Taylor held meetings in his office on Commonwealth Avenue. These were devoted to reading Freud's works from the German, and when translation was too difficult, Miss Taylor, his sister, was called in to assist. I remember only Drs. Peck and Wilbur at these meetings.

"At this time, 1928–29, the important psychoanalytic meetings were held in New York and, through Dr. Peck, I was invited to attend. The meetings were held in Dr. Frankwood Williams' large living room in lower New York and the group numbered perhaps fifteen to twenty. Many came from Philadelphia and the universities and hospitals in the New York area. Dr. Williams was a delightful host and the discussions were lively and stimulating. When Dr. Otto Rank was in town, he chaired the meetings, which were always most exciting. At the close, a sumptuous repast was served in the dining room on the lower floor.

"After this introduction to analysis I felt a Freudian analysis was in order. So, in 1930, after being accepted by Dr. Brill, I began work with Dr. Franz Alexander in Berlin. One of the delights, in contrast to the painful hours of analysis in Europe, at least with Dr. Alexander, was that his analysands traveled with him on his holidays and he was an indefatigable traveler. My analysis took place in Berlin, Herringsdorf, a fishing village on the Baltic coast, Madonna di Campiglio in the Dolomites, Brione, a divine island in the Adriatic, now Tito's private island, Amsterdam, and on the high seas, aboard the SS *Bremen*, when the Herr Professor was not suffering with *mal-de-mer*. In this group (we called it Alexander's traveling circus), were Ives Hendrick, Thomas French, David Slight, Ray Gosselin, Catherine Bacon, and others. In 1932 I joined Drs. Murray, Hendrick, and Kaufman in the struggle which resulted in the birth of an institute.

"One of the important and controversial figures in psychoanalysis in the twenties was Dr. Harry Stack Sullivan, and it was through him that I had first heard about analysis. During 1924 I was at Sheppard and Enoch Pratt and got my early training under him. He was a fascinating and dynamic teacher, somewhat ruthless, awe-inspiring and given to violent tempers, yet tender and compassionate with patients. He believed everyone in psychiatry should be analyzed and it was through him that my interest developed. Later, Martin Peck and Ives Hendrick came under his spell at Sheppard Pratt and were influenced by him in their later work."

DR. GARDNER: We are indebted to Leolia Dalrymple for this statement. We are trying to cover all aspects of psychoanalysis in those early days and indeed, as far up to the present as anyone wishes to go. One aspect is to see its impact upon other institutions. At this time I would like to call on Dr. Paul Howard of McLean Hospital.

DR. HOWARD: I'm a little puzzled about how to approach this subject since the effect of analysts in hospitals was rather an indirect one. They didn't practice psychoanalysis extensively in Boston hospitals. I would like, however, to comment on the influence of analysis on humane attitudes toward individuals in the three Boston hospitals I worked in. The dynamic approach in psychotherapy made the patient seem more meaningfully alive. In many conferences, observation, diagnosis, and prognosis were still machine-like, and deteriorated patients looked like cases of irreversible brain disease. It was most discouraging to work with them, except where there was an occasional spontaneous recovery. Once the analysts brought in a dynamic developmental psychology and pathology, the hospital staff could feel that they were dealing with people who were still human.

At the Boston Psychopathic Hospital, the inpatient resident's job was to do a diagnostic anamnesis and a ten-day disposition. You could get in a little brief therapy with many patients, but C. Macfie Campbell, a small Scotsman with a speedy walk on rounds, was not content with that. He interviewed patients quite carefully, and demonstrated how they developed their ideas in a broad social and experiential context. He was acquainted with psychoanalysis, and spoke frequently with skepticism about such concepts as infantile sexuality, which he felt was not clearly demonstrable. He showed from the literature that others had had these ideas before Freud. I was deeply impressed by his intense and curious sympathy, as he pictured the world as it looked to the patient producing the symptoms. The total effect was human, but he just didn't analyze back far enough. Others at "Psycho," such as Harry Solomon and Esther Cook, the chief social worker who radiated genial understanding, also showed a human interest in patients and their social circumstances.

To show the extensive interest of Campbell in analysis, I might just mention the names of those who were later to become members of the American: Williams, MacPherson, Kenworthy, Menninger, Peck, Herman, Hart (Henry Hart), George Daniels, McFarland, Kasanin, Deming, Biddle, Hendrick, Kaufman, Spurgeon English, Ribble, Noble, Scott, Curran, Leon Salk, George Goldman, Frank D'Elseaux, Edgerton Howard, Abraham Finesinger, Joseph Michaels, Conrad Wall, Pearson, and myself. Hendrick listed twenty-eight appointments of Commonwealth Fellows as house officers at the "Psycho" from 1912 to 1934.

I then went to Boston City Hospital, where we in neurology dealt with more tangible things.

At the Massachusetts General Hospital in 1937, I was a psychiatric resident on one of the first psychiatric wards in a general hospital. This had been started by Dr. Stanley Cobb in 1934. Dr. Cobb had been analyzed, and though he was not to go into practice, he was elected an honorary member of the Boston Society in 1941. The influence of his personality on the hospital was tremendous, as he was able to integrate different points of view. He was a neurologist, but he was so at ease with medicine that he made our humanistic efforts to consider the individual from a functional point of view acceptable to many medical and surgical services that had previously been skeptical. Dr. Finesinger was an analyst studying physiology. Dr. Lindemann's social interests were a vital step in the development of psychiatry in the community and his study of grief proved very important. Helene Deutsch would give the essence of a patient in a few words. Staff conferences were dynamic reviews.

Once in examining a patient I missed a delusion. I had asked him about a hundred, 150, questions and did not find out that he was riddled with cancer. But Felix Deutsch picked it up in a few moments, by listening with his associated anamnesis, which is derived from analytic technique. Just to mention the influence of the movement at the Massachusetts General, there were twenty-one analysts in training there up to 1940, Niels Anthonisen, William Barrett, Ralph Kaufman, Ives Hendrick, Eleanor Pavenstedt, Helene Deutsch, Felix Deutsch, Florence Clothier (who was on the neurological service, and later ran a children's clinic), Robert Young, Stanley Cobb, Jacob Finesinger, my brother Edgerton Howard, Philip Solomon, Erich Lindemann, David Young, Lydia Dawes, Joseph Michaels, Marion Putnam, Milton Rosenbaum, Martin Peck, and Samuel Hunt.

I could say here that before Cobb came to the Massachusetts General Hospital and set up the psychiatric ward, its predecessor was the outpatient Mental Hygiene Clinic, which was manned by six to eight McLean Hospital staff, including four who were or became analysts: Kaufman, Anthonisen, Robert Young, and Ives Hendrick. It was a dynamically oriented clinic with family work and social service.

Going to McLean in 1938, I found that from the beginning there, a spirit of humanity was part of the consideration of patients. This rather broad approach, including the moralistic one, was also bolstered by considerable technical interest in psychology; in 1849 Luther Bell wrote that "The views, feelings and reflections which we do not recognize as our own but which we may spurn as being our own thoughts and sentiments still have come out of the storehouse of our minds as they certainly do in states of aberration." Thus he recognized the unconscious and states of dissociation.

Dr. Edward Cowles continued the advancement of personal consideration for patients, and he established a psychopathological laboratory there. Dr. Hoch began, in 1896, to show the personality factors in mental disease. In 1900, under the direction of Dr. Folin, the laboratory emphasized the biological and physiological factors. Dr. John Whitehorn, who arrived in the early thirties and stayed till 1940, became interested in the patients on the halls and was strongly influenced, I believe, by analysis. He became one of the greatest interviewers and listeners I have ever heard. His skill on rounds at the MGH attracted me to McLean. He was also interested in the style of physicians, how they approached patients, and he once commented that a schizophrenic could be diagnosed by his withdrawal at certain physicians' approach. He was usually able to have patients reveal their antagonisms. A suicidal patient once said after the attempt, "Why, I almost got the wrong man." He skillfully brought out extremely secret thoughts from patients in a way that was most gentle and penetrating.

John Whitehorn was analyzed, but did not seek further training. He became a professor at Johns Hopkins and president of the American Psychiatric Association. Dr. George Gardner, studying for a Ph.D. in psychology in the late twenties, worked at McLean and became excited by Freud's theories. He displayed them on charts, in conversations, and at conferences quite persistently. This was the first psychoanalytic interest there, and it has been continued ever since.

Thus coming to McLean in 1938, I found that only a few cases had had analytic treatment, principally by Dr. Kaufman and Dr. Hendrick. Since that time occasional patients have been referred by their analysts, who could continue their treatment there. Dr. Kaufman came as clinical director in 1931, and was later a consultant. He did research on suicide and Dr. Pavenstedt was also there on that project. Dr. Hendrick was a consultant and attended many conferences. There were other analysts, or candidates in training. Psychotherapy was of high interest, and in 1948 occupied about eighty percent of the staff time outside of research. Since then there has always been a psychoanalytic clinical head.

A list of those who were analysts, does not mean that others were not doing valuable dynamic work. Other names would include Alfred Ludwig, Hughie Varny, Elvin Semrad, Paul Howard, William Peltz, Eleanor Pavenstedt, Lucie Jessner (who came there directly from abroad), Daniel Dawes, Philip Gates, Franklin Carter, Gardner Quarton, Peter Sifneos, and John Lamont. That carries it up through the 1940s.

I think it is historically important that analysts were analyzed, and that this gave a genuine sympathy for the meaning and control of symptoms, and a vision of patients' potential freedom to create attitudes for themselves under special circumstances. Psychiatrists could now work in hospitals and with other diagnostic disciplines conjointly. All the specialists involved could help in their own style. I observed this increasing humanism toward individuals, partly as a result of the analytic movement. However, the individual analyst learned in the history of his own analysis that the person who is the center of creativity, internal and external, is the patient, for illness or for better health. He's his own psychohistory.

DR. GEORGE GARDNER: Thank you very much, Paul. At this point, our final discussion of this session, I'd like to call on Dr. Elvin Semrad.

DR. SEMRAD: It's always good to come late in the program, then you know that everything important has been said and you can only tell some anecdotes that may possibly have some relevance.

I came to Massachusetts in 1935 from my native Nebraska, from a village of 150 people of good peasant stock. I had experience in a grocery store, on the farm, and as a teacher in a one-room schoolhouse. We were known in Nebraska as Bohemians. Later, when I arrived in Boston and got over the culture shock of replying that I was Bohemian, I discovered that somewhere along the way Bohemia and Moravia had become parts of Czechoslovakia, so I've been a Czech ever since.

In 1935, the Psychopathic had a very small group of residents. There were four of us. Two of us became analysts, myself and Mrs. Maxwell Gittelson of Chicago, then known as Frances Hannett. Because of the rumors that Dr. Campbell was against analysis, it took quite a bit of time to get up the fortitude to go into analysis. Dr. Kaufman, Dr. Michaels, and Dr. Hendrick, who were then teaching medical students, were very helpful to me personally. I was the assistant scut-boy, as they say, who arranged the cases and so forth. It impressed me that they talked differently with their patients, to their patients, and about their patients and, being a curious fellow, I wondered how they got to be this way. If it was good enough for them, maybe it was good for me. I finally confronted Dr. Campbell and asked him what he thought of my going into analysis. He said "Well, Semrad, if for ten years you listen to patients, hear what they have to say, then maybe you'll become a therapist." Being young, who could wait ten years? But he said that perhaps it would be all right, and a good learning experience for me, provided I had the money, which I did not have. Nevertheless, the next day I went and arranged for an analysis with Dr. Sachs.—Since I was interested in therapy, I went to McLean after two years at the Boston Psychopathic. Dr. Robert Young, Dr. Niels Anthonisen and Dr. John Whitehorn were very influential people in my career as a therapist-tradesman.—"Well," Dr. Sachs said, "if you still think you want to be analyzed, come back in the fall." So I did.

And we started. We went on for awhile and one day I had the feeling that I was through, and I announced this. He didn't respond, of course. A couple of months later I had the same feeling. This time he said, "We'll stop in the spring," now two springs later. When I left his consultation room, he said, "Come back in the fall and tell me how you are." So I did. Nothing very disastrous happened to me in the meantime. I was a little poorer, being poor to start with. In the fall we talked and he told me about his asthma; he told me about his aches and his pains. I'm sure he hastened the termination process. As I was leaving, he said, "I have spoken to Dr. Murray and he has a case for you." I went home and pondered the question—where I could see a patient, where the money would come from, because I was earning something like $3300 a year and board and room for my family. I went to see Dr. Murray anyway. He listened and he investigated my financial status and said, "Well, Semrad, this patient needs to be analyzed and he's willing to go out to the Metropolitan State Hospital where you are. I'll tell you what I'll do. If you come in at my lunch hour, I'll charge you $5.00 an hour." Well, so I did, and to this day I think that the only thing Dr. Murray eats is soup and ice cream for lunch.

After Dr. Murray came Dr. Hendrick, two cases, and two almost re-analyses. It was good teaching, it was good learning, it was good experience, but it was expensive. As a matter of fact everything didn't go smoothly between me and Dr. Hendrick. On one of the cases, we disagreed, and he suggested that we have a consultation. That's when I met Dr. Edward Bibring. He was the consultant. We had a pleasant fifty minutes, nice talk, nice explanation, and I thought I understood. I wasn't so sure that he thought I understood. As I was leaving his office, he said, "He thinks you're going to rape him." Now he didn't specify who the subject was. Of course that caused me considerable concern, until the patient's associations clarified the issue. Dr. Bibring became a very influential person in the seminars. His seminar on the instincts, and his papers on psychotherapy, analytic technique, and depression were most useful to me. This was particularly so because in my pragmatic interests, I was preoccupied with, and essentially given to applied analysis outside of the couch situation.

After Dr. Hendrick came Dr. Helene Deutsch. She taught me many an important thing. One day I was reporting my patient. This was about the third week of analysis and the patient was talking about oral impregnation and anal delivery. In my fantasy I thought that this would probably be the fastest analysis on record. Dr. Deutsch listened patiently and then she finally said, "Why do you think she's telling you that?" I said, "I don't know." "Well," she said, "why don't you ask her?" So I did. And the patient said, "Isn't that what analysts want to hear?" And then we got to work.

I'm probably the only analyst who stayed in the state service most of his career. I started at the Boston Psychopathic, as a resident for two years. I was not satisfied with the treatment offered here, so I went to McLean instead. Then I started my analysis and had to pay for it, so I got a job at the Metropolitan State Hospital. There I had the distinction, in time, of having the first couch, which Dr. Halloran, the superintendent, had specially built for me and set aside in a special room in the Administration Building. After World War II, when I returned to finish psychoanalytic training, Boston State Hospital was a very fruitful and rewarding experience. No matter what you did, it was better than what had happened during the war years. Success was right around the corner every day. We were fortunate due in large part to analysis, in that young physicians returning from the war wanted a place where they could work and be close enough to Boston to have their analyses. Many people joined us: Drs. James Mann, Doris Menzer-Benaron, Jerry Weinberger, Stewart Smith, Jay Fiedler, John Mackenzie, Christopher Standish, Jacob Swartz, and many others.

An important man in my life was Dr. Felix Deutsch, with whom I had a workshop that went on for about three years, on "The Mysterious Leap from the Mind to the Body." In this workshop, Dr. Mann and I were enabled by Dr. Deutsch to formulate some of the conversion-processes in psychoses that perhaps some of you may have studied. Mrs. Beata Rank helped me in my transition period from associate training analyst to training analyst. I found her empathic, intuitive observations very useful in clarifying the differences between therapeutic and training analyses.

Since I was so intimately associated with state service, and so long with the Mass. Mental Health Center, I thought I might say something about its relationship to analysis in a more precise way than has already been stated. In 1968, when we celebrated our fiftieth anniversary, there was a survey of the residents who had trained with us.*

Seventy-three percent of the graduates had had, or were in, analysis as of that time. Although the proportion varied from era to era, and there had been three superintendents that I knew and worked with, forty percent of our former residents had become practicing analysts. The trend towards personal analysis without clinical training came to my attention when we celebrated our thirty-fifth anniversary at the Boston Psychoanalytic Institute. At that time I surveyed 232 of our residents at the Mass. Mental Health Center.† Thirty-five percent of them had gone into clinical analysis. Another thirty percent had had a personal analysis and had continued their interest in the analytic process and its usefulness in their work.

Dr. Rexford and I are perhaps the youngest on the panel. The institute let us out in 1948. We were the two graduates that year. Besides many personal things that perhaps are best left for the couch, it has been an enriching experience to be involved and associated with these important people. I owe them much.

DR. GARDNER: Thank you, Dr. Semrad, for that very delightful discourse.

The format of this is as follows: we will call upon the other members of the panel, and then we hope that those of you who have been so faithful in listening will also feel free to participate. To begin this afternoon, Dr. Kaufman would like to make an addendum to his morning statements.

DR. KAUFMAN: I should like to add something to what Dr. Bibring said this morning. Actually, I didn't know that I was running the American Medical Association of Vienna with an iron hand; I thought it was a velvet glove. I wanted to tell you where I got this reputation. When I got to Vienna, there was a large organization called the American Medical Association of Vienna, and it was devoted essentially to postgraduate education. After I was in analysis awhile, I was working at the Wagner-Jauregg clinic, doing the kind of things we considered leisurely in Boston, about half a dozen things at the same time. I found that you could come, register as a student, pay your tuition, and then disappear until you were ready to go back, and you got a diploma that was a certificate. There was a group that I called dowry-specialists. A dowry-specialist was a doctor who was recently married and got a dowry of somewhere between eight and ten thousand dollars and decided he wanted to become a specialist. So he went to Vienna. And there you could enroll in a whole series of courses to which you never had to go. Jock and I kept track of those individuals: they'd spend six weeks, three months, a year, never attending any of the courses whatsoever. Then they would get a certificate from the University of Vienna, which they'd go back and hang on the wall. A number of us got somewhat irritated by this lack of standards.

Dr. [Sanford] Gifford sent me a copy of a letter of mine that he found in Ives Hendrick's papers, dated December 16, 1931, and addressed to Dr. Isador Coriat, 416 Marlborough Street, Boston, Massachusetts.

> My dear Dr. Coriat. It has occurred to Hendrick and myself that a solution of the problem discussed at the last meeting might be the following at the present time. In Boston we have a group of some eight Freudian analysts and in the near future this will probably be augmented by three or four other people who are completing their training. Our suggestion would be that we organize a psychoanalytic society composed only of this group. One of the immediate aims of this society will be the definite recognition by the International Psychoanalytic Association. It seems to me that the way to tackle this problem is to go to it fundamentally. I think that Boston is the only city, perhaps in the world and certainly in America, which has already a group of well-trained and accepted analysts who can form the nucleus of a strictly Freudian society. And thus we can avoid in the future any squabbling as to theoretical considerations and the eternal problem, which seems to be coming up at our meetings, as to what constitutes a psychoanalyst. I am also certain that if you accepted the presidency of such a group in Boston it would lead to almost an immediate recognition of this group by the International. There is of course the consideration that the immediate and drastic reorganization of the present society would lead to a certain amount of unpleasantness. To us it seems better to take this one radical step, which will obviate any future difficulties. This is a suggestion to which I would very much like to get your reaction. If you think this plan is at all feasible, we should meet with Dr. Alexander and obtain his opinion and help. We are quite certain that should you think this plan feasible there will be no difficulty in the immediate organization of this group. Our aim of course is to avert the many difficulties which have beset psychoanalytic groups, especially the New York one. I feel this is an excellent chance to rid ourselves in one stroke of all the factors which tend to keep that society in New York in internal difficulty. I hope that you will see your way clear to discuss with us the merits and demerits of the above suggestions.

So, when I said this morning that the reactions to the troika were not altogether transference but a good deal of reality, you can see that this type of situation, which is now forty-odd years old, had at least two purposes, one conscious and the other unconscious. The conscious one is simple. We wanted to raise and keep standards as high as possible. Unconscious ones you can judge for yourself.

There are two people, particularly one, whom I'd like to mention, whom nobody has really talked about. One, of course, is Dr. Edouard Hitschmann, who was one of the first psychobiographers. Many of you are familiar with his work; he contributed a good deal here. The other is a personal memory of one of the fondest friendships that I personally have had, a man who is beloved by everybody in the society, and that's

Martin Peck, our second president. Martin was one of the most modest, gentlemanly people. He knew what he stood for. He didn't behave like a troika and fight and abrade everybody, but he was of tremendous assistance in the formation of our society. We were delighted to have him as a member and when the society-institute formed, our teaching program was exceedingly active. Martin was modest enough not to put on any airs, and participated actively as a student and as a teacher. I had the feeling that we ought to mention him to show that we haven't forgotten someone who was one of the stalwart and really wonderful people in the early society.

Felix Deutsch has already been mentioned. I don't want to add any more to what was said about Felix except, again, that I had the opportunity and privilege of working with him for a number of years. We worked at the Beth Israel together and other places, and somehow or other, I have the feeling that Felix hasn't quite gotten his due not only in relation to analysis, but to his importance to American medicine. He was one of the individuals who made a tremendous contribution in the area that we used to call psychosomatic medicine.

DR. GARDNER: Thank you, Dr. Kaufman. We are glad that you memorialized these important members of the institute. At this point I would like to call on Dr. Florence Clothier.

DR. FLORENCE CLOTHIER: There has been a lot of reminiscing and many nostalgic anecdotes of the early days of the society and institute. All of it was fascinating to me, as a minor participant in that exciting era. I was, however, a little troubled by the impression that may have been left with the audience about my analyst and mentor, Hanns Sachs. Jock, your remarks this morning, while not personally derogatory, indicated that there had been problems between Sachs and the society almost from the beginning. This I knew, but those of us privileged to have been analyzed by him in his early days in Boston dismissed them as irrelevant. Dr. Semrad told us of his analysis with Sachs about ten years after mine. He spoke of Sachs's talking to him about his own asthma and various aches and pains. I want to go on record as stating that, as a somewhat younger analyst, Sachs certainly did not burden his analysands with his own medical problems.

I am one of the candidates who slipped into training early—sort of via the back door. I was never interviewed or approved by any committee. I just went into analysis with Sachs and proceeded to have control cases with Helene Deutsch and Erik Erikson. Analysis with Sachs was a fascinating experience. Those of you familiar with his books and papers are aware of his broad-based, wide knowledge of mythology and the classics. Like Freud, who was his analyst and teacher, he had enormous knowledge of, and respect for, the contributions of wise and creative men over the centuries. There was little chance to discuss these things with him, but material I brought up in analysis was often related to familiar or unfamiliar bits of our cultural heritage. I remember at one point saying that I could never be an analyst because I didn't know enough of mythology (universal fantasies) and the classics. His references, so pertinent and brought out so easily, inspired much reading which has been helpful to me to this day.

I have never thought of myself as a very good analyst, and most of my clinical work has not been traditional psychoanalysis. But my analysis with Sachs, and my subsequent training at the institute seminars and with Helene Deutsch, contributed more than I can say to my personal development and to my effectiveness in working with children and their parents and with college-age adolescents.

Let me tell an anecdote. This occurred in the early or mid-1930s when I was still in analysis. The first time I saw Helene Deutsch was at a meeting of the Boston Society of Neurology and Psychiatry—she had arrived in this country ahead of Felix. Sachs and Helene were seated next to each other and, although I knew nothing of his personal life, I assumed that Helene was his wife. My jealousy of that beautiful woman came out in the next day's session.

I remember very well when Sachs first arrived in this country, probably in 1932–33. David and Muriel Pokross brought him out to our new home in Milton. At that point I had no thought of going into analysis. I was fresh from Johns Hopkins and the strong influence of Adolf Meyer. As a first year medical student, I had written one of those interminable life histories. When I told Dr. Meyer that I was going into analysis, he dug out from the files my life history, written six or seven years before. He asked me if I would keep it and review it as I went through analysis, and to let him know if anything truly significant came out in the analysis that had not been included in the comprehensive life history. When Dr. Meyer handed it to me, his eyes twinkled as he said, "Oh so you are the woman who turned in most of your life history under a man's number." The weekly chapters of the history were turned in by assigned numbers, not by name. I have a tendency to reverse numbers. I still have that now-yellowing history, written in 1927 but never looked at while in analysis or since.

Though Hanns Sachs may have been a thorn in the flesh of those wonderful people, who became my close friends and who were setting up the institute, he made significant contributions to many of us in his own way. He ceased early on to participate in the affairs of the institute and society, but in the years after my analysis he became a valued friend and frequent guest in our Milton home, where our then young children referred to him as "Poppa Sachs with the cigar." You in the audience, and my friends and former colleagues here on the platform, may go away thinking "She never got over her transference." That may be true but I don't regret it.

DR. GARDNER: Thank you, Florence, for that corrective experience that we've all enjoyed. I'd like now to call on Dr. Eleanor Pavenstedt.

DR. PAVENSTEDT: I think I was another person who snuck into the institute under Dr. Sachs's somewhat questionable way of doing things.

I want to talk first about the exciting time that we had in the seminars in 1935–37, when there were very few candidates. As soon as the Deutschs came from Vienna, all the members of the institute attended every seminar, two or three times a week. Florence was reminding me how late we got home in those days, because we really had a wonderful time discussing all of Freud's papers.

I want to talk about the only second-generation analyst in the 40s, that's Marian Putnam, whom we knew as Molly. I don't know of any of the other early analysts that had descendants by that time. Molly came to Boston from Yale, with a pediatric background and a year of analysis in Vienna with Helene Deutsch, following Helene in coming to live in Boston. By then Molly was extremely interested in early child development, the mother-child relationship, and preventive psychiatry by working with young children. She founded the James Jackson Putnam Children's Center, which became a model for nursery schools and child guidance clinics for children under five. I see Betty Cobb down there who shared this wonderful experience with those of us who were privileged to be there with Molly. It really was marvelous, a model not only for the child guidance clinics in this city (almost all of them added a nursery school to their clinics) but throughout the country. Many such institutes were started, and it gave a tremendous impetus to the study of mother-child relationships along psychoanalytic concepts. That's all I have to say.

DR. GARDNER: Thank you, Eleanor. To continue in the field of childhood, I'd like to call on Dr. Robert Young.

DR. YOUNG: Well, I *know* I sneaked in by the back door. I did not apply until after my analysis and supervision. As far as I know, nobody knew I was being analyzed by Hanns Sachs. I appreciate Dr. Clothier's defense of Dr. Sachs because I, too, found him very, very helpful and interested in my career. After my analysis I came back to see him a number of times. He was helpful to me in many ways and gave me literature to read but, unfortunately, most of it was in German.

I had come to McLean Hospital when Dr. Gardner left to go to medical school. He invited me to take his place as psychologist, which at that time meant two or three days at the MGH. Shortly afterwards Dr. Stanley Cobb moved from City Hospital to the MGH, and I went there with him full time. They'd never had a full-time psychologist before and they didn't really know what to do with me. However, I did just as I pleased and I told them that that's what psychologists did. I became interested in the treatment of children, and was encouraged in that by Dr. Cobb. He more or less supervised me, although not on a regular basis. From time to time I had many delightful occasions with Dr. and Mrs. Cobb at their house. He referred private patients to me later on, and I continued to consult him afterwards.

Frankly, I knew nothing about psychoanalysis until the summer of 1934, when I attended a camp at Williamstown run by Dr. Smiley Blanton. He had taken over a fraternity house, and a small group of children with speech difficulties were there. Smiley Blanton had long been interested in children. He had finished his analysis with Dr. Freud in 1930, and had established a number of child guidance clinics throughout the country. He was very free with his time, and I not only got supervision from him for my work but we had many long discussions about Freud. I became interested, and decided then that I wanted to become analyzed. Incidentally, Dr. Blanton died in 1962 at the age of eighty-four. His widow found among his papers something he'd started to write, which he called "The Diary of My Analysis with Sigmund Freud." Apparently he started this with Freud's approval, and Mrs. Blanton finished it up. It was published in 1971 with her comments.

During that summer Blanton had asked me if I would like to be analyzed. I said I would but I had no money. I was getting \$18,000—\$18,000, that's a slip—\$1,800 a year, and I didn't see how in the world I could ever support myself in analysis. In the fall of 1934, I got a telephone call from Dr. Blanton and he said that if I would accept it, he could arrange a Commonwealth Fund scholarship for my analysis. I accepted his offer and started my analysis later in that fall, I think, or possibly winter. I don't know just when, but I continued for two years in analysis with Dr. Sachs. Then, in June of 1936, I told him I thought I would stop the analysis because I was going to get married. There was a dead silence. I wondered what he was going to say and, finally, he spoke up and said he thought that would be good and we could terminate the analysis. And so I did.

I continued my work at the Massachusetts General, and finally Dr. Gardner asked me if I would come to the Judge Baker Guidance Center while he was in the military service. He had invited me for one year only; however, he didn't tell me not to come back, so I've been coming back ever since. Some day I expect they'll tell me not to come back.

When my analysis with Sachs ended, I was still interested in children's work and asked Erik Erikson, who was around here then, if he would supervise some of my work with children. He said he would be glad to, and we made arrangements for that, when I got a letter from the institute. It was the first time I ever knew that *they* knew I existed. The letter said it would be necessary for me to have experience with a couple of adult patients first. I did this, of course, and then later on, when I was ready to analyze children, Erikson had left town. However, during my training period, the Deutsches, Beata Rank, the Bibrings, and the Waelders were all very helpful. I did most of my child supervision with Mrs. Rank, and she was most kind.

Somewhere along the line Dr. Kaufman cornered me, as I remember, at McLean Hospital, and told me that it was nothing personal, but I probably wouldn't be taken into the society in Boston. Now actually I had never thought of becoming a member; I'd never thought of applying. All I'd wanted was training in children's work. But then and there I decided I wanted to become a member. (It's taken me thirty years to be able to say this.) I then attended the seminars, and I do remember 82 Marlborough Street, which was referred to earlier. All the members of the society sat around an enormous oval table, and every other week I presented a child that I was analyzing, under Mrs. Rank's supervision. They all took cracks at me so that, by the end of the evening, I was pretty exhausted. I realize now how important that was, because I got the viewpoints about child analysis of all the people I mentioned before. But I survived. Again, to show how loose the society was at that time, I finished my evening seminars and finally suggested to somebody that it was about time they took me into the society. About a month later, I got a letter saying I'd been accepted. It was certainly easy in those days. Nobody questioned me, nobody interviewed me. Nobody accepted me. I just went.

During my period of seminars, Gibby Dawes was also starting her analysis, at least she was also in the seminars. She was having a difficult time, too. We used to get together and commiserate with each other about our experiences, and that was extremely helpful. Gibby Dawes has hardly been mentioned, but I don't think we should omit her because, at the Judge Baker and at her home, she was a great help to me. I thought she was one of the most outstanding of our child analysts. As I remember, we had no seminars then in child analysis.

When I came to the Judge Baker, there was also Dorothy MacNaughton, and unfortunately she is still living. I say unfortunately because she really doesn't know what is going on. Dr. MacNaughton had a stroke about eight to nine years ago. We used to get together and she was a great help in discussing things. I enjoyed her conferences. She had many likes and dislikes, and she really went all out for the people she liked. The people she didn't much care for, she avoided. Fortunately I was one of the people that she liked, and to me she gave very freely of her time. I think she made a great contribution to psychoanalysis.

I think that's about all of interest. I knew nothing until today about the difficulties with Hanns Sachs. I suppose mine was an early analysis, in 1934. At that time he had only been here a few years, and I certainly never heard anything about his private life, his pains and aches. We were strictly in business. I remember once, at the beginning of my analysis, when I thought I knew the answer to something, he quickly but kindly called my attention to the fact that I was a patient and that such comments would be discussed later, at the end of my analysis. Thank you.

DR. GARDNER: Thank you, Robert, for that overview of your experiences. We're very grateful that you remembered two more colleagues who played such an important part in child analysis. If Dr. Young looks like me and talks the way I do, it's due to the fact that forty-eight years ago this September, I first met Dr. Young at Harvard and we have been more or less together ever since. I've never been able to order him around, and he has always had the ability to make me do what he wanted. He does it quietly and unobtrusively, you see. And now I'd like to call on Dr. Edgerton Howard.

DR. HOWARD: There's little that I can add, although maybe a few reminiscences will help to paint the picture of the thirties. I might say that for me this is an extremely exciting and exhilarating session. It's full of nostalgia, and nostalgic memories. It has taught me a lot of things that I didn't know were going on behind my back. I learned a lot about what happened at the "Psycho," at McLean, which I find stimulating and exciting.

It's a little awkward for a student to get up and talk before his elders, people whom he has revered through the years, looked up to. But time has evened things out a bit, so I'm not quite as embarrassed now as I would have been forty years ago.

Two or three items have come up that puzzled me, about which I'm not quite clear. One's about C. Macfie Campbell. Dr. Campbell was my mentor. I was at the "Psycho" for three years in the early thirties and he was an absolutely superb, unrivalled teacher. I think what little I know about psychiatry in general was learned from him. What puzzles me is that, although I had evidence that C. Macfie held me, I think, in good regard, after every tea at his house, which we attended a number of times a year, the next Monday he would give me hell at staff conferences for some reason or other. This was characteristic of him. It always happened, and it also happened to others, to whom he had expressed some personal, friendly feelings. My third year at "Psycho" was at his request, that I stay on and spend that year teaching medical students, which I did. I wanted to apply for a Commonwealth Fund Fellowship so I could be analyzed. C. Macfie said he would not support this, because too many of his fellows had become analysts and he was not sure that this was the best thing for psychiatry.

I might tell Bob Young the way to become analyzed when you're earning, as I was at that time, $25.00 a month, is to be married to a social worker who is earning $180 a month. Just a couple of other comments. My control analysts were Mo Kaufman and Ives Hendrick, and I couldn't have selected better people. In a light vein, one thing that I learned from Mo was how to conduct a rigid, orthodox psychoanalysis. We both had our offices at 82 Marlborough Street. Mine was up on the third floor and his on the first, right by the waiting room. Many mornings when I came in, Mo was at his door, cigar in his hand, standing at attention. He was looking straight ahead and, as I headed toward the stairs, I'd say, "Good morning." No response at all. There was a patient behind me, and I soon learned not to say good morning to Mo when he was waiting by his door.

Ives Hendrick was an excellent control analyst because he could read every unconscious thought I had. He always did, and he always reported it to me. It did not make it easy, but I learned as much about myself during those control sessions as I learned about patients, which I think is one of the virtues of control. Ives remained a very close friend of mine for years afterwards, though I will have to add that his ability to read my unconscious thoughts made the friendship not always easy. But I understood Ives and always had a tremendously high regard for him, and a great respect.

DR. GARDNER: Thank you very much, Ed.

DR. BIBRING: Ladies and gentlemen, I usurp our chairman's position and call on Dr. Gardner, because it wouldn't be a full day if he didn't tell his tale. Dr. Gardner—

DR. GARDNER: Thank you, Grete, for this invitation to speak at the symposium. I don't want to be too autobiographical, but I will tell you something about my past life and my association with medicine, child psychiatry, and child analysis. To begin at the beginning, I was born in a little village in Plymouth County with an Indian name. There were fifty-two houses in this village. Nothing happened in my life, as far as I know, of an exciting nature until one day when I was in high school. I think it was the second year, and we were all marshalled into the assembly room. I say all, I think there were seventeen people in my class. An impressive-looking gentleman was on the platform and he distributed some interesting documents. It turned out that this man came from the Boston University School of Education. They were seeking to get a base line on the intelligence of children in the rural areas of Massachusetts with their newfangled tests.

We all sat down and took those tests, which seemed to me rather funny. I thought nothing more of them until a few weeks later when the principal came to my house, which was two miles from the school. I couldn't figure out what I had done in school that particular day to warrant his coming. After his visit, the whole climate of the school, and the teachers' attitude toward me, changed. I thought that was rather unusual. I was destined, of course, like my forbears, to be a shoemaker. The principal finally told me that I did so well on that test that he thought I should go to college. I became the darling of the school, and the teachers began desperately trying to prepare me for Harvard College. As far as I know, no one had ever gone to college from that high school.

At any rate, I finally did get to college. You can see why I always pay obeisance to the standardized tests of this world because, if there hadn't been any such instruments, I probably would still be pulling tacks in the McElvin Shoe Factory in Bridgewater. This is enough to show you what identifications I did not have. I will tell you now what identification was thrust upon me which made a great difference in my life.

I went to college and my destiny was to be a teacher. Those of my forbears who went to college were teachers, and the uncle for whom I was named was a teacher. I was supposed to become a teacher of Latin and Greek, so I concentrated on the classics in college. When I entered graduate school, I found that one had to take some courses in educational psychology in order to become a teacher. Then I came under the wing of Dr. Walter Dearborn who, incidentally, was a Ph.D. and an M.D. This is where I met Dr. Young.

I became fascinated with this field of psychology. It would seem that this *should* have been the first time I learned anything about psychoanalysis, but this was not the case. It happened when I was a sophomore in college and I read a book, which I had bought with my limited means. It was entitled *The Unconscious*, by Irving Levine, whom I assume lived somewhere in London because it was published in London. I tried to trace this book a week ago, just to see what it looked like, but I couldn't find it. I had found this a very fascinating book of some 215 pages. It was my first acquaintance with the unconscious, and was one of the first things that interested me in psychoanalysis.

I switched immediately from my ambition of becoming a Latin teacher to becoming a psychologist, with a particular concern about the learning process in children. In this field, I took a Ph.D. at Harvard. However, during my second year of graduate work, in the last course that Morton Prince taught, there was an associate to Prince named Helgy Lenholm, who was a psychologist at McLean. He knew of my interest in educational psychology. He stopped me one day after class and wanted to know if I would come to McLean as a psychologist. I went there, again, as you see, because I knew something about the standardized tests and measures of this world. Without the testing movement I would be an unknown.

I went to McLean, and at that time there were two physicians on the male side, two physicians on the female side, a pathologist, Dr. Whitehorn, and a superintendent whom we never saw, luckily. By this time, I had become thoroughly convinced that the Freudian theory was the only concept that could be applied to the psychoses, as I saw them, and to the neuroses, as I knew them from a distance. Being a frustrated teacher, I began to give seminars at McLean to the staff and what were called residents. These were held in the evening and I can still remember making large charts of the Freudian structures.

I didn't meet with much success and enthusiasm. Most people were organically oriented and wished to remain that way, with the exception of John Whitehorn. I did earn a new name, however. I was immediately dubbed "Sigmund." I stayed there a total of about ten years, including a later residency. I went from there to the Harvard Medical School; the hospital really made it possible for me to go to medical school.

I never lost my interest in the children's field, so I had thirty-two months in pediatrics at the MGH, went back to McLean, and then went to the Judge Baker on a Commonwealth Fellowship. I've been at the Judge Baker ever since.

One item that hasn't been mentioned. When it came time to have an analysis and I was accepted by a committee and by an analyst, the institute had set up the Sigmund Freud Fellowships in Psychoanalysis. Three of us were selected for those fellowships, John Romano, Charles Brenner, and myself. So that made it possible, of course, to have one's analysis with a certain degree of peace.

I attended seminars, did control work, under Dr. [Edward] Bibring in one case and under Helene Deutsch in another. One could not find two more fascinating teachers. In 1944, when I was in the navy, we had the annual meeting of the American Psychiatric in Philadelphia, where I was stationed. Helene Deutsch came to my table at a luncheon and told me that I had been made an associate member of the Boston Psychoanalytic Institute, in those days the first step to membership. Great things were happening at the institute. We began to get together, all of us in the children's field, and we had a lively and impressive group of child analysts. As you probably remember, the Judge Baker was sitting on the side of the hill two streets down from the State House. It had no affiliation with any medical school and was completely out of the mainstream of medicine. This bothered me quite a bit. I began to put out not too subtle suggestions to my friends at the MGH and at Children's Hospital: wouldn't they like to have a vigorous affiliate, namely the Judge Baker, associated with them? At the MGH, which was my home base in pediatrics, there was little interest in setting up an affiliation of this sort, at least on the part of the chief of pediatrics, at that time. However, Children's Hospital was quite receptive, and the affiliation was established in

1953. We were fortunate to have some money given then to the Judge Baker, and we moved to the Longwood Avenue area, across from Children's Hospital.

Before that, child psychiatry at Children's Hospital began, as far as psychoanalysis goes, with Dr. Lydia Dawes. Dr. Dawes was the first analyst on the staff, under Dr. Carruthers, and she continued for many years in an unpaid position, establishing a good rapport with the pediatricians and neurologists. There had already been good groundwork established there, not only through Dr. Dawes but also through other students who had been there with her, particularly Dr. Dane Prugh, who is now in Colorado. Dane Prugh, if I remember correctly, was an analysand and student of Dr. Grete Bibring. She can correct me if I'm wrong. (People didn't usually divulge who their analyst was in those days; there was something highly secret about it.) Dane had established a decent department, and had a training program going, when the Judge Baker came as an affiliate across the street. From then on things developed; analysis of children developed; we had our child analysis hours; we had our seminars and case presentations.

This, in general, is the background of my association with the Boston Psychoanalytic Institute. However, I want you to know that I was once an officer of the Boston society-institute; for four years I was vice president, but I never made the presidency. Dr. Felix Deutsch was president, and my job, as I saw it, was to keep Felix healthy so that I wouldn't have to take over the onerous job of being president, because those were tumultuous times, shall we say. Everything came out all right in the end, in large part due to the fact that Felix kept healthy. Thank you very much.

DR. FLORENCE CLOTHIER: In regard to the early days of child analysis in Boston, I particularly remember Erik Erikson. I think the first continuing case in his seminar was one of my cases—a little girl named Margot Johnson who lived with a real, wicked, and cruel stepmother and was alternately withdrawn and aggressively hostile. Erik guided me through the resolution of Margot's transference onto me of her relationship to her stepmother. For almost a year she remained at the New England Home for Little Wanderers, where I was then the staff psychiatrist. Eventually she was successfully placed in a foster home. I have never been sure whether the major credit should have gone to her therapy or to the foster family, probably both. Erik remained in the Boston area only for a few years, but I believe he had planned to stay. He talked of setting up a program of working with small children and seeing them on a regular periodic basis, much as a dentist carries out his prophylactic work. If, in these play sessions or in interviews with the mother, he detected cause for alarm he would be in a position to avert trouble before attitudes, symptoms, or behavior became crystallized. He discussed with me whether it would be possible to make an annual charge for trying to prevent problems. If they occurred, he would conduct therapy without charge. It seemed to me an innovative idea but was never carried out. He did see in play sessions a number of normal young children, including my oldest son, now forty-one, but then of kindergarten-age. I believe that his early paper, "Configurations of Play," published in the *Psychoanalytic Quarterly,* was based on these play sessions.

DR. GARDNER: Thank you, Florence, for mentioning that; I'm sorry that I did not mention his name. When Erik Erikson was here, I was still a medical student. I can state immodestly, however, that Dr. Erikson's appointment at Harvard, a permanent professorship, was initiated by me. It was engineered by others, but initiated by me, so that takes care of the fact that I forgot to mention him.

At this point I would like to involve the audience, which has been so faithful in listening. We would like to get on record, if possible, any data, anecdote, or experience pertinent to the Boston Psychoanalytic Society and Institute. I will take the liberty, at this point, of calling on Betty Cobb.

MRS. ELIZABETH COBB HALL: I would like to tell the story, that some of you may have heard, about Stanley and the Harvard Tercentenary Committee. In deciding on honarary speakers, Stanley suggested Sigmund Freud but others suggested C.G. Jung. Finally Jung, not Freud, was invited. Then we were asked to invite Jung to stay with us, and it was quite an experience. It must have been four or five days. I remember particularly the night before he was to receive an honorary degree, and he had to hire a top hat and tails. It seemed to me he spent the evening before prancing in front of the hall mirror with his dress clothes on. But the particular story was when Stanley took Jung into his clinic—I believe it was told as if it happened in front of the whole Tercentenary audience, but that was not true—and in front of his clinic Stanley introduced him as Dr. Freud.

DR. GARDNER: Thank you, Betty, very much. Now I would like to call on Dr. Valenstein.

DR. VALENSTEIN: This is an extraordinary experience, to sit here and feel earlier parts of one's life, one's prehistory which one didn't know about, dovetail into where one begins in Boston. I came here in 1939, to the Boston Psychopathic Hospital, and I'll start a little bit with Macfie, whom I can see in my mind's eye just as clearly as his white jacket and his highly flushed forehead and neck, walking behind him on rounds. I was there for two years. I came for my psychiatric residency, and then he invited me back to be chief of service. By that time I had become reasonably adept at the thumbnail case presentation or I shouldn't have been invited back.

I think there are answers to the paradox of what he was like, and why people speak on both sides about him. There are those who remember him with a great deal of appreciation, as an extraordinarily important and stimulating man in their careers. And there are those who thought that somehow he didn't leave his mark, or that he stood even as a detriment. He was, in a sense both. You see, I came at the end of his career and he was older and, I think, a changed man. It was no secret. I learned a lot from Esther Cook, who had been there for many years. She talked about the halcyon days of the Boston Psychopathic when things were—I wouldn't say gemütlich—more friendly, in a way. He had given up his teas, for one thing. His wife had died and he'd been dependent on her and on the family. It was thought that he'd had a depression, but because he was a very formal, prideful man, a very correct man, I suppose he hadn't acknowledged it and simply retreated even further into his formalistic character. He was a paradox. I ended up with an ambivalent feeling because, on the one hand, he was a model. He was a professor-scholar. He knew the library like no one else. His office opened into the library and in his spare time he would go and open all the books. He was in no sense an entrepreneur. He was not a corporate man and at that time, fortunately—or maybe unfortunately—he wasn't tempted to expand psychiatry into the extraordinary panacea-like position, as it came to have.

I remember that it was a rigorous training in clinical perspicuity, in the careful and indefatigable doing of the mental status and in the recording of it, so that we became exactingly observant. Campbell could be quite brusque and quite sharp on rounds if you weren't on your toes; it was important to learn how to be nimble. Once when I was chief of service, I think one of the juniors was flustered and obviously fuzzy, which got us all restless. He described his patient as being bewildered and Macfie turned on him and said, "Be careful not to construe your bewilderment into the patient's expression."

One more word about him and then I'll come to something about analysis which I think may be relevant. I started in 1946, in uniform still. There was something about the atmosphere that those of us who came fresh out of the military, terribly enthusiastic and terribly needful, found in analysis. Macfie would make rounds exactly at 11, in a fresh white coat, very trim and correct, in his somewhat *geheimrat* fashion. He wasn't German but he was very correct, and he would interview every patient. I don't doubt that he was enormously interested in man in general and extraordinarily knowledgeable. But he was on the other hand, I would say, limitedly empathic. He was empathic, but it had what we would today call a certain out-of-it quality. While he was interested in humanity, there was something lacking in his empathic immediacy for patients. This would explain, I think, why he could be open to analysis as a scholarly tradition (and he probably knew a great deal from his reading in the early days), but at the same time he could have his reservations about the personal experience of analysis, the transference in the clinical sense.

We were interested in analysis by that time, but we weren't a large group. To go into psychiatry was suspect, of course. Either you were a missed divinity student or some kind of a crackpot. Nonetheless, if you dared and went into psychiatry from medical school, there was a certain frustration. For what do you do after you've magnificently classified all those people, which we did endlessly, day after day? I began to have the feeling, as did a few others, I think, that if this was all there was to psychiatry, I'd better take up plumbing. We were curious about analysis, and there were murmurs about some kind of an institute in town. I thought it must be like a masonic order, because there was a feeling of barriers. I well remember one breakthrough, which was, I think, exceedingly important. Mo Kaufman gave an elective in medical psychotherapy, and on some evenings gave lectures at the Psychopathic. Somehow it was exciting. Not everybody came, and those who did had the feeling that here was somebody who thinks beyond Kraepelinian classification, and thinks of human beings and of patients from another point of view. It was just a taste, mind you. We stumbled onto trying to have our own seminar, which didn't get very far. Helen Tartakoff was there, the war had just begun, and I wanted very much to have some exposure to analysis. I had heard there were seminars, and you, Helen, were going to them and also having some ritualistic daily meeting with your control case, back in some curious room on the corridor, which was all very unusual and protected, so that one wondered what went on. I wanted so much to come to the seminars and I asked if some of us who were interested could come. She tried in her nicest way to explain that there were, well, certain formal procedures, and that it just wasn't permitted. I found this very frustrating, and somehow a paradox, that someone who was interested couldn't come. I think you'd said some thing about how one had to work through one's resistances, goodness knows what. In any case, it didn't happen.

Now let me take it another way. It was felt that Macfie was, in a certain sense, a marvelous example of a true professor and scholar. On the other hand, there was the frustration that one couldn't quite reach him and that he no longer reached out to his residents. The Commonwealth Fellowships were a thing of the past. There was the time when one could either hope to go to Queens Square for neurology or for an analysis perhaps to Vienna. By that time, however, Campbell was down on it and, if one went so far as to ask, he was discouraging and reluctant to allow time to be taken.

Let me take it beyond the war a bit. Many of us were in the service, and there, of course, the analyst and the analytic point of view had something to offer that excited all of us who didn't have it. Some of us had had some exposure to the air force program, or to other military psychiatry programs, and we came back already inquiring about where to get analytic training. Finding the money seemed an impediment, but there was no suggestion, as yet, that this would mean prestige or money or patients. The joke was—I think Edward Bibring once told it—"The difference between analysis before and after the war is this: before the war the analyst chased the patients, and after the war the patients chased the analysts." We didn't know that yet, and we didn't know it would be as rewarding as it was in those two decades, 1945 to 1965. It may be fortunate, in some ways, that analysis has lost some of its charisma and golden frame. We had come back very excited, because there was something new to explore. There was some intimation that analysis might be the way, was the keystone to the arch.

The early seminars and training gave us an enormous sense of fulfillment. We took up the slack that was left by the physiological approach of Adolf Meyer and Macfie Campbell. Nobody resented it when I started. Even the formalistic requirements, I didn't think much about. When I was accepted by the institute, I was still in uniform but on terminal leave, and I didn't know how to choose an analyst. I asked one or another of my acquaintances who knew analysis, whom shall I go to? And one person said, "Maybe you should go to someone who does ego-analysis." I didn't know what that meant. But I was aware of certain possibilities and directions rather than others. Let me give you an example. It was an experience with an early control case, supervised by one of the senior, marvelous clinicians. I began to talk about my patient defending himself this way and that way, and using this and that defense, and was met with: "Why do you say defense? You mean the patient resisted." So I said, "Yes, the patient resists," and I soon learned that if I meant defense I should say resistance. I soon gave up the word defense, and always spoke of the patient's resistance.

It has been a day of very amiable reminiscences. There is a great deal which is enormously satisfying about the institute—it stayed together, even though there were things that weren't altogether smooth, from a scientific point of view and, of course, there were other currents. I think I'll leave it there. Thank you.

DR. GARDNER: Thank you very much, Val. As I mentioned at the beginning, I'm anxious to hear from everyone with something to contribute. I'm also interested in the institutions and the effects of psychoanalytic personnel on the institutions. We have not heard from the Peter Bent Brigham Hospital, and I'd like to call on Henry Fox to tell us something about the introduction of psychoanalytic concepts at the Brigham and what has happened since.

DR. FOX: I think the work at the Brigham is an example of the many ways in which Boston analysts have contributed to areas outside the immediate psychoanalytic situation. I myself am a training analyst, but at the Peter Bent Brigham our idea was not to train nonpsychiatrists to be analysts, but somehow to share with them the kinds of insights, the things that we had learned through analysis, which they could use in their everyday work with patients. I can't help but give some of my own background to going there, because it has a bearing on what I have tried for twenty-five years to do in a general hospital. I went to Harvard College, where I was particularly interested in William James. Then I decided that I couldn't be a philosopher because I liked to work with people, and I picked Johns Hopkins because Adolf Meyer was there.

I do feel that in the discussion so far, both William James and Adolf Meyer have been rather underplayed. People have said that Henry James wrote novels like a psychologist but that William James wrote psychology like a novelist. Certainly, William James had the vigor and breadth and the pragmatic approach that interested us all.

But when I went to Johns Hopkins and worked with Adolf Meyer—I found that my own background fitted in, in an extraordinary way, with his. I think this had something to do with the way in which psychoanalysis was received in the United States. It had a more enthusiastic reception here than in Europe.

Dr. Valenstein spoke of the Kraepelinian approach; this is one thing that Dr. Meyer himself always tried hard to combat. He was not interested in disease syndromes; he was interested in the flexibility of people. Coming from Switzerland, it was natural for Adolph Meyer to think in terms of families and the canton, what they were like, and what kind of experiences they had during their lives, instead of trying to classify them using the Kraepelinian system.

I worked with Adolf Meyer for six or seven years at Johns Hopkins. I became his chief resident, then assistant professor. He was a great figure, a great teacher for me. Eventually, I felt it might not be a bad idea if I looked into psychoanalysis a little. As you know, Meyer was one of the founding members of the American Psychoanalytic Society, but he never became an analyst himself. There was a somewhat reserved quality about him that went all the way through his work. I had my office next to his at the Phipps Clinic, and I went to see him one day. I said, "You know, Dr. Meyer, I'm wondering whether it mightn't be a good idea for me to be analyzed." He looked at me for awhile and said, "Do you have a girl friend?" and I said "Yes." He said, "Well, what would she think of your being analyzed?" "Well, I don't think she'd like it very much," I replied. "Well, there you are," he said.

So I didn't. I went overseas, in charge of psychiatry for the Hopkins unit, but, as Dr. Valenstein has said, we all became tremendously interested in the experiences that the ordinary person has and in the way he reacts. We got far beyond any set disease categories. When I came back to this country, I was invited by George Thorn to come [to the Brigham] and help him out with psychiatry. I got the letter as I was leaving the Philippines, and so I came.

My idea was to work within the department of medicine as much as possible, and that's what I've tried to do all along. It was challenging and difficult, and after awhile I decided that it was so difficult that maybe it would be a good idea if I had a little analysis myself. While I was in the Philippines, a man was sent by the government to investigate what we were doing in psychiatry. His name, I think, was John Murray, and I rather liked him, even though I resented somebody sent to quiz us. When I came to Boston and found he was in Boston, I thought he might be the person to have an analysis with. Then the question of becoming a member of the institute arose. Why not work there? I didn't see any point in it but thought I might as well. I thought you could get a cheaper analysis that way too, with the government helping to pay for it. So that is what I did.

Aside from a certain—I hope—modification of my own narcissism, which is a specialty of any analyst, I was particularly interested in the kind of things that Dr. Meyer had left out at Hopkins. They were, specifically, the transference and counter-transference, as well as the primary and secondary process, I mean the primitive and the less primitive. These were the main things, the main issues, which had to be dealt with in a general hospital, and in teaching people who were not psychiatrists. I think that is the kind of thing we have been working with all along, and still try to work with, to help the nonpsychiatrist to be a little more aware of his patients and how he feels toward them. Also to be aware in a more immediate way of what patients feel toward the doctor, and to take this into account. I think we've only started on what's known as psychosomatic medicine, which I learned so much about from Felix Deutsch. The whole business of body language, what it means in primitive terms, still requires a tremendous amount of exploration. We haven't yet begun to find out what that can mean, in understanding the causes of illness and the way illness must be treated.

DR. GARDNER: Thank you very much, Henry, for that contribution. Dr. Valenstein alluded to military experiences, and I think we should get some highlights on the impact of psychoanalysis on the military, and vice versa. I'd like to have Dr. Murray comment on that.

DR. MURRAY: Dr. Valenstein has mentioned the tremendous impact that the war experience made on younger physicians who were connected with the military, and who got a firsthand experience with the psychiatrists in the military who had psychoanalytic backgrounds. There is no doubt that the impetus of war gave psychoanalysis a tremendous boost. When we came back from the war, there were so many people eager for psychoanalytic training because of what they had seen during the war. There were a great many people who contributed to this impact of Freudian psychology on the etiology of neuroses, psychosomatic disorders, character pathology, and what have you. Some were consultants, some were military-area consultants; others were connected with units in the field.

Three people in particular stand out. The first one is Roy Grinker. The second one is Mo Kaufman. And, if you will permit me, the third one is myself. I'm a little embarrassed to say this, but as Mo said, we'll stick to the facts. First let's take Mo. Mo went down to Atlanta and set up a preparation course for psychiatrists who were going into the military, based upon his psychoanalytic background. This had a great impact on those people who were participants. Even after he left, and Colonel Porter took over, what Mo had planted there was carried on. Again, Mo made another important contribution in the South Pacific, through his firsthand contact with the immediate anxiety-producing situation of combat, and the manner in which he handled it. This spread around among the military personnel and again reflected the importance of psychoanalytic thinking.

While I was chief psychiatrist in the air force, with headquarters in the Pentagon, I received a manuscript from North Africa written by Roy Grinker and John Spiegel, *War Neuroses in North Africa, The Tunisian Campaign*. This was published after the war under the heading of *Men Under Stress*. The book came into the air surgeon's office and I recommended its publication. My boss, Major General David N.W. Grant, said "No, this book can't be published." When I asked why not, he said, "Well, in the first place, it's critical of the air force. In the second place, how do we know that some of these case histories won't be presented over the radio the way Orson Welles did, creating the same kind of a panic state that Orson Welles's program did? And, in the third place, the Army and Navy Press has so many publications ahead of it that it can't be published for eighteen months. Why do you want it published?" I said, "Because this book presents the fact that the psychological impact of traumatic events can be just as important an etiological factor in disease as bacterial invasions, new growths, and what have you. As I go out and make contact with the various hospitals, the doctors are just hungry for the facts that this book of Grinker's and Spiegel's presents. As for publication, I'll just go to my very good friend, Frank Fremont-Smith, who is medical director of the Macy Foundation, and he will publish that book for us."

To continue, I said to Grant, "We'll classify it, so that it won't be broadcast over the radio, and I will edit the book and take out all the critical remarks about the air force." General Grant said "All right, I give in." And so the book was published, and 45,000 copies were distributed. It had a tremendous impact on the psychoanalytic implications of anxiety states.

Now we come to Murray's contribution. It was my idea, when I went in the service, that flying personnel would suffer from their war experiences and would need definitive treatment when they returned to this country. This idea was not well received by my superiors in the air force, but I worked under Colonel Paul Holbrook who was in full agreement with this. So we were able to set up, as Val mentioned, the hospital in St. Petersburg, Florida, where I sent Roy Grinker to set up his techniques of treatment. We had a number of these convalescent hospitals in the air force, which gave treatment to those returning with what we call flying fatigue, or war neurosis, treatment that was based on psychoanalytic concepts of the origin of neurotic illness. I think these were the things that spread diffusely through the service and were responsible for what Val has mentioned, the tremendous upsurge in the interest in Freudian psychology that followed after the war and gave such a boost to analytic training at that time.

DR. GARDNER: Thank you very much, John. Dr. Kaufman would like a few words.

DR. KAUFMAN: There are a number of things I think must be emphasized that analysts did in the military service. There was no analysis, as such, in the service, but we did demonstrate how an analytically trained psychiatrist could meet certain situations, from the individual at an airfield in the States to an individual who was under combat conditions and suffering from a war neurosis. This also demonstrated what Henry was talking about, mainly, that the ordinary medical officer who was not a psychiatrist, who might have been completely out of sympathy with psychiatry, nevertheless did the job when there was a job to be done. He saw it work, and it awakened his enthusiasm, and there was this tremendous surge of interest. God works in very wide fashion with limited means. As it happened, when I first decided to get into the service, General Hillman, who was chief of professional services, promised me that the first overseas assignment would be mine. My wife Betty never knew this. We went down to Atlanta, and we set up a school with a very simple idea. We were going to take the civilian psychiatrists who enlisted, put them through one month's service, and orient them to the problems they were going to meet as military psychiatrists.

One day, about ten months later, after we had found a house with a leaky cesspool in Atlanta, I got my orders to go overseas. I was ordered to report within ten days, but they didn't know my wife. She said, "To hell with you. We've come down to Atlanta. We've moved down, bag and baggage, twenty-eight cases of books among other things, and they aren't going to order my husband overseas in ten days." So she called Washington. Fortunately Halloran was the chief and we knew him, so my target date to go overseas was delayed. Then I rushed to San Francisco to go overseas, but I spent three delightful weeks, mostly with Jake Kasanin at Fort Mason, because the boat needed the engines fixed. It was October 26 when I arrived in the South Pacific, at New Caledonia, I remember. I knew the names of the other consultants, because they had been picked from Hopkins and Yale, but they weren't all there. After about two days, when our surgeon, General Maxwell, decided that I'd been cleared, he told me, "They're going up on a campaign." The only reading matter I had was the book that Jock was talking about. This was about the treatment of combat conditions in Africa, in Tunisia. I found out twenty years later that these were acute combat reactions who had been flown 500 miles from the combat situation. Most of you are familiar with that book. It talked about the use of sodium pentothal, so the only thing I took was as much sodium pentothal and benzedrine as I could get aboard the plane, and hit for Guadalcanal, which was our staging area. Eventually we landed in Bougainville, I hunted around, and asked if there was a psychiatrist with the division. Finally the surgeon of the division directed me to him. He was a battalion-aid surgeon, actually. Being a psychiatrist, he was assigned to a battalion aid station. He took me right in and set up a program of treatment. We used sodium pentothal. Then, very fortunately, one day I filled up a syringe and, before I had an opportunity to push the plunger (I still don't know how to find a vein), the patient was already reacting as if I'd given him the sodium pentothal. So I said, "To hell with this, what do I have to waste sodium pentothal for?" So we started to use hypnosis.

Fortunately, once you left the United States you had no responsibility. You didn't have to do a damned thing they had told you to do in the States, which was a very good thing, depending, of course, on who the surgeon of that area was, because he had complete control. Our surgeon was General Maxwell who, in civilian life, was "Regular Army." He was a nose and throat man, he didn't know very much, and he let me do what I wanted.

As a result of this experience, we were able to set up a total program for the whole theater. The group was made up of three units, the Colorado, the Yale, and the Harvard units, to begin with. We were able to do a job for which psychiatry, out of all the medical specialties, was particularly fit and could take the whole situation in. This was a demonstration of psychiatry in action, and I'm very proud of the fact that I was part of it. This excited even the surgeons, by the way we set up schools and were able to do all kinds of things. We succeeded because we had sufficient knowledge that we could transmit in a way that the medical officers could understand. We weren't just magicians, we were doing something practical. I think this was a tremendously important factor in the large number of doctors who were in the service and became trained in psychiatry before going back to private practice.

DR. GARDNER: Thank you, Mo. Dr. Semrad has requested time for a few remarks. You get these old servicemen going and there's no end to it. Wait till I tell you about the navy.

DR. SEMRAD: I never did get overseas, but, as one of my assignments, I was exiled to Georgia for some time, where I had a mental hygiene clinic and was a psychiatrist to an infantry training center. To emphasize the value of a psychodynamic, analytic orientation, let me tell you about a problem that existed there. The general told me that he had 500 men in the compound who had been overseas, who had good service records, had rank, but couldn't function as training cadre. They had all sorts of neurotic reactions, startle-reactions, a whole series of reactions. The general asked, what could I do about it. I said, "I don't know." Those three words have saved me so many times. I went down to my clinic and talked with my chief personnel consultant, Dr. Donald McNassor, who had worked with Fritz Redl at Wayne State University. He was a teacher by training and he said, "Let's put them in groups." How were we to do that? What did you do in groups? Well, we'd find out. We tossed it around a bit and decided that we could probably face fifteen men at a time. There were groups in the morning, groups in the afternoon, groups in the evening. McNassor took half of them, I took half of them, and we learned. It was very exciting to see these unhappy, anxious, troubled men walk away from the group meetings together, to go to the Enlisted Men's Club, to socialize and exchange their war experience. The first thing you knew, they were back in the training center in cadre positions. This was also the time of the Battle of the Bulge, when the demand for training cadre was very great.

I thought that this was a terrific tool for helping people get over difficulties. Of course, I didn't realize at that time that I was dealing with healthy men who were just overburdened. This was to be learned later, as was so often the experience in the observations of the men in the service.

One day we had a visitor from the surgeon general's office. He stayed one day, he stayed two days, he stayed three days. He went down to the battalions and on the third day he said to me, "You know why I'm here?" I said, "I haven't the slightest idea." To myself I was wondering what did I do that I shouldn't have done. He said "Well, we got a report through Command that there was a successful experiment here, and I was sent out to find out if you were a charlatan or not." In this instance again psychoanalysis showed its usefulness.

DR. GARDNER: Thank you, Elvin. Dr. Kaufman tells me that for those interested in the history of psychiatry in the military service, a book is about to come out. At this point I would like to ask who wishes to volunteer information about psychoanalysis in Boston, of a personal nature or related to any of the institutions in which psychoanalysts have practiced in the last forty years.

BARBARA ROSS: In his own circles, I would guess, George Gardner is not usually seen as the man of wisdom that he is in the teaching of academic psychology. His course at the University of Massachusetts, Boston, on Psychopathology in Childhood, Normal and Abnormal, is absolutely one of the most popular, one of the most profitable experiences for our undergraduates over the last few years. This is simply another instutional note I wanted to add.

DR. GARDNER: After that, as Mo Kaufman said, I should close the meeting while I'm ahead. Thank you very much, Dr. Ross. And now, Dr. Weinberger.

DR. WEINBERGER: During the war, I was with Dr. Kolb in Atlanta as a part of my tour of duty, but after the war, we all got our Commonwealth Fellowships through the VA. I think the VA should be mentioned here, as a great training center for so many of our psychiatrists who went into analysis. At the Boston VA clinic there was: Phil Gates, Arthur Valenstein, Morrie Adler, Martin Berezin, and any number of us. At the VA hospital there was Bill Murphy, and so on. The Veterans Administration did a great job taking us in, when we couldn't go back to the state hospital system. They gave us refuge and enabled us to get analytic training. Thank you.

DR. GARDNER: Is there anyone else who wishes to make any remarks? One aspect that has not been touched by this symposium will have to be done by an individual investigator, to make the record complete. That would be an extensive overview of the research contributions of the psychoanalysts of Boston in the past half century. I think this should be mentioned here, to be added to the records of our profession and the institutions in which we served. At this point I'll call on Dr. Sanford Gifford.

DR. SANFORD GIFFORD: I hadn't planned to close the discussion. I have enjoyed listening quietly to our members who have given us their early experiences, so openly, frankly, and good-humoredly. But I have a couple of thoughts brought to mind by the last discussion.

One is Dr. Kaufman's mention of Dr. Jacob Kasanin, which brings to mind a correspondence I've come across between him and Dr. Hendrick. This was an exchange of letters after Dr. Kasanin had left Boston for Chicago, to continue his analytic work at Michael Reese Hospital. In this correspondence, Dr. Hendrick confided his distress about the birth pangs of the institute, and questioned the drastic reorganization of the society, which took place at the expense of so many hurt feelings.

Later, Dr. Kasanin went to San Francisco. And there I encountered psychoanalysis for the second time, in the study group that Dr. Kasanin held at his house once a month. In Dr. Dalrymple's reminiscences, Dr. Coriat's study group reminded me of the meetings at Dr. Kasanin's house, not that we sat at his feet. We were like the group that met at Dr. Coriat's in the 1920s, because everyone who was interested in analysis was invited, from his own residents, medical students, to almost anyone in the city. There were about ten or fifteen people usually. We read *Totem and Taboo* and other things, and discussed them. Since I attended Dr. Kasanin's meetings in 1942, this brings me somehow within the scope of this symposium.

The other thing I wanted to comment on was a sub-theme that kept recurring during the discussion, one that I hadn't really expected—what might be called the economic interpretation of psychoanalytic history, the theme of people living on $25 a month or $1800 a year. It even occurred to me that this partly answers one question that we had posed in putting this meeting together. Was there something special about the

Boston scene that made the medical orientation of analysis stronger here than in other cities?—studies by Michaels and Levin in the 1950s, pointed out the extent to which Boston analysts held hospital and university positions. The economic theme that came out today gives a simple answer: that it was necessary to take jobs in hospitals in order to support one's analytic training. This is a simpler answer, than looking for continuities from the days of James Jackson Putnam, seeking some connection between the early traditions of medical psychotherapy in Boston and the receptiveness of Boston to analysis. I throw this out just from my offhand impressions of what has been said. And, in closing, I'd like to thank everyone who participated, the audience as well as the speakers, the discussants and the members of the panel.

DR. GARDNER: Thank you, Dr. Gifford. And with that I declare the symposium closed.

References

* M.R. Sharaff, D.J. Levenson, and M. Greenblatt, "The Psychiatric Alumni of 'Psycho,'" presented at the semicentenary, Massachusetts Mental Health Center, 1962.

† E.V. Semrad, *Psychoanalysis, Boston 1968*. Presented on the occasion of the thirty-fifth anniversary of the Boston Psychoanalytic Society and Institute, at a joint meeting with the Western New England Psychoanalytic Society, MIT Faculty Club, October 26, 1968.

Illustrations

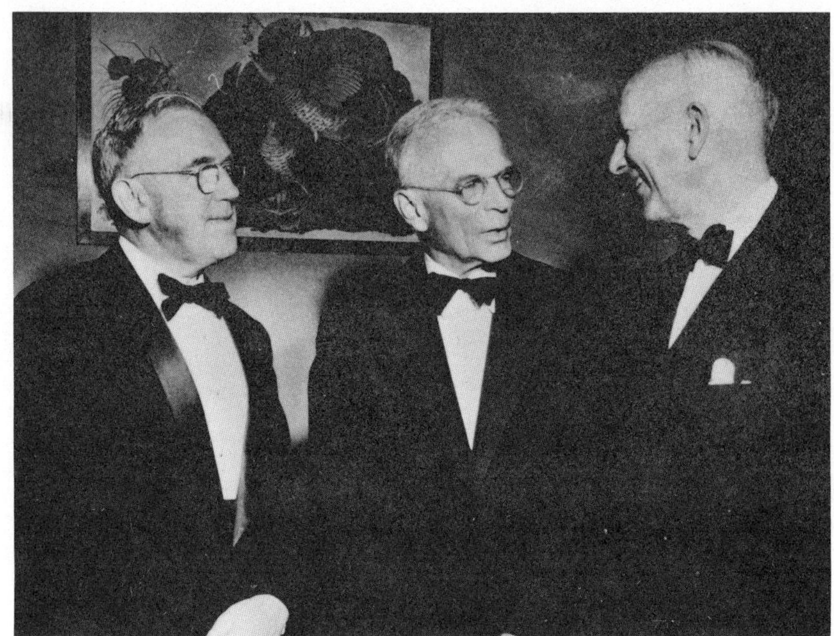

33. Photograph taken in 1960 at the twenty-fifth anniversary of the Massachusetts General Hospital psychiatric service. This psychiatric service, the first set up in a general hospital in 1934, was established by Stanley Cobb. *From left to right:* Erich Lindemann, Stanley Cobb, and Frank Fremont-Smith. *Archives of the Boston Psychoanalytic Society and Institute.*

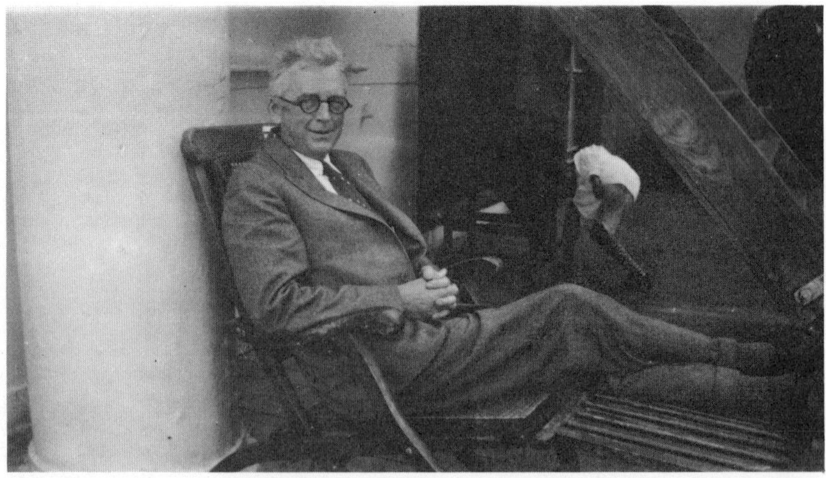

34. Martin W. Peck, Ile de France, August 1929, returning from the International Psychoanalytic Conference in London. *Archives of the Boston Psychoanalytic Society and Institute.*

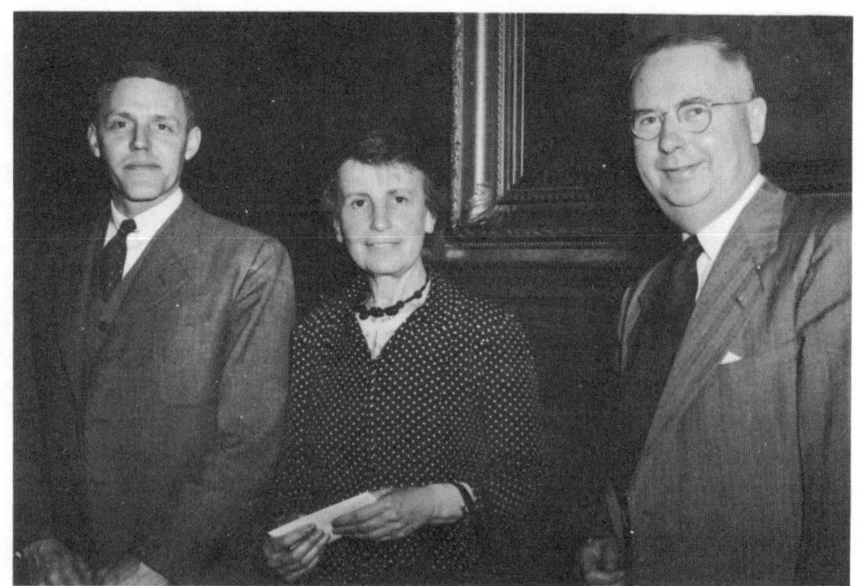

35. Photograph taken in April 1950 at the Judge Baker Guidance Center. *Left to right:* Phillip Adler, chairman, board of trustees, Anna Freud, and George E. Gardner, director of the Judge Baker Guidance Center. *Courtesy of Nancy Staver, Judge Baker Guidance Center.*

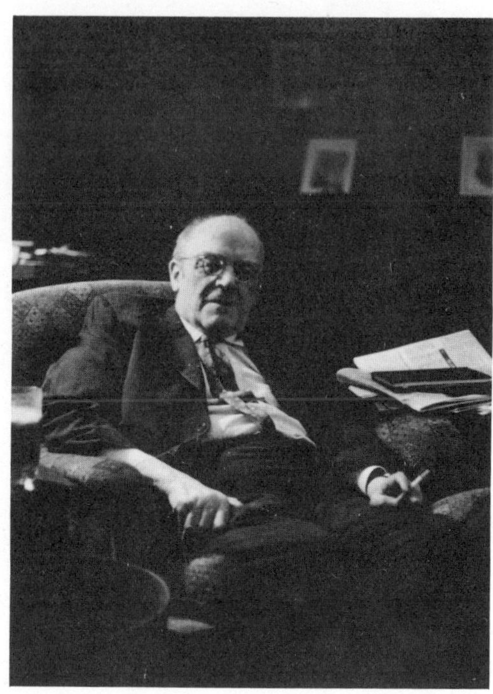

36. Ives Hendrick in the late 1960s. *Archives of the Boston Psychoanalytic Society and Institute.*

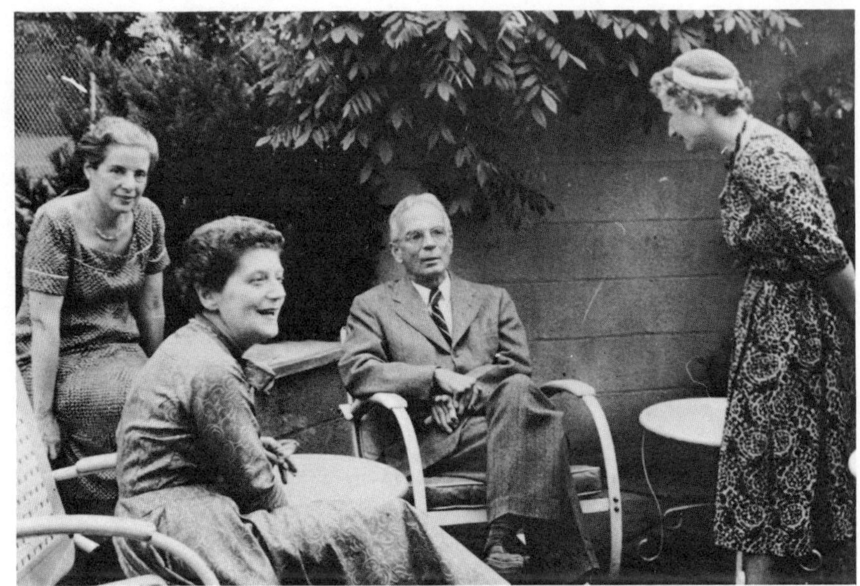

37. *Left to right:* Elizabeth Zetzel, Lucie Jessner, Stanley Cobb, and Eleanor Pavenstedt in the early 1950s. *Courtesy of Mrs. Elizabeth Cobb Hall.*

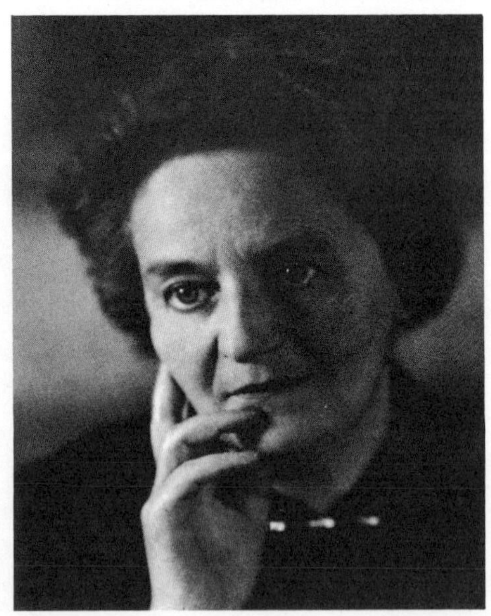

38. Helene Deutsch in the early 1930s. *Archives of the Boston Psychoanalytic Society and Institute.*

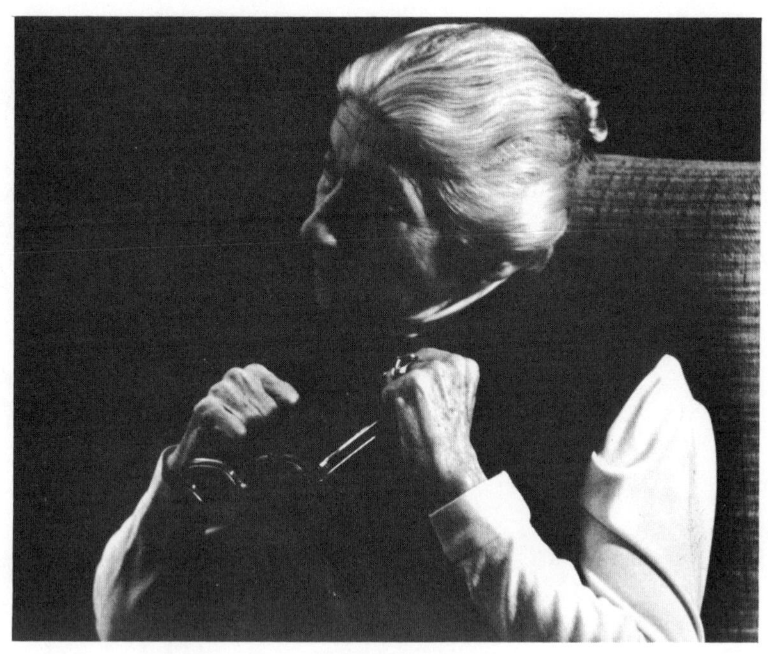

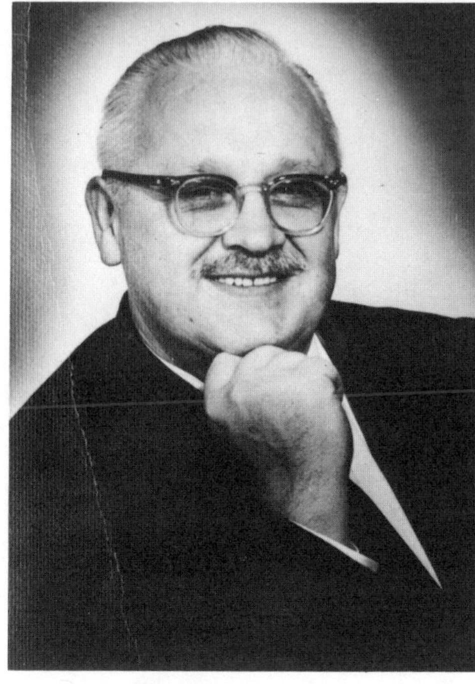

39. Grete Bibring, 1974. *Rick Stafford, photographer,* Harvard Gazette.

40. Elvin Semrad, 1970. *Courtesy of Mrs. Elvin Semrad.*

Contributors

1. DANIEL AARON, Ph.D., is a professor in the English department of Harvard University. His most recent work is the *Unwritten War: American Writers and The Civil War* (Knopf, 1973).
2. BARBARA ROSS, Ph.D., is associate professor of psychology, University of Massachusetts at Boston. She has published primarily on the history of psychology. She is editor of the *Journal of the History of the Behavioral Sciences.*
3. DOROTHY ROSS, Ph.D., is assistant professor of history and John and Buellah Rollins Bicentennial Preceptor, Princeton University. She is author of *G. Stanley Hall: The Psychologist as Prophet* (University of Chicago Press, 1972).
4. DAVID SHAKOW, Ph.D., is senior research psychologist, National Institute of Mental Health. He was chief psychologist and director of psychological research, Worcester State Hospital, 1928–1946.
5. HENRI F. ELLENBERGER, M.D., is professor, department of criminology, University of Montreal, and psychiatrist at the Hôtel-Dieu Hospital, Montreal. He is the author of the *Discovery of the Unconscious: The History and Evolution of Dynamic Psychiatry* (Basic Books, 1970).
6. JULIUS SILBERGER, JR., M.D., is assistant clinical professor of psychology, Harvard Medical School. He is at work on a biography of Mary Baker Eddy.
7. SANFORD R. GIFFORD, JR., M.D., is associate clinical professor of psychiatry, Harvard Medical School, and librarian of the Boston Psychoanalytic Society and Institute.
8. NORMAN DAIN, Ph.D., is professor of history at Rutgers University (Newark), and research associate, department of psychiatry, Cornell University Medical College. He has authored, *Concepts of Insanity in the United States, 1789–1865* and *Disordered Minds: The First Century of Eastern State Hospital in Williamsburg, Virginia, 1766–1866*. He is currently completing a biography of Clifford W. Beers.
9. EUNICE ALLAN, D.S.W., has been professor of social work, director of treatment methods, and clinical coordinator in the program of advanced study, Smith College School for Social Work, since 1949. From 1943 to 1949 she was chief of psychiatric social service, Massachusetts General Hospital.
10. NATHAN G. HALE, JR., Ph.D., is associate professor of history at the

University of California, Riverside. He is author of *James Jackson Putnam and Psychoanalysis* (Harvard University Press, 1971) and *Freud and the Americans: The Beginnings of Psychoanalysis in the United States, 1876–1917* (Oxford University Press, 1971).

11. OTTO MARX, M.D., was professor of psychiatry at Boston University School of Medicine, who, in 1969, was a visiting professor of medical history at Harvard University. Presently he is psychiatrist at the Veterans Administration Hospital in Palo Alto, California.

12. BARBARA SICHERMAN, Ph.D., was from 1967 to 1973 assistant professor of history at Manhattanville College. Formerly a Fellow of the Radcliffe Institute, she is now editor of *Notable American Women*, Radcliffe College.

13. ROBERT H. SHARPLEY, M.D., is clinical instructor in psychiatry at Harvard Medical School and president of the Solomon C. Fuller Institute.

14. JOHN C. BURNHAM, Ph.D., is professor of history and lecturer in psychiatry at Ohio State University. He is the author of *Psychoanalysis and American Medicine, 1894–1918: Medicine, Science, and Culture* (International Universities Press, 1967).

15. GEORGE E. GIFFORD, JR., M.D., is clinical instructor in psychiatry, consultant to the historical collections, Countway Library, Harvard Medical School; head, history of medicine section, and associate professor of socio-medical sciences, Boston University School of Medicine.

16. PAUL G. MYERSON, M.D., is professor, chairman of the department of psychiatry, Tufts University Medical School, and former president of the Boston Psychoanalytic Society and Institute. He is the son of Abraham Myerson, M.D.

17. GEORGE E. GARDNER, Ph.D., M.D., is professor of psychiatry, emeritus, Harvard Medical School. He was psychiatrist in chief at Children's Hospital Medical Center, 1947 to 1953.

18. EDGERTON MCC. HOWARD, M.D., was a staff member, 1941 to 1947; associate medical director and consultant, 1947 to the present; and chief of the clinic, 1946 to 1964 at the Austen Riggs Clinic.

19. BENJAMIN C. RIGGS, M.D., is a professor of psychiatry at the Medical University of South Carolina. He is the son of Austen Riggs, M.D.

20. MILTON GREENBLATT, M.D., is assistant dean, School of Medicine, and professor of psychiatry, University of California at Los Angeles, and chief of staff at the Veterans Administration Hospital, Brentwood, California. He was assistant superintendent and director of research and laboratories at the Boston Psychopathic Hospital from 1946 to

1963, professor of psychiatry at Tufts University from 1963 to 1973, and Commissioner, Massachusetts Department of Mental Health, from 1967 to 1973.

Moderators

Otto Marx and Sanford Gifford have been noted under Contributors. William Malamud is listed under Participating Invited Discussants.

21. JEANNE L. BRAND, Ph.D., is chief of the international programs, the division of the National Library of Medicine. Prior to this she was on the extramural programs of the National Institutes of Health. *Psychiatry and its History: Methodological Problems in Research* (Thomas, 1970) was co-edited by George Mora and Jeanne L. Brand.

Participating Invited Discussants

22. JOHN A. ABBOTT, M.D., a practicing psychiatrist, is on the Board of Consultation, Massachusetts General Hospital. A graduate of Harvard Medical School in 1931, he worked in Henry Murray's Harvard Psychology Clinic in 1936 and 1937, and was assistant resident during the first year of Stanley Cobb's psychiatry service at Massachusetts General Hospital.
23. S. SPAFFORD ACKERLY, M.D., is professor and chairman of the department of psychiatry, emeritus, at the University of Louisville, School of Medicine. His early training in psychiatry was at the Worcester State Hospital in the 1920s. He was an early staff member at the Judge Baker Guidance Center and was associated with the Boston Psychoanalytic Society and Institute in its very early years.
24. J. SANBOURNE BOCKOVEN, M.D., is superintendent of the Dr. Harry C. Solomon Mental Health Center in Lowell, Massachusetts, and area program director of the Lowell Mental Health Area. He is author of *Moral Treatment in American Psychiatry* (Springer, 1963) and *Moral Treatment in Community Mental Health* (Springer, 1972).
25. G. COLKET CANER, M.D., now retired from the private practice of psychiatry, was associate in neurology, Massachusetts General Hospital, and psychiatrist in the department of hygiene, Harvard University. He

was a friend of George A. Waterman, M.D.

26. The late JEAN A. CURRAN, M.D., was the former dean and professor of medical history, emeritus, State University of New York, Downstate Medical Center. He is the author of *Founders of Harvard Schools of Public Health, 1909–1946* (Josiah Macy, Jr., Foundation, 1970).

27. HENRY M. FOX, M.D., one of Adolph Meyer's last residents, is now physician emeritus, Peter Bent Brigham Hospital and clinical professor of psychiatry, emeritus, Harvard Medical School.

28. BARDWELL H. FLOWER, M.D., was Assistant Commissioner, Department of Mental Health, Commonwealth of Massachusetts from 1938 to 1941 and superintendent, Worcester State Hospital from 1941 to 1969. In 1970 he was awarded a D.Sc. honoris causa by Assumption College, Worcester, Massachusetts.

29. MRS. FRANCIS C. HALL (ELIZABETH ALMY COBB HALL), the widow of Stanley Cobb, M.D., describes herself as "a self-made psychotherapist—with the aid and support of Stanley Cobb, Helene Deutsch, and Marian C. Putnam." She has been associated with the Judge Baker Guidance Center, the department of abnormal psychology with Dr. Henry Murray at Harvard University, the Boston City Hospital outpatient department with Dr. William Herman, The Shady Hill Growth Study, the Hecht House Nursery School since 1945, the James Jackson Putnam Child Guidance Center from 1943 to 1955, and the Cambridge Guidance Center from 1955 to 1967.

30. LESTON L. HAVENS, M.D., is professor of psychiatry, Massachusetts Mental Health Center, Harvard Medical School. He is author of *Approaches to the Mind—Movement of the Psychiatric School from Sects Toward Science* (Little Brown, 1973).

31. EDNA HEIDBREDER, Ph.D., is professor of psychology, emeritus, Wellesley College. She is author of *Seven Psychologics* (Appleton-Century-Crofts, 1933). *Historical Conceptions of Psychology* edited by Mary Henk, Jullian Jaynes and John Sullivan (Springer, 1973) is dedicated to her.

32. WILLIAM MALAMUD, SR., M.D., was professor of psychiatry at Tufts College Medical School from 1939 to 1946, chairman of the department, and professor of psychiatry at the Boston University School of Medicine from 1946 to 1958. He is author of *History of Psychiatric Therapies: One Hundred Years of American Psychiatry* (Columbia University Press, 1944).

33. The late JOHN A.P. MILLET, M.D., was professor of psychiatry and assistant dean, New York School of Psychiatry from 1959 to 1964, and a professor emeritus at the time of his death. A graduate of the Harvard Medical School in 1914, he became "Assistant in the Nerve Room" at

Massachusetts General Hospital that same year. He was physician to the Austen Riggs Foundation from 1923 to 1930.

34. CHARLES PINDERHUGES, M.D., is professor of psychiatry at Boston University School of Medicine, and lecturer at Harvard Medical School. A practicing psychoanalyst, he is director of psychiatric research at the Boston Veterans Administration Hospital. He is a member of the Board of Directors of the Solomon C. Fuller Institute.

35. LILLIAN SALTMAN has a master's degree from the Simmons College of Social Work and is working on a dissertation, "Psychiatric Social Work and Society" as the final requirement for the degree of doctor of social welfare at the Columbia University School of Social Work.

36. ROBERT I. WATSON, Ph.D., was professor of psychology, University of New Hampshire. He is founder and past editor of the *Journal of the History of Behavioral Sciences* and author of the *Great Psychologists—Aristotle and Freud* (J.B. Lippincott, 1971). He is now adjunct professor of psychology, University of Florida at Gainesville.

Participants

S. Spafford Ackerly

Dr. Ackerly was born in 1895, in Brooklyn, New York, and attended Wesleyan University. He was wounded during military service in the United States Infantry (1917–1920) and completed his studies at Wesleyan in 1921. He studied medicine at Yale, where he first became friends with Ives Hendrick, and they both graduated in 1925. After interning at New York Hospital, he sought postgraduate training abroad, in London and Vienna, where he was analyzed by Dr. Alfred Adler and studied with Paul Schilder (1927–1928). He became clinical director at Worcester State Hospital in 1928, carried out research on delinquency with Drs. Healy and Bronner, and was a research associate at the Yale Institute of Human Relations (1930–1932). From 1932 until 1962 he was professor of psychiatry at the University of Louisville (Kentucky), and distinguished professor until his retirement in 1973, as more or less psychiatrist in residence. He is best known as a child psychiatrist, and for his influential role in initiating programs for training and research in child development. He belongs to the Orthopsychiatric Association, the Academy of Child Psychiatry, and other child study groups, as well as the American Academy of Psychoanalysis, the American Psychoanalytic Association, and the American Board of Psychiatry and Neurology.

Grete L. Bibring

The late Dr. Grete Lehner Bibring was born in 1899, in Vienna, the youngest of four children. Her family belonged to the Jewish *haute bourgeoisie*, free-thinking (*Konfessionslos*) and politically liberal, that played an important part in the intellectual life of the city, and in the history of psychoanalysis. Her father was a successful manufacturer and a man of cultivated tastes—a lifelong student of Hegel; one brother became an engineer and another brother a writer and theater critic. Dr. Bibring attended the "Humanistic Gymnasium for Girls," where her first interests were in Latin and Greek literature, then in botany, and finally in medicine. After her *baccalauréat* in 1918, she enrolled in the medical faculty of the University of Vienna, where her anatomical studies, under the celebrated Professor Julius Tandler, proved to be a passionate, deeply esthetic experience. In medical school she developed a lifelong interest in internal medicine and differential diagnosis.

Though she had read several of Freud's books at sixteen, when her curiosity was aroused by her *gymnasium* psychology class, her development as a psychoanalyst began during her first year of medical school. She was sitting between Edward Bibring and Wilhelm Reich in anatomy class, when a fellow student, Otto

Fenichel, announced a meeting for anyone interested in analysis. These four students formed a study group, reading Freud's papers together and attending meetings of the Vienna Psychoanalytic Society. She married Edward Bibring in 1922, and all four became members of the psychoanalytic society in 1924, the same year that Dr. Grete Bibring graduated from medical school. She had undertaken a didactic analysis with Herman Nunberg during medical school, and a *Nachanalyse* after several years as a practicing psychoanalyst. During the Nazi occupation of Austria in March 1938, she and her husband, who was then chairman of the Education Committee, helped many colleagues to leave the country. They then emigrated to London, with their two sons. After several years as members of the British Psychoanalytic Society, they emigrated to Boston in 1941, at the invitation of their Viennese colleagues, Jenny and Robert Waelder.

Edward Bibring held a part-time teaching position at Tufts Medical School, but he remained primarily a full-time analyst and one of the foremost teachers at the Boston Psychoanalytic Society and Institute, admired for his lucid interpretations of analytic theory and technique. He was president of the society in 1947–1949, and he continued to publish the kind of theoretical papers for which he was already well known in Vienna, until his death in 1959 of Parkinson's syndrome. Grete Bibring was also active in the teaching, training, and committee work of the Boston Psychoanalytic Society and Institute, being elected president in 1955–1958, and president of the American Psychoanalytic Association in 1962. She was also well known for her contributions to general hospital psychiatry, for her collaborative research on normal pregnancy, and as the first woman professor at Harvard Medical School. In 1944 she was invited by Dr. Herrman Blumgart, chief of medicine at the Beth Israel Hospital and a brother of the New York analyst Dr. Leonard Blumgart, to reestablish a department of psychiatry, after the hiatus left by Dr. M. Ralph Kaufman during the war years. She hesitated to accept this post, lacking administrative experience, but her gifts as a teacher of medical students, house officers and psychiatric residents, her analytic understanding of general hospital patients, and her excellent relations with medical and surgical colleagues attracted an exceptional group of psychoanalysts who trained several generations of devoted followers.

Dr. Bibring's interest in pregnancy, as a normal maturational phase of development, was a natural outgrowth of these interests. Her work, in collaboration with others, has appeared in several books and many published articles, including *The Teaching of Dynamic Psychiatry* (International Universities Press, 1968) and *Psychological Aspects of Pregnancy*, with Arthur F. Valenstein (Harper and Row, in press). After her retirement from Beth Israel Hospital in 1965, she remained active in analytic training, and wrote two books and ten articles, including "Old Age: Its Liabilities and Assets," and "Freud and the Understanding of Human Nature." For seven years she taught an unusual elective seminar at Radcliffe College, on the changing role of women today, and made an educational television film with Dr. Oliver Cope, directed by Mary Feldhaus-Webber.

Florence Clothier

Dr. Clothier was born in 1903, in Wynnewood, Pennsylvania. She graduated from Vassar College in 1926 and from Johns Hopkins Medical School in 1930, where she studied under Adolf Meyer and Ester Richards. After an internship at Philadelphia General Hospital and her marriage to Dr. George B. Wislocki (later professor of anatomy at Harvard), she settled in Boston, and took an externship in psychiatry at Boston Psychopathic Hospital. In 1932 she became the first director of the Massachusetts General Hospital child guidance center, under Dr. James Ayer, professor of neurology, prior to the establishment of the new psychiatry department by Dr. Stanley Cobb. In 1934 she began her analytic training at the Boston Psychoanalytic Society and Institute, including a didactic analysis with Hanns Sachs and control cases with Helene Deutsch and Erik Erikson, and she became a member with Dr. William Barrett, in 1939. She served on the Board of Trustees of the society and, taught an early seminar for nursery school teachers at the institute.

During this time Dr. Clothier held a part-time position at the Beth Israel Child Guidance Clinic (1934–1940) and joined the staff of the New England Home for Little Wanderers, to which she devoted a major part of her professional life, from 1933 to 1956. She helped transform the New England Home, originally a privately endowed "shelter" for runaway children, into an unusual residential center for child study, combining the traditions of nineteenth century New England philanthropy with the most advanced methods of child analysis. She was also active as lecturer and consultant at Harvard and Tufts Medical Schools, and the Cushing Veterans Hospital.

In 1957 Dr. Clothier became assistant to the president of Vassar, and consultant to the student health services. Upon her retirement from academia, in 1969, she returned to her summer residence in Little Compton, Rhode Island, where she continues to work as chief psychiatrist at the Fall River Community Health Center. Active in many public service capacities, Dr. Clothier served on the Milton, Massachusetts Board of Public Welfare (1940–1956), as director and president twice of the Planned Parenthood League, as a board member of the Euthanasia Educational Council, and as vice president of the Society for the Right to Die. She has published over thirty papers on the emotional disturbances of children and adolescents, child development, and problems of adoption, illegitimacy, education, and euthanasia.

Leolia A. Dalrymple

Dr. Dalrymple was born in 1894, in Toronto, and graduated from the Toronto School of Medicine in 1925. Though her maternal grandfather was a doctor, her mother was religious, disapproved of psychiatry and psychoanalysis, and believed that mental illness was caused by the devil. She introduced Dr. Dalrymple to her friends as a "brain surgeon." Nevertheless Dr. Dalrymple began her medical career with a psychiatric residency at Sheppard and Enoch Pratt Hospital where her interest in psychoanalysis was aroused by Harry Stack Sullivan. After further psychiatric study at the Tavistock Clinic in London, she became chief of the women's service at Butler Hospital, Providence, Rhode Island (1929–1939), and staff psychiatrist at Pembroke College (Brown University). Dr. Arthur Ruggles, the director of Butler Hospital, was sympathetic to analysis, inviting Gregory Zilboorg and others from New York to lecture. She was analyzed by Martin Peck in 1927, joined his Rankian colleagues and became a member of the second Boston Psychoanalytic Society in 1930.

During 1930 to 1931 Dr. Dalrymple undertook a training analysis with Dr. Franz Alexander in Berlin, and became a founding member of the reorganized Boston Psychoanalytic Society and Institute of 1935. She settled in Boston and practiced as a full-time analyst, without academic or hospital appointments, except for a short period in the Beth Israel Hospital outpatient clinic, (1941–1945). Dr. Dalrymple sought a fuller didactic analysis with Dr. Helene Deutsch (1939–1941), and finally became a training analyst. She served faithfully on many institute committees, and as treasurer and trustee to the society, until her retirement in 1969.

Helene Deutsch

Helene Rosenbach Deutsch was born in 1884, at Przemysl, Poland, the youngest of four children, in a cultivated non-religious Jewish family. Her father was a lawyer and local magistrate, with whom she strongly identified, but she struggled to free herself from her provincial background, studying in Lwów and Zürich to obtain her *Abitur.* In Zürich she met and admired revolutionary figures like Rosa Luxembourg and Vera Figner, and attended several international socialist congresses. In 1907 she passed her entrance examinations and enrolled in the medical faculty of the University of Vienna, one of seven women in her class, only three of whom completed their studies. She graduated in 1912 and married Dr. Felix Deutsch, whom she had met the previous year in Munich, while studying psychiatry and experimenting with the word association test under Kraepelin. After graduation she joined the University of Vienna psychiatric clinic, under Wagner-Jauregg, who was sceptical of analysis but respected her clinical skill. Meanwhile her husband continued his busy practice in internal medicine, and in 1917 their son, Martin, was born.

Helene Deutsch had been interested in psychoanalytic theory since 1907, when a friend gave her *The Interpretation of Dreams*, but this interest remained latent until her association with Paul Schilder and Otto Pötzl at the Wagner-Jauregg clinic, and some social contact with Freud. In August 1918 she began a didactic analysis with Freud, which was interrupted after one year, to enable him to resume his treatment of the "wolf-man," already a classic study in the analytic literature. At this time she left the Wagner-Jauregg clinic, to devote herself entirely to the practice of analysis. She spent a year in Berlin (1922–1923), with Freud's encouragement, to obtain further analysis with Karl Abraham and to study the organization of the Berlin Psychoanalytic Institute, which had been established in 1920, the first training center of its kind. On her return she introduced some of its procedures to the Vienna Psychoanalytic Society, creating the first "control seminar" (or continuous case presentation), and remained director of training until she and her husband emigrated to Boston in 1935.

During her years in Vienna, Helene Deutsch was well known as a leading training analyst, for her many papers on character-analysis and the "as if" personality, and for her special interest in feminine psychology, which later flowered in her celebrated volumes on *The Psychology of Women*. Her husband Felix had become increasingly interested in analysis; he was eventually to pioneer in psychosomatic research. He began attending meetings of the society in 1919 and presented his first analytic paper there in 1921. The following year he undertook a didactic analysis with Siegfried Bernfeld and became Freud's personal physician, at the time Freud's mouth cancer was discovered. In 1927 Felix Deutsch was the first to introduce the term "psychosomatic" in its present-day sense, at the General Medical Congress for Psychotherapy at Bad Nauheim.

In 1930 Helene Deutsch was invited to the first International Congress on Mental Hygiene in Washington, D.C., and in 1933 her husband visited this country on a lecture tour, where he became more aware of the Nazi threat than any of their Viennese colleagues except Robert Waelder. They also considered emigrating to the United States because of the radical political activities of their son, then a student at Dr. Tschurlock's academy in Zürich. The decision was made in 1935, in response to an invitation to Felix Deutsch from Dr. Stanley Cobb, to continue his psychosomatic research at the Massachusetts General Hospital. Helene Deutsch and her son arrived in Boston in September 1935 and Felix joined them three months later. As the second European training analyst in Boston, after Hanns Sachs, Helene Deutsch immediately became active in teaching at the Boston Psychoanalytic Society and Institute, and Felix joined the faculty somewhat later. Both served devotedly on various institute committees, and both were elected president, she in 1939–1941 and he in 1951–1954. Although both were already recognized for their separate areas of special interest in Vienna, their most productive work occurred in this country. Felix Deutsch died in 1964. Helene Deutsch has published three books since her retirement, including studies of the Dionysus myth and adolescence in changing times, and her autobiography, *Confrontations with Myself* (W.W. Norton, 1973).

Henry Morgenthau Fox

Dr. Fox was born in 1907, in New York City, graduated from Harvard in 1928 and from Johns Hopkins Medical School in 1933. After a medical internship at

Johns Hopkins Hospital, he began his psychiatric training at the Phipps Clinic, under Adolph Meyer, with whom he was closely associated for the next eight years, as chief resident and associate and assistant professor. In 1942, when the Johns Hopkins military unit was formed (118th General Hospital), Dr. Fox became chief of the neuropsychiatric service, as lieutenant colonel, and served overseas for forty-two months in Australia and the Philippines. After leaving the military service in 1946, he was invited by Dr. George W. Thorn, an associate from Hopkins, to reestablish a psychiatric service at the Peter Bent Brigham Hospital. Although there was no direct continuity between Dr. Donald J. MacPherson's original psychiatric teaching rounds on the medical wards at the Peter Bent Brigham Hospital (1920–1939), or Dr. John Romano's energetic consultation service when Dr. Soma Weiss was chief of medicine (1939–1941), Dr. Fox's unit continued the tradition of psychiatry as a part of the medical service rather than an independent department. Dr. Fox began his psychoanalytic training at the Boston Psychoanalytic Society and Institute in 1946, graduating in 1951. He became a training analyst, instructor, and chaired the Education Committee (1973–1974).

Always a prolific writer, from an early study on thalamic syndrome at Phipps through his papers on military psychiatry, Dr. Fox published forty-five articles on general hospital psychiatry, psychosomatic research, and psychoanalysis, including chapters on psychiatry in Harrison's *Principles of Internal Medicine* (1954). Dr. Fox's work is best known for a long-term psychophysiological study of the "normal personality," correlating certain ego-characteristics with patterns of pituitary-adrenocortical response, first in healthy college-age volunteer subjects and then in comparable healthy identical and fraternal twins. He and his associates at the Peter Bent Brigham Hospital published some early observations on the psychological effects of ACTH and cortisone, and patterns of adrenocortical secretion in racing crews, cyclothymic personality disorders, and during the psychoanalysis of a patient with peptic ulcer. Dr. Fox's years as director of the Peter Bent Brigham Hospital's psychiatric unit, from 1946 to 1973, reflected the rise and decline of federal support for psychosomatic research and training by the Commonwealth Fund, the Army Stress Committee, and the National Institutes of Mental Health.

George E. Gardner

Dr. Gardner was born in 1904, in West Bridgewater, Massachusetts. He graduated from Dartmouth in 1925, took a master's degree in education at Harvard in 1926, and a Ph.D. in educational psychology at Harvard in 1930. After a few years as a clinical psychologist, he enrolled in Harvard Medical School, graduating in 1937. He did an internship and residency in pediatrics at Massachusetts General Hospital, a year of psychiatry at McLean Hospital, and joined the staff of the Judge Baker Guidance Center as a Commonwealth Fellow (1939–1940).

That same year he applied for psychoanalytic training and was awarded a Sigmund Freud fellowship by the Boston Psychoanalytic Institute. He completed his training in 1947, interrupted by military service (1943–1946). In addition to serving on many committees of the Boston Psychoanalytic Society and Institute, Dr. Gardner was elected vice president in 1951–1954. Since, 1941 his principal energies have been devoted to the Judge Baker. As its director he engineered its transformation from a small unaffiliated private institution on Chestnut Street to a greatly enlarged center, integrated with the psychiatric service of Children's Hospital Medical Center and occupying its own building on Longwood Avenue. In 1953 he became chief of the new combined department and later professor of child psychiatry at Harvard Medical School, where he had been teaching since 1946. He was an enthusiastic teacher of child development to medical students, and he also taught a course in the social relations department that was popular with Harvard undergraduates. He belongs to the Group for the Advancement of Psychiatry and to many child psychiatry associations, and has published over seventy-five papers, as well as contributed to many books, and edited the first two volumes of *Case Studies in Childhood Emotional Disabilities* (American Orthopsychiatric Association, 1953 and 1956).

Milton Greenblatt

Dr. Greenblatt was born in Boston, in 1914, and attended Tufts College and Tufts Medical School, graduating from both with highest honors in 1939. After interning at the Beth Israel, he took a psychiatric residency at the Boston Psychopathic Hospital, to which he devoted the major part of his career. Beginning as director of the fledgling EEG lab in 1942, he became director of research, of clinical psychiatry, and assistant superintendant over the next thirty years. In 1963 he became professor of psychiatry at Tufts, superintendant of Boston State Hospital and commissioner of the Massachusetts Department of Mental Health, a position he held during the difficult years of 1967 to 1973. He then became chief of staff of the Veterans Administration Hospital at Brentwood, California, and is now assistant dean, School of Medicine, and professor of psychiatry at UCLA. Dr. Greenblatt has held high offices in innumerable professional organizations, local and national, including the American Board of Psychiatry and Neurology, the American Psychiatric Association, and the Group for the Advancement of Psychiatry. He was associate editor of the *American Journal of Psychiatry* and chairman of the publications board of the Group for the Advancement of Psychiatry.

During this full career in academic and institutional psychiatry, Dr. Greenblatt has written over 260 articles and eighteen books or monographs. Their titles reflect many major currents in the treatment of hospitalized mental patients, within our lifetime, and the evolution of the Boston Psychopathic Hospital into the Massachusetts Mental Health Center. Beginning his research during the last years of fever therapy, Dr. Greenblatt published the first definitive studies of lobotomy (*The Frontal Lobes and Schizophrenia*, with Harry C. Solomon, 1953). From a broad interest in the "dynamic" treatment of hospitalized patients, he became a leader in recent trends towards "de-hospitalization" (*The Patient and the Mental Hospital*, 1957; *Mental Patients in Transition*, 1961; *The Prevention of Hospitalization*, 1963; *The Dynamics of Institutional Change*, 1971).

Leston L. Havens

Dr. Havens was born in Brooklyn, New York, in 1924. He attended Williams College and Cornell Medical College. On the staff of the Massachusetts Mental Health Center (Boston Psychopathic Hospital) since 1954, he is at present professor of psychiatry at Harvard Medical School. A graduate of the Boston Psychoanalytic Society and Institute, he is on its faculty and is also the director of medical student and second-year resident teaching at the Massachusetts Mental Health Center. Dr. Havens has written *Approaches to the Mind: Movement of the Psychiatric Schools from Sects toward Science* (Little Brown, 1973) and *Participant Observation* (Jason Aronson, 1976).

Edgerton McC. Howard

Dr. Edgerton Howard, the brother of Paul Howard, was born in 1902, in Albany, New York. He graduated from Williams College in 1926 and completed his medical studies at Columbia in 1930. During medical school he undertook a personal analysis with Dr. Frankwood Williams, a prominent American follower of Otto Rank. After an internship in Albany, he became a resident in psychiatry at the Boston Psychopathic Hospital in 1931, and chief of service, 1932–1934. After a residency in neurology at Boston City Hospital, he joined the new psychiatric service that Dr. Stanley Cobb had established at the Massachusetts General Hospital. In 1934 he began a didactic analysis with Dr. Hanns Sachs and completed his analytic training at the Boston Psychoanalytic Society and Institute in 1938. He was psychiatrist to the Northfield School, Smith College, and Williams until 1941 when he joined the staff of the Austen Riggs Center, just after the death of Dr. Riggs. As associate and the acting medical director, and as the first fully trained analyst on the staff, Dr. Howard played a major role in a difficult transitional period and the beginning of a new era. Robert P. Knight became director in 1947, and brought Erik Erikson, David Rapaport, and other eminent analysts from Topeka; this Riggs group joined the New Haven analytic group to form the Western New England Psychoanalytic Society and Institute.

Dr. Howard continued as associate medical director at Riggs until 1968, and served in other important positions—director of the Berkshire Mental Health Center (an affiliate of Riggs) and teacher and training analyst in the Western New England Psychoanalytic Society, with two terms as president of the society and one term as president of the institute. He participated in various activities concerned with public affairs and mental health: the Joint Committee of 1949 (with Erich Lindemann), the 1962 Governor's Conference on Mental Health Centers, and the Governor's Committee to Implement Chapter 735. He also served eight years on the Stockbridge Board of Health and was regional director of mental health, 1968–1973.

Paul M. Howard

Dr. Paul Howard, the brother of Dr. Edgerton Howard, was born in 1905, in Albany, New York. Following graduation from Williams College in 1926, he worked for two years as a journalist in New York before undertaking an analysis with Dr. Marion Kenworthy. He embarked on medical school at the University of Pennsylvania, graduated in 1933, and began a series of residencies in psychiatry and neurology at the Boston Psychopathic, Boston City, and the Massachusetts General hospitals, during the early years of Dr. Cobb's service there. In 1936 he began his analytic training at the Boston Psychoanalytic Society and Institute and had a didactic analysis with Dr. Helene Deutsch. He became a member of the Society in 1943, served as secretary, 1946–1949 and as instructor 1956–1957. He had joined the staff of the McLean Hospital in 1938, to which he has devoted the major part of his professional life, serving in every capacity from resident to acting clinical director. Dr. Howard is now on the senior consulting staff of McLean Hospital, where he is best known as a therapist and teacher.

M. Ralph Kaufman

Dr. Kaufman was born in 1900, in the small Bessarabian town of Beltz, and emigrated with his family to Toronto at an early age. He graduated from McGill Medical School in 1925, and interned at Manhattan State Hospital (Ward's Island), where psychoanalysis had been flourishing under Adolf Meyer and August Hoch since the turn of the century. After a residency in neurology at Montefiore Hospital and in psychiatry at the Boston Psychopathic Hospital, he obtained a Commonwealth Fund fellowship for analytic training abroad. During his two years in Vienna, 1928–1931, he was analyzed by Wilhelm Reich and studied anatomy and psychiatry at the University of Vienna. There he met Dr. John Murray and Dr. Margaret Ribble, who were also to settle in Boston. On his return here, he became an instructor in psychiatry at Harvard Medical School and, as a fully trained analyst, he joined Ives Hendrick in the reorganization of the Boston Psychoanalytic Society and Institute. For the first two years he was in Boston, he was clinical director at McLean Hospital, and from 1933 to 1942 he established the first psychiatric unit at the Beth Israel Hospital. With Lydia Dawes in child psychiatry and Felix Deutsch in psychosomatic research, he created the kind of department of general hospital psychiatry, with teaching and training for medical and surgical house officers, that Dr. Stanley Cobb established at the Massachusetts General Hospital in 1934. At the same time, Dr. Kaufman was active in the affairs of the Boston Psychoanalytic Society and Institute. He taught many seminars, served as chairman of the Education Committee from 1936 to 1942 and was elected president (1937–1939).

In 1942 Dr. Kaufman departed for military service. He became neuropsychiatric consultant to the Sixth Army Division and to the South Pacific and Pacific Ocean Areas. He was later a teacher and administrator at the Lawson General Hospital training center for military psychiatry in Atlanta. Like John Murray, William Menninger, Roy Grinker, and John Spiegel in North Africa Dr. Kaufman contributed to the vast expansion in military psychiatry that created a new climate for psychiatric and psychoanalytic training in the postwar decade. He returned from these military experiences to New York, where he was professor of psychiatry at Columbia from 1946–1967, and chief of psychiatry at Mt. Sinai Hospital until his retirement in 1971.

From his early neurological papers in 1928 to his history of military psychiatry in 1973, Dr. Kaufman wrote over eighty papers. Their titles and co-authors provide a capsule history of many major trends in psychoanalytic research during the past fifty years, spanning an early interest in psychoses and in clinical psychosomatic studies (including a classic paper on anorexia nervosa with Felix Deutsch) to the highly sophisticated team research on patients with gastric fistula that he conducted with Dr. Sydney G. Margolin at Mt. Sinai Hospital. In the late 1950s he contributed to psychopharmacological studies of LSD and rauwolfia, and throughout his career he has written enthusiastically on general hospital psychiatry, problems of psychiatric teaching, and the history of psychiatry.

John Milne Murray

Dr. Murray was born in 1896, in Concord, New Hampshire, a descendant of Scottish stone-cutters who had worked in the granite quarries of that region. He attended Dartmouth College and the University of Pennsylvania School of Medicine, graduating in 1921. After a residency in psychiatry at the New Hampshire State Hospital, he entered general practice in Concord. Here he became interested in analytic training abroad through his friendship with Dr. Smith Ely Jelliffe of New York. With the help of a Commonwealth Fund stipend, arranged by Dr. Arthur Ruggles of Butler Hospital, he studied analysis in Vienna from 1929 to 1931, where he joined Dr. Kaufman, Margaret Ribble, and Spurgeon English in weekly meetings with Wilhelm Reich. Returning to settle in Boston, he belonged to the group of young reformers led by Ives Hendrick and M. Ralph Kaufman, and became a founding member in the reorganization of the new Boston Psychoanalytic Society and Institute in 1935.

He remained active in the affairs of the institute, twice serving as chairman of the Education Committee and twice as president of the society (1942–1943 and 1949–1951). He taught some of the first clinical seminars to candidates, and to social workers at Smith College and Boston University. He was also active in the American Psychoanalytic and the American Psychiatric Associations, director of the American Board of Psychiatry and Neurology, and consultant in psychiatry to Dartmouth College, MIT, and St. Paul's School. During the war years he was chief consultant to the army air force, retiring with the rank of lieutenant colonel. After the war he became a member of the advisory committees on medical education to the Surgeon General and the Veterans Administration. He played an important part in establishing the psychiatric training programs of the New England Veterans Administration, which enabled so many younger veterans to become analysts. He wrote many analytic papers on clinical topics, the best known on "entitlement" in the narcissistic character. He was professor of psychiatry at Boston University School of Medicine from 1946 until his retirement in 1961.

Eleanor Pavenstedt

Dr. Pavenstedt was born in 1903, in New York City and lived there until she finished high school. In 1920 she moved to Europe with her family (her parents were German), studied medicine at the University of Geneva and graduated in 1929. In Switzerland she became interested in child psychiatry, and with this in mind she took an internship in pediatrics at Bellevue and a neurological clerkship at Queen's Square Hospital in London. She completed a psychiatric residency at the Phipps Clinic, Baltimore, in 1934 under Adolf Meyer, and sought special training in child psychiatry there and at the Philadelphia Child Guidance Clinic. In 1934 she moved to Boston, to be director of the child psychiatry outpatient clinic at Massachusetts General Hospital. She came at the invitation of Dr. Stanley Cobb, who was establishing his new department that year, and she was a fellow at Harvard Medical School until 1937. During this same period she obtained further experience in child psychiatry at the Judge Baker Guidance Center with Dr. William Healy and at the Habit Clinic with Dr. Douglas Thom. In 1935 she began her analytic training at the Boston Psychoanalytic Institute with Dr. Hanns Sachs and later with Dr. Helene Deutsch. After a year consulting at Wellesley College, she joined the staff of the James Jackson Putnam Children's Center in 1943. With Dr. Marian C. Putnam and Mrs. Beata Rank, she did research there on early childhood schizophrenia and "children with atypical development," which remained at the center of her professional interests until 1954. She began teaching child psychiatry in 1949 at the Boston University School of Medicine, and was professor of child psychiatry at Boston University (1949–1965). She also taught at the Simmons College School of Social Work (1936–1949). At the Boston Psychoanalytic Society and Institute she was a training analyst, taught child development seminars, and served on many committees, including a term as chairman of the Education Committee. She belonged to the American Orthopsychiatric Association, the Academy of Child

Psychiatry, and the American Psychoanalytic Association, where she was chairman of subcommittees on early developement and social problems. She published over a dozen papers on the atypical child and early development, including a longitudinal study on the effects of maternal immaturity on child development. She edited and contributed to two books, *Dynamic Psychopathology of Childhood*, with Dr. Lucie Jessner, editor (Grune and Stratton, 1959) and *The Drifters: Children of Disorganized Lower-Class Families* (Little Brown, 1967), based on her research with Dr. Charles A. Malone and others.

Eveoleen N. Rexford

Dr. Rexford was born in 1911, in Corning, New York, and attended Keuka College, graduating in 1930. After taking a master's degree at Cornell, she studied medicine at the University of Buffalo and graduated in 1935. She was an intern and psychiatric resident at Buffalo City Hospital, and a medical and neurological resident at Central Islip State Hospital. In 1942 she became a Commonwealth Fellow in child psychiatry at the Judge Baker Guidance Center, and was on the staff for five years. Dr. Rexford practiced as a part-time psychiatrist in Wellesley for a year and then joined Dr. Putnam and Mrs. Rank at the James Jackson Putnam Children's Center. She began her analytic training at the Boston Psychoanalytic Society and Institute in 1943 and became a member in 1948. From 1949 to 1965 she was director of the Douglas A. Thom Clinic for Children, and for the past twelve years she has been director of child psychiatry and professor of psychiatry at Boston University Medical School. In 1972–1973 she was a Commonwealth Fund medical scholar.

Besides the part-time practice of child analysis, Dr. Rexford has been unusually active in different teaching, training, administration, and editorial positions. She has been instructor, lecturer, and visiting physician at Harvard Medical School, Simmons College of Social Work, Boston University, and Boston City Hospital. She was a member and chairman of several committees of the American Academy of Child Psychiatry, and editor of its journal. She was a committee member and president (1967–1969) of the American Association of Psychiatric Clinics for Children, and a member of the Board on Professional Standards and chairman of the Child Analysis Committee of the American Psychoanalytic Association. She has held many important offices in the Boston Psychoanalytic Society and Institute, including librarian, secretary (1955–1958), and chairman of the Faculty Committee and the Committee on Child Analysis. She has taken part in innumerable national planning commissions and conferences, and in local committees on mental health planning and special education for emotionally disturbed children. She has published a dozen papers on psychoanalysis and child psychiatry, including chapters in *Psychiatry in the General Hospital* (Bernard Bandler, editor, 1966) and the *Handbook of Psychiatry* (S. Arieti, editor). She is currently working on a monograph about attitudes toward children in American society, to be called *An American Mythology: How We Care for Our Children.*

Benjamin C. Riggs

Dr. Riggs was born in 1914, in Stockbridge, Massachusetts, the fourth child of Dr. Austen F. Riggs, and grew up on the grounds of the Austen Riggs Center. He attended Harvard College and Columbia Medical School, graduating in 1940, and took internships and a medical residency at Bellevue and the University of Pennsylvania Hospital. He was engaged in the study of gastroenterolgy and biochemistry, from 1943 to 1945, publishing a dozen papers and book reviews on experimental medicine during a five-year period. Between 1943 and 1948 he trained in clinical psychiatry, with residencies at Baldpate, Massachusetts General, and Metropolitan State hospitals, and in psychoanalysis at the Boston Psychoanalytic Society and Institute, 1956–1964. After some years of teaching at Tufts and Harvard, and a year as superintendant of Metropolitan State (1949–1950), he moved to Atlanta in 1966. For four years he taught at Emory Medical School and was a charter member of the Atlanta Psychoanalytic Society. Since 1973 he has been professor of psychiatry, and acting chairman of the department, at the Medical University of South Carolina, in Charleston. His recent papers, besides his memoir of his father, have approached the clinical interview from the standpoint of general systems theory.

Elvin V. Semrad

The late Dr. Semrad was born in 1909, in Abie, Nebraska, and attended Peru State Teachers College and the University of Nebraska, graduating in 1932. He completed his medical studies at the University of Nebraska, interned at the University Hospital in Omaha and took residencies in psychiatry at the Boston Psychopathic Hospital (1935–1937) and at McLean Hospital, the following year. He began an analysis with Dr. Hanns Sachs during his years at the Boston Psychopathic Hospital, was accepted for training at the Boston Psychoanalytic Society and Institute in 1939, and graduated in 1948. He had joined the staff of Metropolitan State Hospital in 1938, served four years in the military service (1942–1946), and then became clinical director at Boston State Hospital. Here he influenced many young veterans, who were inspired by his analytic understanding of psychoses and his pioneer work with group methods in the treatment of psychoses, to become analysts. In 1953 he became clinical director at the Boston Psychopathic Hospital, where he continued to influence several generations of psychiatric residents. From 1938–1952 Dr. Semrad was on the faculty of Boston University Medical School, and from 1940 until his death in October 1976, he was professor of psychiatry at Harvard Medical School. He also taught at the Boston School of Social Work, Simmons College, and in the social relations department of Harvard College. As a training analyst at the Boston Psychoanalytic Society and Institute, he served on many committees, and as secretary of the society (1953–1955) and president (1968–1970). He published seventy-two papers and chapters of books since 1936, some with co-authors, that reflect every aspect of his career. The best known deal with psychotherapy of the psychoses (with Doris Menzer, Christopher Standish, and others) and the application of group therapy to psychotic patients (with John Arsenian, Standish, and others).

Helen Herlihy Tartakoff

Dr. Tartakoff was born in 1906, in Chicago, the daughter of a well-to-do engineer. She first attended parochial schools, though her family was tolerant about religion, and then the University of Chicago, where she studied English literature and philosophy, graduating in 1927. For the next few years she worked as a writer, in journalism and advertising and on an unpublished novel. A German professor at college had interested her in Freud, and in the early thirties, soon after Franz Alexander had established the Chicago Psychoanalytic Institute, she enrolled in a course that was open to teachers and other laypersons. In consulting Alexander about a family problem, she was encouraged to consider becoming an analyst, and after meeting Margaret Gerard, the future child analyst, she went to Vienna in the fall of 1933. After a consultation with Helene Deutsch, Dr. Tartakoff began her analysis with Jenny Waelder, and a year later she was admitted to the Vienna Society as a candidate for full training. At the same time, after discussions with Helen Ross and Mary O'Neil Hawkins, she decided to undertake medical training at the University of Vienna, as part of her preparation for becoming an analyst.

She recalls her life as an analytic candidate in Vienna as "the golden years, in the twilight of the gods," until the Nazi occupation in March 1938 made further analytic practice impossible, and interrupted her medical training as well. After helping her Viennese friends with visas and money, she returned to the United States that summer. She settled in Boston where a fellow- candidate, the late Dr. Joseph J. Michaels, had suggested that she complete her medical studies at Tufts, from which she graduated in 1940. Though she resumed her training analysis with Dr. Waelder, who had also settled in Boston, she was not admitted to the Boston Psychoanalytic Society and Institute until she had graduated from medical school. She became a member in 1944. During those years she married Dr. Joseph Tartakoff, who had been her instructor in hand surgery. She interned at Michael Reese Hospital, took a psychiatric residency at the Boston Psychopathic Hospital, and had the first of their two children. She completed both medical and analytic training in ten years, and encountered no unusual obstacles as a woman. By the time she entered the University of Vienna, in fact, over forty percent of its medical students were women.

Since 1944 Dr. Tartakoff has been a full-time analyst and training analyst, active on many committees of the Boston Psychoanalytic Society and Institute and the American Psychoanalytic Association. She remains one of our foremost teachers, long remembered for her seminar on analytic technique. She has also held academic appointments at Harvard Medical School and the Beth Israel Hospital, written many articles and book reviews, and served on the editorial board of the *Journal of the American Psychoanalytic Association.* Her best known paper is "The Normal Personality in our Culture and the Nobel Prize Complex."

Robert A. Young

The late Dr. Young was born in 1900, in Wilton, New Hampshire, and attended Boston University, graduating in 1923. He took his master's and doctoral degrees in education at Harvard, in 1926 and 1935. He was clinical psychologist at Massachusetts General Hospital (1931–1943) and assistant professor in psychology at the Boston University Graduate School of Education and the School of Social Work (1936–1962). Since 1942 he has been on the staff of the Judge Baker Guidance Center, serving as assistant director (1957–1965) and as director of its Manville Residential Center (1958–1971). He began his training analysis with Dr. Hanns Sachs in 1934; a Commonwealth Fund fellowship enabled him to complete full clinical training, with supervisory work under Beata Rank and Helene Deutsch, and in 1940 he became an affiliate member of the Boston Psychoanalytic Society and Institute.

Dr. Young was active in many other part-time teaching and administrative positions, including the Cambridge-Somerville Youth Study (1941–1946), and as director of the New Hampshire Child Guidance Center in Manchester (1947–1957). He taught clinical psychology and education at Harvard and Tufts universities, the Smith College School of Social Work, and the Boston University School of Nursing. Besides the part-time practice of analysis and child psychotherapy, he was the founder and director of an experimental summer camp for the residential treatment of disturbed boys, from 1949 to 1969, which was the subject of a documentary film by Dr. Edward A. Mason. He holds memberships in the American Psychoanalytic Association and the American Psychological Association, the American Association for Child Psychoanalysis, and the American Group Psychotherapy Association. He is a Fellow of the American Orthopsychiatric Association, and served as a board member (1960–1962). Between 1938 and 1971 he published a dozen papers on child psychiatry and child analysis, including an introductory chapter in *Therapeutic Camping: Its Past and Future* (South Carolina Division of Community Health Service, 1971).

Index of Names

Numbers in italics refer to illustrations.